RELAX, THIS WON'T HURT

T0089869

RELAX, THIS WON'T HURT

Painless Answers to Women's Most Pressing Health Questions

Judith Reichman, M.D.

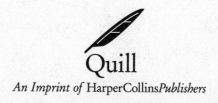

Quill

An Imprint of HarperCollins*Publishers*

A hardcover edition of this book was published in 2000 by William Morrow and Company, Inc.

First Quill edition published 2001.

Designed by Jam Design

The Library of Congress has catalogued the hardcover edition as follows:

Reichman, Judith.
    Relax, this won't hurt : painless answers to women's most pressing health questions / Judith Reichman. — 1st ed.
        p. cm.
    Includes index.
    ISBN 0-688-16301-7
    1. Gynecology—Miscellanea.   2. Women—Health and hygiene—Miscellanea.   I. Title.
RG121 .R43 2000
613'.04244—dc21   99-053257

ISBN 0-06-095932-0 (pbk.)

    02   03   04   05   WB/RRD   10 9 8 7 6 5 4

I dedicate this book to the physicians
whose research, teaching and caring for
women has allowed us to make such
enormous advances in our health care.

CONTENTS

Acknowledgments

THIS BOOK, LIKE the body, is composed and driven by multiple biological systems. The heart that pumped it with oxygen and nutrients for all its metabolic processes was Dana Points, executive editor of *Self* magazine. We sat together for days and weeks at a time at the computer, surrounded by files, articles, books and chocolate, and came up with answers to the questions that my patients (and we as women) felt were important to our care and well-being. We laughed a lot, sometimes we cried, and we drank far too many cappuccinos. Although the two of us graduated from Barnard College decades apart, we share an obsessive compulsiveness (that, as yet, in my clinical judgment, does not require medication) and a can-do attitude that was fostered by this wonderful women's institution. Dana, you are the best cardiovascular system and soul mate a woman could ever have. Thank you.

The musculoskeletal system of this book was provided by my publisher, William Morrow, and, most particularly, by my editor, Meaghan Dowling. Thank you for your support and for pushing me aerobically (with your scheduling) and building my confidence muscles by making sure I knew you were solidly behind the development and promotion of this book.

The growth hormone for *Relax* came from my literary agents, Maureen and Eric Lasher, who pushed me into publishing puberty and enabled my writer's growth spurt.

The book's central nervous system (or, more specifically, its brain) comes from the hundreds of physicians and scientists whose current research and articles gave me the neuronal connections upon which I rely to diagnose and treat women. I am especially indebted to the specialists who read sections of the manuscript and provided guidance and corrections. Thank you to Drs. Daniel Berman, Glen Braunstein, Yzhar Charuzi, Alan DeCherney, Cal Hobel, Ron Leuchter, Gerald Levey, Brian Meckelberg, Alan Metzger, Joel Pannish and Barry Rosenbloom. Neurological fine-tuning was added by Pam LaBarbiera, whose graceful copyediting kept me grammatically correct without altering my voice, which, as most readers my have noticed, is rendered in very long, breath-defying sentences (smokers beware).

The dermatologic system of this book, which holds together and protects the inner contents, comes in the form of the wonderful jacket, which was designed by Bradford Foltz. And the greatest dermatologic wonder is the jacket photo that made my skin look so great, taken by Lynn Goldsmith. Thank you, Lynn. You're a wonderful woman and a great photographer, and you made me feel like a rock star for one glorious day.

Additional emotional support was provided by two extraordinary women whom I am fortunate to have as friends, and who read the manuscript and made invaluable suggestions. Thank you, Lynne Wasserman and Francis Rothschild.

The true endocrine system for the book—the hormones that gave me my sense of well-being—was provided by my husband, Gil Cates. He encouraged me to tell my story at the end of the book because he felt it would help other women. He patiently accepted my book-writing-related absences, and was there to welcome me back when they abated. Gil, you are not just the testosterone in my life—you provide me with my thyroid and adrenal hormones (which, we know, oversee all other hormones) as well as the all-important neurochemical stimulation of wisdom, humor and love. My system (forget the book at this point) is lucky to have you.

The genetic basis for the book comes from my first-degree relatives, my parents, daughters and sister. We share some amazing genes. They may not as yet have been officially mapped by the Human Genome Project, but I know they exist—I've named them gene S1 and gene S2 (support and stubbornness), gene L (love), gene I (inquisitiveness) and gene H (hypochondriasis).

The gastrointestinal system, or at least the initial feeding of information for *Relax*, was provided by the Cedars-Sinai medical library staff and my

ACKNOWLEDGMENTS / xi

office manager, Ana Tabares. Debbie Craig helped with the digestion of the facts, while other members of my office staff, Rose Perry and Judy Casanova, calmed, nursed and protected my patients and me from the frenzied schedule encountered during the completion of this book.

The reproductive system for *Relax* developed from several sources. Many of the questions that were implanted and successfully gestated originated with the *Today* show. Stephanie Saft, my segment producer, was the inspiration for the topics covered in the Thirties and Forties chapters and made me translate my answers from medical gibberish to understandable English.

Linda Finnell and Jeff Zucker astutely keep their fingers on the pulse of what millions of women want to know and shared their gift of grasp of these queries with me. Thank you. And finally, I want to express my appreciation to Katie Couric. Her medical curiosity, concern, tremendous intelligence and great personal empathy have kept me trying harder to produce the eggs of medical information that become fertilized on television, on the Web and in this book—and grow into a better awareness of women's health.

On a more personal health note: I want to thank the team of physicians who have helped me: Drs. Jim Brenner, Edward Phillips, Barbara Hayden, Ron Wender, Barry Rosenbloom, Richard Gold and Irene Davos. Your compassion was as great as your expertise, and I am forever grateful.

Judith Reichman, M.D.
Los Angeles
September 15, 1999

A Letter to the Reader

I REALIZE THAT in the current world of Web medicine, you may wonder whether a traditionally published book will provide you with the answers you need to guide your health choices and medical care. Before you jump to your mental "delete" key, I want to put in a quick "save." A vast number of studies and opinions are presented to us at the speed of DSL, but unless we have advanced degrees in medicine, statistics, epidemiology, and computer science, we sorely need doctor-patient explanations and recommendations. This book will, I hope, continue to fulfill this mandate.

There are some new questions and revised answers that have emerged. I would like to take the next few pages to "cut and paste" them into the book. There is a growing hormone credibility crisis that has, of late, caused more anxiety attacks among my patients than both Y2K and the stock market corrections. The Women's Health Initiative Study, which is currently following 27,000 postmenopausal women on estrogen or combined estrogen and progestin, found that in the first two years, there was a slight increase in risk of heart attack and stroke with hormone use. *But* (and the *but* did not always appear in the reports you read), the total number of these "adverse" events was less than expected for the population. More important, the researchers felt that it could take more than two years for hormone replacement to exert any beneficial effect on the risk of plaque formation and heart disease.

Two other studies raised the specter that the progestin in HRT could cause breast cancer. The first, published in the *Journal of the American Medical Association* (JAMA), looked at the history of hormone use in more than 46,000 women. After four years, there was an 8 percent increase in yearly risk of breast cancer for thin women (note *thin*, not over-weight) using estrogen and progestin. Estrogen was cleared of culpability—with just a 1 percent increase for those who took estrogen alone. Again, we have to look between the lines and numbers. According to the statistical mavens, these percentages are not statistically significant. Moreover, only 4 percent of all the women took estrogen with progestin throughout the study, and they were not even asked which or how much progestin they took. A second study from the University of Southern California clarified some of these issues. It was a retrospective or "look back and remember" questionnaire (and memories will certainly be jarred by the subsequent development of cancer). Eighteen hundred postmenopausal women with breast cancer were compared to a similar number of healthy women. Those who took progestin cyclically (10 to 14 days a month) showed a 24 percent increase in their risk of breast cancer after five years when compared to non-users. This risk was not present if they took progestin contin-uously—that is, on a daily basis. Progestins may change breast cells and put them in a state where they are less likely to divide, so perhaps the cells become confused and are more likely to become abnormal during monthly cycling. I do not advise a woman on HRT who still has her uterus to simply stop progestin. This could, after one year, cause her to risk devel-opment of uterine cancer. Instead, whenever possible, I now recommend using continuous low doses of progestin or natural progesterone. Two new products combining estrogen and progestin in one pill have recently been FDA approved. Femhrt is like a very mini–birth control pill containing just one-fourth the amount of the synthetic estrogen (ethinyl estradiol) and a low amount of progestin. The second product is Ortho-Prefest, which alternates tablets containing estradiol (estrogen the ovary makes) to be taken for three days, followed by three days of a tablet combining a very low dose of progestin with the estradiol.

If you can't or won't use HRT and your hot flashes are making you mis-erable, in addition to the therapies I give you in the book you might con-sider using certain antidepressants. Paxil and Effexor have been medically tested and shown to help decrease the intensity and frequency of that mis-erable flushing and sweating.

A LETTER TO THE READER / xv

One more addition: A new medication is available for the treatment and prevention of osteoporosis. It's a biphosphonate called Actonel and, like Fosamax, it helps prevent bone-eating cells from chopping out those tiny cavities that cause our bones to become fragile. Finally, a deletion: In the "Your Fifties" chapter, I write about the possible risk of liver damage when the drug Rezulin is prescribed for Type II diabetes. This drug has now been taken off the market.

Now that the human genome has been deciphered, I'm sure that in future books, I will have to devote huge segments to the prevention, diagnosis, and therapy of disease based on genetic science. I, and all of your doctors, reserve the right to update and, hopefully, improve our advice about your medical options and care. But, for now, the answers I give you in the upcoming chapters are the best I can offer to help take away the hurt.

Judith Reichman, M.D.

PROLOGUE

Why "This Won't Hurt"

MY FATHER IS a theoretical physicist who has always felt that mathematical order is the divine foundation of the world and, as such, should form the basis of my education. I dropped math (among other things) at the age of 18 and turned on to the biological. Fortunately, that included college courses in biology. But the number systems instilled in my young, impressionable brain have created some irreversible synapses, and when I ponder the ultimate question "Who am I?" I do so mathematically, calculating and weighing my various personal parts (fat not included). The greatest percentage of me is woman. In this woman fraction, I am subdivided into mother (I've done that twice), wife (also twice), daughter, friend and a consumer of whatever it takes to feel great, look good and live longer. The second part of me is physician, and that, too, is subdivided into listener and observer (of women's ailments and problems), diagnostician (I find out what has medically gone wrong), dispenser of medications (I make it right), surgeon (when all else fails, I cut, laser or excise), therapist (I separate the psychological from the organic) and gatekeeper (I open doors so we can all enter the realm of medical knowledge).

This book, like me, is a synthesis of woman, medicine and health information. We've all listened in fear, mistrust or grudging hope to the phrase "Relax, this won't hurt," which has patronizingly been pronounced by many of our doctors. I first heard this when I was 16 years old, and our family internist decided that it was time for me to have a pelvic exam.

Without explaining why, he had his nurse position me in the requisite stir-rups, and upon discovering that, for obvious reasons, he would have difficulty performing said exam, he uttered the greatest lie of my second decade: "Relax, this won't hurt"—and proceeded to try to feel my uterus and ovaries by doing a rectal exam!

I have co-opted this declaration as a title and as a promise. Knowledge about our bodies and the medical facts we need to keep ourselves healthy can be accessible, easy to understand and, yes, painless. I've been told there are 25 standard plots for theater and movies. We've done better in medicine. There are more than 100 basic questions that women ask their doctors. I'll answer these questions in the ensuing chapters. I promise not to give a huge compilation of studies, statistics and medical facts that need to be sorted or explained, then qualified and quantified. I've already absorbed the shock of medical literature bombardment and have come out of the ordeal unharmed and ready to go. Here are the medical answers and the advice that I take myself and feel comfortable dispensing to my patients.

So please just relax, sit back and take your time. You don't have to rush through a 10-minute appointment with the doctor. You can get your questions answered by all of me—woman, physician, mother, daughter, friend and patient—at your own pace. And what you do with the answers can change your life.

YOUR TEENS

PUBERTY IS THE most tumultuous and wonderful hormonal change your body will ever go through. The Latin root of the word, *pubescere*, means "to become hairy, come to maturity." But this transition represents much more than the need to shave or wear a bra. Let's go over the good stuff first: You're growing breasts, getting taller, developing curves. Your reproductive organs—your vagina, ovaries and uterus—are maturing, which will make it possible for you to have sex when you're ready. Your periods begin, which of course will permit you to get pregnant and bear children in the future.

On the downside, these periods can be messy and cause painful cramps and moodiness. You're also growing hair in strange places (under your arms, in the pubic area). Your skin is getting oilier, and you're sprouting pimples. You perspire and develop body odor. And for some of you, weight gain is an issue.

WHY IS THIS ALL HAPPENING?

It all starts with our XX sex chromosomes, which are present in the nucleus of each one of our cells and contain the instructions for our body's development. Note: The male sex is chromosomally challenged. They're missing a little piece of the second X chromosome and as a result are XYs. Only we XXs are capable of developing ovaries, which contain millions of eggs (also known as follicles) that will produce female hormones and that ultimately can be fertilized and cause pregnancy.

There are three major hormone systems that cause our bodies to change. Each system or *axis* is composed of a central brain control, several hormonal messengers and glands that produce additional hormones. The adrenal axis is the first to mature. At the age of eight or nine, the center of our brain, called the hypothalamus, produces a hormone that directs the brain's pituitary gland to prompt the adrenal glands (which sit on top of our kidneys) to get going. As a result, we begin to produce several malelike hormones. It's the testosteronelike qualities of these adrenal hormones that prompt so-called sweet little girls (ponytails and barrettes included) to start sweating, emitting body odor, growing body hair and developing acne. (And, oh yes, becoming interested in boys.) This phase is called the *adrenarche*.

The second source of hormonal upheaval is due to the activity of the *somatotropic axis* (*soma*=body, *tropic*=growth) and the production of growth hormone. This complicated axis interacts with many other crucial hormones such as insulin, thyroid adrenal hormones and sex hormones, and, indeed, if one of these hormones is missing, the axis is thrown off and our development may be delayed or absent. If all the hormones do their job, our organs and bones grow. During our growth spurt, we gain about three and a half inches in height every year from the time our breasts begin to develop until we get our period. Once our cycles are regular, we'll probably add just two more inches to our height, and we'll stop growing somewhere between ages 16 and 18.

This brings us to our ovarian hormones, which are produced by the follicles in our ovaries. Believe it or not, we're born with a million eggs. But they're very fragile, and more than half die before we even get to puberty. The ones that make it will slowly be stimulated and start to produce the very hormones that cause us to mature from girls to women. As we get into our teens, the hypothalamus begins to put out a hormone called GnRH (gonadotropin-releasing hormone). "Gonad" is the generic term for sex glands, in our case, ovaries.

Initially, our less-than-mature brains start to secrete GnRH in spurts during the night. With time, these pulses become steady, occurring day and night, and finally they are strong enough to cause production of another brain hormone, FSH (follicle-stimulating hormone). FSH is the final instructor for the development of our follicles, and as they mature, they produce estrogen, the hormone that will rule our development and other important aspects of our lives.

Estrogen causes our breasts to develop and contributes to our female physique, prompting fat to accumulate in our breasts, hips, thighs and derrieres. It also changes the lining of the vagina, converting it from smooth, shiny and inflexible to wrinkled, pink and pliable. At the same time, this hormone causes the uterus to mature so that its walls thicken and the glands of its cervix, or opening, produce mucus, which is secreted into the vagina. As a result, a light, yellow-tinged discharge often stains our underwear.

Even though our follicles are producing estrogen, they have not reached maturity until they produce a second female hormone, progesterone. We need critical amounts of estrogen to tell our brain that it's time to produce LH, or luteinizing hormone. LH then instructs the follicle to release the egg from the ovary (ovulation) and produce progesterone. This hormone causes the lining of the uterus to thicken and become a lush, welcoming abode for a potential pregnancy (if—heaven forbid, at your age—the egg is fertilized). If the egg isn't fertilized by the sperm, 14 days after its release, the leftover follicle, called the *corpus luteum*, collapses and dies. There's no more estrogen and progesterone to nourish the uterine lining, so it too collapses and is shed, causing a period. Our first period is so important it's been given its own name: *menarche*. Knowing all this will not only explain what's happening, but should also get you an A in biology!

AM I NORMAL?

I hate the word "normal" because it implies that those of us who don't fit into a very specific category are medical misfits in need of treatment or change. We can blame the doctors and scientists. They have a professional need to condense facts into charts and graphs, and this can be misleading. For example, if the age at which 100 girls get their first period is plotted on a graph, the bulk of the group falls on the number 13. But there are still many girls who start their periods at 12 or 14, while others fall on the numbers 9 or 16. If you were to draw a line between these numbers, it would look like a small hill. This is called a "Gaussian curve"—I've renamed it a "lousian curve" because those of us who fall on the beginning or the end of it may be considered outside the norm. But this doesn't necessarily mean we're abnormal. Nature simply has a range that we have to accept and work with.

Even though a large number of girls get their first period at age 13 (or an average age of 12.8, to be precise), you could still be considered perfectly normal if you start as early as age 8 or as late as 16. Don't be alarmed if your first few periods aren't regular—they can come as frequently as every two weeks or be months apart. It often takes two years after your first period before your cycles are regular and you get a period every 21 to 45 days. Even if all your friends have started to compare notes on pads versus tampons, you don't have to run to the doctor as long as your breasts and pubic hair have started to develop by age 14 and you begin to menstruate by age 16.

Breast development can vary as well. It starts at an average age of 11 but can range from age 8 to age 15. First you'll develop breast "buds." Don't be concerned if they feel like lumps or one is bigger than the other—with time, the glands grow and fat will accumulate, making your breasts softer and fuller. Your nipples will also become larger and darker. The ultimate size of your breasts depends on your genes (so look at your mom), your weight and how much you exercise. Both breasts will never be exactly the same size—none of us have completely symmetrical bodies. But occasionally, one breast grows noticeably larger than the other. If this happens, your doctor will probably want you to wait until your breasts have stopped growing (usually around age 16) before you consider evening them out with either an implant for the underdeveloped breast or surgery to reduce the overdeveloped one. Pubic hair tends to appear a couple of months after breast development starts. In the beginning it's soft, babylike hair, but within two years it should thicken and become curly and dense.

None of this occurs in a weightless vacuum. As you grow taller, you nearly double your amount of body fat. The net result is an average weight gain of 15 to 20 pounds over a two- to three-year period. Despite what the skinny images you see in magazines and on television would have you believe, you're not getting fat, you're simply acquiring the curves that nature intended you to have. During this time, it's natural for you to be larger—both in height and in weight—than the boys. They don't start their hormonal development and growth spurt until around age 14, and unlike girls, they *lose* body fat during this time period. By the end of puberty the average adolescent girl has twice the body fat of the average adolescent male. Since boys' growth spurt lasts longer, they'll end up taller.

WHY AM I AN EARLY BLOOMER?

Don't think of yourself as an early bloomer—think of yourself as part of a trend. In general, American girls are going through puberty earlier than they did 100 years ago. This is largely because of improved nutrition. We know that we need a critical amount of body fat, 17% of our total weight, in order to start menstruating. For example, a 15-year-old who is 5'5" should weigh at least 96 pounds before her menstrual cycles would be expected to begin. We need even more body fat (22%) in order to maintain regular cycles. In general, by the age of 16, our bodies are 27% fat, and by age 18 we're at 28%. Our stored fat is there to provide energy during pregnancy and breast-feeding. It also makes some of our estrogen and helps us process the estrogen we make in our ovaries.

Your race could also be one of the reasons you're maturing faster than your friends. African-American girls tend to begin to develop breasts and grow pubic hair at around age nine, while Caucasian girls tend to develop a year later. But it's not unusual for these changes to start as early as age seven.

SO WHAT SHOULD I DO ABOUT BEING AN EARLY BLOOMER?

Probably nothing. Early puberty simply means that your hormones are coming out faster and at higher levels than other girls' are, and the impact on your present and future health should be minimal. The one thing your parents (and perhaps you) might worry about is your height. Growth hormone makes your bones grow longer, but it's estrogen that eventually stops your bones from lengthening. So it stands to reason that if you get your first period two years earlier than your friends, your growth spurt will be shortened by two years and your adult height may be five to seven inches less than that of other women your age. There are doctors who feel that this is sufficient reason to administer medications that can shut down the production of the hormone that stimulates the ovaries and causes this early development. These drugs are called GnRH analogs and can be administered as shots (Lupron) or nasal spray (Synarel). Another therapy, synthetic growth hormone, is sometimes used to promote stature, but this is for kids who are genetically predisposed to be very short, and it is not generally used for normally developing girls with early puberty.

So much for the medical answer. Even though I've reassured you that there's nothing physically wrong, you, your friends—and even your parents—may have problems dealing with this. I remember when my daughter started to develop breasts, I remarked at breakfast, "Oh my God! What's that I see under your shirt?" She wore sweatshirts to breakfast for the next six months. I probably should have prepared both of us by sitting down with her and discussing the changes she could expect in her body long before they happened. (Actually, most psychologists feel that second or third grade is the time to start.)

I've subsequently apologized for my lack of forethought. It's hard for moms to see their little girls begin to "bud" at any age, but especially before their teens. We're just not ready, and, unfortunately, we may convey this, adding to their fear that something's wrong. But the wrong is on our part: A daughter's adolescence triggers a mother's concerns about sex, drugs, driving and independence—and it is the ultimate reminder of our own aging.

The natural thing for most early-maturing girls to do is to search for a group of friends who are more like them—in other words, an older crowd. You may feel pressured by these more experienced friends to drink, use drugs or have sex. But developing sexual organs at an early age—and producing hormones that make you interested in sex—doesn't mean you're ready to do it.

Wow, are there a lot of dilemmas. No wonder so many girls who have to deal with early maturity become depressed. It doesn't seem fair: Boys who mature early feel they have a social edge because they're taller and better at sports. Girls just feel awkward and embarrassed. We have to reeducate ourselves so we can reap the same benefits as boys. Just because you're shopping for bras and your friends aren't doesn't mean that where it counts—in your head and your soul—you're different. Stick with friends your own age and don't be ashamed of who you are. Remember, you're now the leader and can show them or tell them what to expect. Case in point: Even though I'm a gynecologist, my daughter learned to use a tampon from a more developed friend.

ALL MY FRIENDS HAVE HAD THEIR PERIOD EXCEPT ME. WHAT'S WRONG?

That depends on how old you are and what else is going on with your body. As long as you have some breast development and pubic hair growth, you can patiently wait without worrying until you're 16. After that age, if you still haven't gotten your period, you should see a doctor. Moreover, if by the age of 14 your body doesn't appear to be developing, a visit to the doctor would not be premature. The most common cause of delayed puberty is low body fat. This occurs in girls who diet excessively, engage in very vigorous exercise or do both. Remember, you need 17% body fat to begin your period and 22% to keep it regular. And for every year you spend doing vigorous exercise as a child, you'll delay the onset of your first period by an average of five months.

Even though menstruating may feel like a nuisance, not getting a period may be hazardous to your health. If you don't have enough estrogen to produce a period, you don't have enough to maintain bone mass, and you risk developing stress fractures. You're also likely to develop osteoporosis. Your bones become old decades before you do, causing you to lose height, become hunched over or even break a hip.

There are other conditions that can delay puberty and prevent our getting our period. Thankfully, they're rare.

Turner's syndrome: Some girls are born with only one normal X chromosome. The other is either missing or incomplete. As a result, their ovaries may not develop, they lack estrogen and puberty is arrested. They also can have developmental abnormalities in their hands, arms and neck, and remain very short. This is serious and requires treatment with a combination of estrogen and progesterone to encourage sexual development, normal height and normal periods.

Testicular feminization: This is a condition in which the actual chromosomes are the male ones, XY, and testes are present. But because a crucial enzyme that is necessary for the body's cells and tissues to recognize testosterone is missing, the body develops like a female—complete with vagina and breasts. However, because the second X chromosome needed to make a genetic female is not present, the uterus never develops and there is no period. Nor is there underarm or pubic hair. This diagnosis is made by physical exam and chromosomal testing. The therapy should include the removal of the testes after they have done their thing and produced enough sex hormone to achieve a normal growth spurt. (Because the testes are in the abdomen where the ovaries usually sit, they are exposed to abnormal amounts of heat and can eventually become cancerous.) Once they are removed, estrogen is given to maintain female sexual characteristics and strong bones. The good news is that this condition is associated with a slim, strong body and no cellulite. The bad news is that it will never be possible to bear children.

Genital malformations: In order to get a period, you need a functioning uterus that opens into a vagina. On rare occasions, the uterus can be absent, in which case you obviously won't get a period. If the uterus is there but closed off from the vagina, blood will collect and the uterus will swell. This causes severe monthly pain but no bleeding, and can create a tumorlike mass. There is also a condition called *imperforate hymen*, in which the hymen, a thin membrane at the entrance to the vagina, is completely closed so that blood can't pass through. Once more, blood will accumulate in both the uterus and the vagina, causing pain. The treatment for both conditions is surgery to open the pathway.

HOW DO I KNOW IF MY PERIOD IS NORMAL?

Let's define *normal*. In our teens, this means getting a period every 21 to 45 days (counting from the first day of one menstrual period until the first day of the next). The exact number of days between periods can vary from cycle to cycle.

Also, remember that it's perfectly normal to have irregular periods for up to two years after you start menstruating. Ovulation—release of the egg and subsequent progesterone production—is a very sensitive process, and every hormone has to come at the right time and in the right amount in order for it to occur. The communication links between your brain and your ovaries are not yet well established, and it takes a while for them to get in sync. If you don't ovulate, you may miss a period or get an early one. Half of all adolescents do not ovulate regularly for the first two years after menarche, and 20% still aren't regular when they reach the five-year mark. The later you start your periods, the longer it may take for you to ovulate regularly. Being stressed out or underweight, exercising intensely or having an eating disorder can cause you to miss periods.

If in addition to having irregular periods you are overweight and develop acne, abnormal hair growth or both, you may have a condition called *polycystic ovarian syndrome*. This is accompanied by excessive production of male hormone and insulin. It should be treated with birth control pills and possibly a glucose-lowering diabetes medication (see page 247).

MY CRAMPS ARE REALLY PAINFUL. WHAT SHOULD I DO?

Take comfort in the fact that you're not alone: 75% of teenagers suffer from *dysmenorrhea*, or painful menstruation. The first line of defense is to use an over-the-counter painkiller, specifically an antiprostaglandin such as ibuprofen (Advil, Motrin, Pamprin-IB, or Nuprin) or naproxen (Aleve). These drugs are used because cramps are due to uterine contractions caused by the production of a substance called prostaglandin. These contractions close the vessels inside the uterus that are bleeding. On one hand, this protects you from excessive blood loss. On the other, it hurts.

Don't wait until your cramps become severe to start taking a painkiller. The goal is to prevent excessive prostaglandin production in the first place, so take a pill at the first sign that you're getting your period, and repeat the dose every four to eight hours to maintain active levels of the medication in your system (the label will give you this information). If ibuprofen is your drug of choice, you may need more than one tablet at a time. Some of my patients take 600 milligrams at once, but you should ask your doctor before exceeding what's recommended on the label. Never take these medications on an empty stomach.

If over-the-counter remedies aren't working, don't assume there's something radically wrong. You may simply be extraordinarily prostaglandin-sensitive, and it's time to consult your doctor, who may prescribe birth control pills. Even though you may not need contraception, the Pill is very effective at limiting prostaglandin production and is God's gift (or at least medicine's gift) to those of us who suffer from bad cramps. You'll also be blessed with periods that are predictable and light. If your cramps are still bad despite using the Pill, there is a chance you have a condition called endometriosis (see page 91). So if you don't get pain control with this type of birth control, your doctor may need to do additional tests to check for this disorder.

CAN I USE TAMPONS?

Yes. The tampon will not break or otherwise harm the hymen, nor will it get lost or stuck in your vagina. Choose the lightest absorbency tampon available (these are also the thinnest). Read the instructions that come in the package, and try putting a little Vaseline on the tip of the tampon to make insertion easier. It's also helpful to squat or put one leg on the toilet seat during insertion. The vagina tilts backward, so aim for your tailbone. The first time you pull the tampon out, you may feel as if you're going to take your insides out with it. Relax—there's no chance this will happen. It's easier to insert and remove a tampon during the heaviest-flow days of your period. Change the tampon three to four times during the day. It's okay to leave it in overnight. When your flow is light, you can use a thin pad instead of a tampon.

WHAT SHOULD I KNOW ABOUT SEX?

Sex is an important expression of romantic love, but only when it takes place between two committed grown-ups who are both ready to engage in intercourse and who trust each other completely. You should know that it carries a tremendous price. It can cause you to get sick (sexually transmitted diseases, or STDs), it can lead to cervical cancer and, obviously, it can bring about an unintended pregnancy. Sex when you're not ready, with the wrong person or against your will can also have devastating psychological consequences, such as future problems with intimacy or sex and even chronic pelvic pain.

That's my adult, medically oriented introduction to this very complicated subject. Now let's get down to the specific questions that most of my teenage patients ask.

WHAT'S THE "RIGHT" TIME TO START HAVING SEX?

If you're my daughter, the answer is, "Either at age thirty or after you've finished graduate school, whichever comes later . . ." But to answer this seriously, I have to separate your body's physical preparedness for sex from your psychological readiness for it. You won't start feeling a real desire (not to be confused with the longings you're told to feel by movies, books and your friends) until your adrenal glands start to produce male hormones. This is the *adrenarche* that causes you to develop acne, body hair and body odor—not exactly changes we associate with being sexy.

So now you're seeing boys in a whole new light. But are you physically prepared for sex? Probably not. There is a delay between male hormone production and the secretion of female hormones at levels that are sufficient to make the vagina elastic enough so that it won't be torn during intercourse. Even after you start your period, your cervix remains vulnerable. The younger you are when you expose it to unprotected intercourse, and the more partners you have to bombard it with harmful viruses, the greater your risk of cervical cancer later in life. From the physical point of view, once your periods are regular, your reproductive organs are probably up to the physical challenge of sex. But that doesn't mean you'll really enjoy it. For women, true sexual pleasure—and the orgasms that everyone talks about—comes with time, practice and a caring partner.

AM I THE ONLY ONE NOT HAVING SEX?

No. But I wouldn't be telling the truth if I didn't give you the following statistics: By age 14, almost one-quarter of teens have had intercourse, and by age 18, 70% have done so. But this doesn't mean that they're having sex frequently. It just means they've done it once.

I'VE FOOLED AROUND "DOWN THERE" BUT HAVEN'T ACTUALLY HAD INTERCOURSE. AM I STILL A VIRGIN?

Masturbation (by yourself or with a partner) or oral sex will not tear the hymen. Penetration with anything larger than a finger can. But even without penetration, you can contract a sexually transmitted disease—maybe even get pregnant. If sperm are deposited near the vagina, on the outer lips or even the inner thighs, they are capable of swimming up and making contact with an egg.

MY BOYFRIEND WANTS US TO HAVE SEX. WHAT SHOULD I DO?

First you need to decide what *you* want to do—a decision that should not be made in the heat of passion. If you are ready to have intercourse because you feel it's an expression of your emotional commitment to one person, then you need to take responsibility for the consequences. That means protecting yourself from STDs and from pregnancy (more advice on this below). If you don't want to have intercourse, you'll have to discuss it with him and give him fair warning. If he pressures you and makes you feel inadequate, it's time to reevaluate the relationship. Who you are and what you're worth as a person are not dependent on access to your vagina.

ONCE I'VE DECIDED TO HAVE SEX, HOW SHOULD I PROTECT MYSELF AGAINST PREGNANCY AND STDS?

There's no foolproof method that can do either. Although doctors, teachers, parents and even your peers are all preaching "condoms, condoms, condoms," this method of protection is less than 90% effective in preventing pregnancy and less than 80% effective in blocking sexually transmitted diseases. The younger and less experienced your partner, the more likely that accidents will occur. Condoms have to be placed on the penis when it's erect and before it comes in contact with your body. The first few drops of semen that are secreted before ejaculation are enough to get you pregnant or give you an infection. That's why withdrawal before ejaculation (signaled by that famous phrase "Don't worry, I won't come") fails to prevent pregnancy 18% of the time. It's also important that you or your partner grasp the rim of the condom and keep it on the penis when he withdraws to avoid spills.

Even if you do all this right, condoms can tear or leak. So be prepared to request emergency contraception (see page 15 for more about this) if this should happen. Most condoms contain spermicide, but to improve your chances of protection from both pregnancy and STDs, you might want to put extra spermicide, in the form of a gel, suppository or vaginal film, into your vagina. You can also use a diaphragm with spermicide. Double the protection may not mean double the fun, but it can double your peace of mind. Don't be tempted to use the spermicide alone, however. Used solo, it fails at pregnancy prevention 21% of the time. You won't do much better with the diaphragm plus a spermicide. This combination fails to provide contraception 18% of the time, nor does it provide adequate protection against STDs.

For maximum contraception, you should consider birth control pills, which protect against pregnancy 97% of the time—perhaps even more often if you are diligent about taking your pills at the same time every day. The Pill works by overriding your body's own production of estrogen, temporarily shutting off secretion of hormones that trigger ovulation (the release of an egg). This applies to a pill that contains both estrogen and progestin. A progestin-only pill is not as effective at shutting down ovulation, but it makes the mucus produced by the cervix thick and hostile, which helps prevent sperm from gaining access to the egg. This type of pill has twice the failure rate of combined estrogen-plus-progestin pills, and is even more likely to be inadequate if you don't take it at the same time every day. But because the Pill does not safeguard against STDs, you should still use condoms. This is as close to protection perfection as you can get—outside of abstinence.

If you think that you're not going to be consistent in taking the Pill, you might want to consider Depo-Provera, a long-acting injectable contraceptive. The shot is given every three months and is 99.7% effective at preventing pregnancy. It can cause your periods to become irregular, even stop, and you may develop spotting. On occasion it can also trigger weight gain, headaches and depression (although nothing leads to weight gain, headaches and depression like an unwanted pregnancy). Depo-Provera certainly will not protect you from STDs.

HELP, THE CONDOM BROKE! (OKAY, WE DIDN'T USE IT IN THE FIRST PLACE.) WHAT SHOULD I DO?

This is an emergency, and it's time for emergency contraception. Any doctor can provide you with the high dose of oral contraceptives that, taken within 72 hours of the accident, can decrease your risk for pregnancy by 75%. (This doesn't mean that 25% of women who use it will get pregnant. Let me explain: If 100 women were to have unprotected intercourse during the most fertile part of their cycle, 8 would get pregnant. But if those same 100 women used emergency contraception, only 2 would conceive. That's a 75% reduction in risk.)

If you already happen to have a package of birth control pills at home and you're not on the Pill, you can immediately take either four low-dose pills or two high-dose pills and repeat the same dosage 12 hours later. A low-dose pill is one that contains 35 milligrams of estrogen; high-dose pills contain 50 milligrams (the package label will say how much estrogen a pill has). If you're on a triphasic pill such as Ortho Tri-Cyclen, Triphasil or Tri-Norinyl, use the pills in the pack (four at a time) from day 14 through day 21.

There is also a special packet of emergency contraceptive pills sold under the brand name Preven. You can call your doctor for a prescription in an emergency, or preorder one to keep at home just in case. If you don't have a regular doctor, call 1-888-NOT-2-LATE for the name of a health care provider near you who will prescribe this product.

Emergency contraception is truly contraception: It prevents release of the egg or fertilization. If the egg becomes fertilized before you take the Pill, you're more likely to be among the 25% of women for whom this method doesn't work. (This type of morning-after contraception is not an "abortion pill" and should not be confused with RU-486, an antiprogesterone that can prevent implantation or induce miscarriage.) The most common side effect is nausea, so many doctors will prescribe an antinausea pill along with it. Don't worry: Even if you vomit, the pills will probably work. They may bring on an early period if you take them during the first half of your cycle, or a late period if you take them in the second half.

HOW CAN I GET PROTECTION WITHOUT
MY PARENTS KNOWING?

You can walk into any drugstore and buy condoms—no one should ask questions, and there is no law that prevents selling them to minors. If you'd like to explore all your contraceptive choices, call your local chapter of Planned Parenthood. All Planned Parenthood clinics offer free examinations, STD testing and advice on and access to contraception. In some states, their health care providers will allow you to pick up free or low-cost birth control pills without even having a pelvic exam. If you fear that you are pregnant, you can be tested and obtain confidential information about your options. In these situations, the law considers you to be an "emancipated minor." In other words, your parents don't have to be informed, nor must they consent to your use of contraception.

HOW CAN I BRING UP THE SUBJECT
OF CONDOMS WITH MY PARTNER?

The time to discuss condom use is well before the two of you are engaged in a moment of deep passion. Just in case he fails as the designated condom buyer, carry your own. Then, when a condom is needed, you can simply say, "I brought this so we don't have to worry." If he says he doesn't need or like condoms or just says "trust me," you can declare that you trust that he really cares about you, and that's why you know he'll agree to use a condom. You might point out that it's for his benefit as well as your own. If he still refuses, you should do the same. Chances are he'll reach for that package. What aroused man would not realize that sex with a condom is better than no sex at all?

I HAVE A STEADY BOYFRIEND.
WHEN CAN WE STOP USING CONDOMS?

My recommendation is that each of you get tested for HIV, the virus that causes AIDS, at the beginning of your relationship. After six months, if you've been monogamous and used condoms religiously, you should be tested again. If you both test negative both times, the only thing you can be sure of is that you will not contract HIV if you stop using condoms and neither of you has sex with anyone else. But a word of warning: I can't begin to tell you how many of my teenage patients have found that their so-called exclusive boyfriends were actually cheating.

Even if your mate is truly a one-woman man, there are a huge number of viruses and bacteria that can be shared once you stop using protection. The adage that you sleep with every partner that your partner ever slept with is absolutely true. There is a virtual epidemic of human papillomaviruses (HPV), viruses that cause venereal warts and precancerous changes in the cervix, herpes, chlamydia and gonorrhea, which can lead to infertility, as well as hepatitis and trichomonas, which causes irritating discharge. This is not just an adult problem: Each year, 25% of new STD cases are diagnosed in teenagers. Despite what your friends may have told you, you cannot look at your partner's genitals and tell whether he has any of these infections. (Please note: Only 10% of those who carry the herpes virus develop visible lesions and just 1% of those with HPV develop external warts.) If you stop using condoms, be prepared to share *everything* with your boyfriend.

WHEN SHOULD I START SEEING A GYNECOLOGIST?

You should have your first visit at the age of 16 or when you become sexually active, whichever comes first. If you are 16 and have not had sex, you should still see the doctor to discuss your gynecologic health, although you may not need a pelvic exam. You also need to see the doctor if your periods are extremely painful, if you have not gotten a period by age 16, or if you have not started to develop breasts and pubic hair by age 14. Your family doctor may be the one to see you, or you might ask your mother if it's okay for you to see her gynecologist.

My patients know that after an initial visit they can call me with questions or pop in for tests or advice and that it's always confidential. But other doctors might want to share important information about your health with your parents, so ask the physician how she handles confidentiality for teenagers. If you're not happy with her response, or if you are uncomfortable sharing a doctor with your mother, make your own appointment at Planned Parenthood or a local family planning clinic.

WHAT'S THE POINT OF HAVING A PAP SMEAR, ANYWAY?

The Pap smear has revolutionized women's health. Cervical cancer used to kill tens of thousands of young women annually. But with a quick turn of a tiny brush at the opening of the cervix, doctors can take a sample of cells that, when examined under the microscope, can show precancerous changes. This allows us to treat you with simple office procedures so that you never get the cancer. As great as the Pap smear is, it will only check for cervical precancer and cancer. It will not detect a sexually transmitted disease or other infection. That requires using a swab to gather cells from the cervix and checking to see if bacteria or viruses are present. It certainly cannot check to see if you're pregnant.

I THINK I'M PREGNANT. WHAT SHOULD I DO?

If your period's late, you can do a simple home pregnancy test. If the results are negative, wait a week and, if you still don't have your period, repeat the test. It's very common to miss periods for the first couple of years after you start menstruating. Stress, crazy diets, weight loss or extreme exercise can be the culprit. If your period was fairly regular and you've now missed three cycles, it's time to talk to your doctor. She may prescribe progesterone (Provera or Prometrium) to bring on your period. If that doesn't help, she may recommend taking the Pill to regulate your cycle and make sure you have enough estrogen to protect your bones.

Now to the problems of a positive pregnancy test. This will probably be one of the most stressful and confusing issues you will ever face, and you need to be able to talk to a sympathetic and understanding adult. It may be a parent, but if you feel that you can't confide in your mom or dad, at least not initially, you can talk to counselors at a family planning clinic such as Planned Parenthood. They will go over your options with you. These include continuing the pregnancy and either keeping the baby or giving it up for adoption, or terminating the pregnancy. If you decide on the latter, talk to the counselor about whether or not you will need a parent's consent to get an abortion. If you live in a state that requires parental consent and you can't get it, your counselor may be able to help you obtain it from the court system or leave the state to have the procedure. The sooner you deal with this, the easier it will be from a medical point of view. Currently, there are a number of Planned Parenthood clinics that perform medical abortions (those done with drugs instead of surgery) if you are less than seven weeks pregnant. Because this form of termination is still in the testing stages, these clinics may be reluctant to give you the medication if you're under 18, or they may require a parent's consent.

Early surgical abortion (before 12 weeks of pregnancy) can be done as an office procedure. It involves dilating (opening) the cervix and scraping and vacuuming the uterine lining. The patient is usually awake but is given an intravenous medication that dulls pain and causes drowsiness, as well as a local anesthetic to numb the cervix. The whole procedure takes about five minutes and patients can go home in a couple of hours, after the medications wear off. Antibiotics are usually prescribed afterward to prevent infection.

If a surgical abortion is performed by a competent physician, the chance of complications is minimal (less than 0.5%). But let's not forget that this is a procedure that nobody wants to have, and it should never be considered a form of contraception.

Unfortunately, 10% of terminations have to be performed when a woman is more than 12 weeks pregnant. If she has irregular periods she may not realize she's pregnant for several months, or making the decision to have an abortion and then getting consent for one may result in a delay. These procedures are more difficult, have higher complication rates and sometimes require a general anesthetic and even a hospital visit. So if your period is late, don't ignore it. Pregnancy is not something that will go away on its own.

SO WHAT'S THE BIG DEAL IF I SMOKE? ALL MY FRIENDS DO.

You're almost right—if we look at the stats on teen smokers, the number is probably closer to one in three. But for those who do smoke, it's a huge deal, so huge that I don't even know whether to start with the issue of addiction or with the facts about smoking's devastating effect on your health. Because I'm addicted to giving advice, let's start with the former.

It's as easy to get hooked on nicotine as it is on cocaine. Nicotine raises levels of several brain chemicals so that you either feel relaxed or invigorated, and it takes the edge off of anxiety and depression. When you try to stop, the high levels of these brain chemicals plummet, and initially you feel lousy. The impact of those cigarettes on your health is so severe that if you do take up the habit you will eventually be faced with a choice: quit or be sick or even die. And stopping is so tough that it's a lot easier never to start in the first place.

Now let me tell you why I'm so sure you'll face this choice. There are 2,500 chemicals in tobacco smoke (more than in the exhaust of a car— would you inhale that?). These chemicals are responsible for 29% of all cancers in women, including the leading cancer killer, lung cancer.

Women who smoke are 12 times more likely than those who don't to die from lung cancer. Thirty percent of cervical cancers are due to exposure to chemicals in cigarette smoke that decrease your immunity to the sexually transmitted human papillomavirus. You're also more likely to develop venereal warts.

Smoking is also to blame for 55% of fatal heart attacks and strokes in women under the age of 65. And the risk of being maimed or dying from one of these conditions is highest among those who begin smoking before age 15. The chemicals in cigarette smoke also suck the calcium out of your bones, putting you at risk for fractures at a relatively young age.

Then there's the cosmetic issue. Tobacco smoke stains your teeth and gives you bad breath. It damages small blood vessels in the skin, especially around your lips and eyes, and can age your complexion by 10 years or more.

Because 91% of women who smoke as adults had their first cigarette in their teens, and very few women begin smoking after age 20, you can beat this addiction forever if you stay away from cigarettes now. Your body will thank you for the rest of your life.

SOMETIMES I DRINK SO MUCH AT A PARTY THAT I CAN'T REMEMBER WHAT HAPPENED THE NEXT DAY. SHOULD I WORRY?

You bet you should. The minute you lose awareness you put yourself at risk for sexual assault, a fatal car accident or choking on your own vomit. You also risk alcohol poisoning, coma and brain damage.

Don't kid yourself into thinking you can keep up with the guys. Because of your smaller size, the estrogen you produce and differences in the way women and men metabolize alcohol, you absorb it more rapidly and break it down less efficiently. Finally, alcohol travels to your brain faster. So one drink for you (a drink is defined as a bottle of beer, a glass of wine or 1.5 ounces of hard liquor) equals two for a man. Despite this gender inequality, up to 45% of women in college binge on alcohol, downing six or more drinks in a sitting, as often as three nights a week.

Many of these binge drinkers are using alcohol to self-medicate for anxiety, to get them into a party mood and to make sex easier. The truth is that alcohol actually inhibits desire and sexual response. Unfortunately, it also inhibits your vigilance about choosing a partner and protecting yourself against pregnancy and STDs.

Bingeing may also start you on the road to alcoholism. Most female alcoholics begin drinking at age 13. You're especially at risk if you have low self-esteem, severe PMS, an eating disorder, depression or a history of sexual abuse. If either of your parents is an alcoholic, genetics could also be working against you: You stand a 50% chance of having inherited a susceptibility to alcohol abuse. Since alcoholism is the third leading cause of death among women 35 to 55 and shortens a woman's life span by 15 years, anything that leads you to chronically abuse alcohol is a major concern at any age. A final word about the possible finality of drinking: Nearly half of motor-vehicle-related deaths, half of suicides and homicides and one-third of fatal drownings and boating accidents involve alcohol. The more, the deadlier!

WHAT TESTS SHOULD I HAVE?

These are the examinations, tests and procedures I recommend to my teenage patients.

Examination/test/procedure	How often
Blood pressure	Every two years
Pelvic exam and Pap smear	Annually after age 16 or first sexual activity, whichever comes first
STD testing	Chlamydia testing with each Pap test if sexually active; other tests at your/your doctor's discretion
Immunizations	Tetanus booster every 10 years; hepatitis B vaccine if not given in childhood
Eye exam	Once at puberty

WHAT CAN GO WRONG AT MY AGE?

Acne

Nearly 85% of teens suffer from acne. Contrary to popular belief, this is not due to your consumption of french fries and chocolate, or a reflection on your personal hygiene habits. Rather, it is because puberty starts with an awakening of the adrenal glands, which pump out increasing amounts of male hormone. These androgens promote oil secretion by the skin, which sets up the process of pimple formation. It takes two months to make a pimple. An oil gland in your skin is activated and secretes excessive amounts of oil called *sebum*. The gland gets clogged and bacteria trapped within it multiply, resulting in inflammation, otherwise known as a zit.

For many teens, this is more than just a cosmetic issue. Acne can be disfiguring and cause permanent scarring that can leave you feeling self-conscious, depressed and inadequate. That's why it is a major problem that warrants medical attention.

Treatment involves some combination of the following: slowing oil production, stopping glands from becoming clogged and halting infection. Nonprescription products containing benzoil peroxide or salicylic acid can prevent clogging and infection. If they don't work, your doctor might prescribe an antibiotic such as clindamycin or erythromycin that's applied to the skin to block formation of new pimples. Or she may recommend tretinoin (Retin-A), which will do the same. If you still break out, the next step would be to use antibiotic pills, including tetracycline, erythromycin, minocycline or trimethoprim-sulfamethoxazole. These can suppress bacteria and reduce inflammation. Adding a tretinoin cream to your regimen may help these antibiotics work.

If you really want to nip pimples in the bud, you might want to ask your doctor about taking birth control pills. The Pill's estrogen will counterbalance your male hormones and help prevent oil accumulation in the glands. One pill, Ortho Tri-Cyclen, even has the Food and Drug Administration's approval for use in treating acne.

If all else fails and you're still plagued by severe acne, your doctor might recommend the drug Accutane. This will dry your skin and prevent clogging, infection and inflammation. If you take this drug, you'll need to be carefully monitored with blood tests to check your liver function. Because Accutane can cause birth defects, you must either be completely celibate or use a reliable contraceptive (usually the Pill). Even after you stop taking the drug, you should not get pregnant for at least a month.

Depression

Being a teenager is tough even under the best of circumstances. You're trying to figure out who you are, where you fit in and how to deal with your parents and other authority figures. You're expected to perform at school, compete at sports, develop relationships (and decide if they should become sexual) and set the course for your future. On top of all this, you're coping with the

biggest hormonal upheaval of your life and a body that's growing and changing before your eyes. So of course there will be times when you feel down.
But being a teenager also means that you're at risk for a far more serious form
of depression, one that can seriously disrupt or even end your life.

As we go through puberty, we become women, and one in five women
will, at some point in her life, develop clinical depression. We're twice as
likely as men to have this disorder, in part because the estrogen and progesterone we produce affect levels of mood-regulating brain chemicals
such as serotonin. True clinical depression entails persistent feelings of sadness, unhappiness or emptiness; loss of interest in things that previously
gave you pleasure; low self-esteem; negative thoughts; difficulty concentrating; as well as suicidal thoughts, even hallucinations. If this occurs, you
may feel agitated or exhausted, cry for no apparent reason, withdraw from
your friends or family, have trouble sleeping (or staying awake) and lose (or
gain) appetite or weight. Fifteen percent of women who are clinically
depressed kill themselves, making this truly a matter of life and death. So if
any of these symptoms sound familiar, let your family and your doctor
know. You're at greater than average risk for depression if you have a family history of it, if you've been sexually abused, if you have attention deficit
disorder (ADD) or if you smoke or abuse alcohol or other drugs.

Even if you are not clinically depressed, you may experience premenstrual syndrome (PMS), which could leave you feeling blue for one to two
weeks before you menstruate. In some cases, you may feel so down that
you are unable to cope with your daily activities. This is called premenstrual dysphoric disorder (PMDD). Having either of these conditions places
you at increased risk of clinical depression.

Listen to your feelings and don't feel that you have to cope on your own.
There are very effective therapies for all forms of depression (see page 65),
and seeking help now can ensure that your present—and future—are
much happier.

Eating Disorders

Just being a teenager puts you at risk for an eating disorder. It's understandable. You went from a childlike, lean, flat-chested physique to that of a
heavier, bustier and more curvaceous young woman. Suddenly people are
looking at you as a sexual being—which can be scary. Everything you watch
on television or read in magazines tells you that gaining weight is a sin, that
you should fight fat with all your might and that if you don't succeed in
regaining your prepubertal body, no one will love or admire you. And these

changes occurred without your permission; your surging hormones simply took control of your body! You're left feeling that if you can regain control by whatever means necessary, you will not only stay slim (and like yourself better) but will be able to control other aspects of your life as well.

The eating disorders most likely to strike in adolescence are *anorexia* and *bulimia*. Anorexia is defined as a refusal to maintain the lowest weight considered normal for your age and height, together with a horrendous fear of becoming fat, a distorted body image and three consecutive missed menstrual periods without pregnancy. Anorexics may memorize the caloric content of every morsel they put in their mouths and concoct eating rituals, such as avoiding certain combinations of foods or dissecting what they eat into dozens of small pieces. They are also likely to become vegetarians. Up to 1% of girls between the ages of 14 and 19 develop this condition.

Bulimia, which literally means "ox eating," is characterized by recurrent binge eating (two episodes per week for at least three months). It is accompanied by a loss of control while bingeing; the regular use of vomiting, laxatives, diuretics, strict diets, fasting or vigorous exercise to control weight; and an overwhelming concern with body shape and weight. One to five percent of girls fit these criteria, but many more girls binge: Up to half of adolescent girls overeat and then vomit to control their weight.

An eating disorder is more likely to occur if you've been teased about your weight in the past or are driven (by yourself or your parents) to excel in a physical activity, especially gymnastics, ballet or running, where weight affects performance. Having a perfectionist personality, low self-esteem or difficulty communicating with others or being separated from your family during camp or boarding school will also put you at risk. Living at home isn't easy, either. If members of your family are rigid and demanding of perfection, or if they have trouble communicating or displaying their feelings, they may give you the sense that you were and should continue to be a perfect little girl, with a little girl's body.

When you don't feed your body, it slows down. A serious eating disorder and weight loss can cause your blood pressure to fall, your breathing to slow and your periods to stop. Your skin may become dry, your hair can fall out and your nails get brittle. You may feel cold and lightheaded, become bloated, constipated and suffer from joint pain. Add to all this disturbed sleep, and depression is sure to come. If you're bulimic, you are also likely to develop bad breath and decayed, yellow teeth. Ultimately, an eating disorder can kill you.

The longer you let these symptoms go on, the more likely it is that the damage will be permanent. If your family has not figured out what's going on, it may be up to you to reach out for help. If your symptoms or psychological problems are life-threatening, you will need hospitalization. But if you're in no immediate danger, most of your therapy can be done while you live at home and continue your school or work routine. This entails a combination of psychotherapy, nutritional counseling, behavior modification and participation in self-help groups. Although there are no drugs specifically approved to treat anorexia and bulimia, doctors often prescribe antidepressants, which can help. Therapy lasts a year or more, but even after your weight has stabilized, you are vulnerable to future bouts with eating or other psychological disorders and so may have to be on the alert for life.

MY TOP 10 LIST FOR STAYING HEALTHY IN YOUR TEENS

1. Don't smoke.
2. Use a seat belt. The number one cause of death for teenagers is automobile accidents. Never drive drunk or get in the car with a drunk driver.
3. Don't use drugs or abuse alcohol.
4. Avoid drastic weight changes.
5. Do some form of moderate exercise—as little as three hours a week will lower your future risk of breast cancer.
6. If you choose to have sex, limit your number of partners, always use condoms and add birth control pills (or some other additional form of protection).
7. Limit your sun exposure and use ample amounts of a sunscreen with a sun protection factor of at least 15. There's no such thing as a healthy tan, and you should never allow yourself to burn.
8. Get at least 1,000 milligrams of calcium per day, either from dairy products or a calcium supplement. Take a multivitamin that contains 400 micrograms of folic acid each day.
9. Have five servings of fruits and vegetables per day. Even three-quarters of a cup of juice, a small piece of fruit or half a cup of cooked vegetables counts as a serving.
10. Cultivate a close relationship with your parents, a teacher or another adult whom you respect and trust to help you make difficult decisions in your life.

YOUR TWENTIES

PUBERTY WAS A time when your glands had to learn how to interrelate and function on cue. Your periods weren't always on time, you were acquiring fat in new places and your skin was a battlefield for male and female hormones. But by your early twenties your endocrine system, which includes your pituitary and adrenal glands, thyroid, ovaries and pancreas, should be set on its course and working at full speed. This means that your hormonal system now knows how to control your body. Most of you can count on getting your period every month, and your fertility has never been better. If you get acne, it tends to be cyclical rather than continuous.

The setpoint for your natural weight has been established in your brain's center, and this will regulate how you use or conserve calories in the years to come. At this point in your life, if you eat too much your body usually accommodates this lapse of eating control and burns the excess calories; while if you eat too little, it slows down to conserve energy. That explains your wonderful and unique ability to recklessly eat those hamburgers and french fries and not notice the results on your hips. (But remember, this is a temporary reprieve!) During this decade, your dress and shoe size stop changing and you can finally spend the money on a designer outfit without worrying that you'll outgrow it. If you leave your body alone at this age, it will usually do great. Many of your queries at this time will relate to your sexuality and the concomitant issues of contraception, pregnancy and infections. Here are the answers.

I'M SUPPOSED TO BE REGULAR. I'M NOT. WHY?

First let's define "regular": It's a period that comes every 21 to 45 days (count from the first day of one period to the first day of the next). A normal flow lasts 3 to 7 days, and you can expect to soak 10 to 21 tampons or pads per cycle.

The process that brings on a period begins in your brain in the hypothalamus and pituitary gland, continues on to your ovaries and ends with the thickening and shedding of the uterine lining. Anything that affects this pathway can throw your cycle out of sync. To complicate matters, overriding hormones produced by the thyroid can interfere with or cancel out the signals generated along this pathway.

When you start to produce estrogen in the ovary, the lining of the uterus begins to thicken and prepares for the progesterone surge that comes after ovulation to further boost its growth and development. Normally, in the absence of pregnancy, estrogen and progesterone levels fall and the lining sloughs. This is your period. When there is too little estrogen produced in the ovary in the first place, the lining never builds up and there is nothing to shed. Another possibility is that estrogen is produced but there is insufficient progesterone because of faulty or absent ovulation. In this case, the lining can shed early, late or not at all.

So what can affect the first signal in the hormonal cascade that originates in the hypothalamus? Stress, that catchall term for all the physical or psychological stimuli that bombard this brain center, is the most common reason for early or late periods. Stress from a hypothalamic point of view includes extreme exercise, radical dietary changes, sudden weight loss, travel across time zones, illness, emotional upheaval and anything else that you personally find puts pressure on your body and soul.

As we travel down the endocrine pathway, the next stop is the pituitary. This gland is instructed by the hypothalamus to secrete follicle stimulating hormone (FSH), which then signals the ovary to start producing estrogen.

After sufficient estrogen is made, the female hormone bathes the pituitary and coaxes it to put out luteinizing hormone (LH), which goes down to the estrogen-primed ovary and causes ovulation and subsequent production of progesterone.

This process can be interrupted by a tumor in or near the pituitary. Any tumor in the brain sounds horrendously scary, but there is actually a relatively common, benign growth called a *pituitary adenoma* that may be present in as many as 10% of women. (We know this because it's been found during autopsies.) Occasionally, this tumor becomes large enough to affect pituitary function and, as a result, cycles can be thrown off. Because this adenoma also triggers an increase in production of the hormone prolactin, which causes our breasts to make milk after childbirth, women with this type of tumor often secrete fluid from their nipples. This has been given the fancy medical name *galactorrhea*. (You've probably noticed that when your doctor does a breast exam, she squeezes the breast to check for galactorrhea.) If your periods are irregular and you're experiencing nipple discharge, an MRI is warranted to see if the pituitary is enlarged (a pituitary adenoma). This condition rarely requires surgery. It usually can be treated with medication that reduces prolactin secretion and controls tumor growth.

Now on to the ovaries. These glands must be sensitive and receptive to higher signals. But sometimes they aren't. When their own hormonal milieu is off, as can occur in a condition called *polycystic ovarian syndrome* (PCO), the follicles don't go "all the way" and release an egg or produce adequate progesterone. Instead, in their state of confusion, they make lots of small, painless cysts. This is a very complex and not yet completely understood condition that probably involves abnormal amounts of FSH and LH from the pituitary as well as excess production of male hormones and insulin. Full-blown PCO comes with the classic symptoms of irregular or widely spaced periods or no periods at all, together with excessive malelike body hair, weight gain and subsequent infertility. If not treated, it can lead to some serious medical conditions such as diabetes, endometrial cancer, breast cancer and heart disease.

In up to 10% of women, PCO can also appear in a milder form, causing only irregular periods, slightly increased body hair or acne, with or without a tendency to gain weight, especially around the waistline. Once you understand why PCO happens, the therapy is logical: Birth control pills shut down abnormal signals from the pituitary and take over for the misbehaving ovary, providing even amounts of estrogen and progesterone. They also block male hormones. In some women, medications that treat early diabetes and lower insulin levels may help control this disorder and its associated weight gain.

On very rare occasions, the ovaries can fail 20 years before their expected time. This can be due to chromosomal abnormalities in which part of the second X chromosome is missing (Turner's syndrome). Some women may also have a diminished number of eggs in their ovaries from birth. This can be genetic and their mothers and sisters also tend to experience a very early menopause. If delayed or absent periods are accompanied by hot flashes, it's worth checking for premature menopause. This is done with blood tests that measure FSH and estrogen. (When the ovary fails and is not producing estrogen, the pituitary works harder to try to prod it into action and FSH levels rise.) At present, there's no way to "restart" failed ovaries, and treatment for premature ovarian failure involves replacing the missing hormones with estrogen and progesterone (hormone replacement therapy, or HRT).

Our final stop on our cycle pathway is the uterus, or more precisely its endometrium. If this lining is scarred, it can't respond to the signals from the ovary to thicken and shed, even if all the hormones are there in the right amounts at the right time. Scarring can occur as a result of severe infection after dilation and curettage (D&C), which is performed following incomplete delivery of the placenta in childbirth, after a miscarriage or to terminate a pregnancy. Treatment for this condition, called Asherman's syndrome, is only necessary if you plan to have children. In that case, attempts are made to surgically remove the scar tissue and restore the lining with high doses of estrogen and progesterone.

A gland that isn't considered part of this pathway but is important in determining regularity is the thyroid. I call the thyroid the "mama gland" because if it produces too much or too little thyroid hormone, it can throw off many of the body's other hormonal systems. So one of the first things that needs to be assessed if your periods go awry is thyroid activity. Like ovarian hormones, thyroid hormone production is under the direction of the pituitary and its thyroid stimulating hormone (TSH). This is what should be measured in blood tests to establish levels of thyroid function. If your thyroid is underactive, the pituitary will work harder and thyroid stimulating hormone (TSH) will be elevated. In this case, your late or missing periods may be accompanied by a general slowing of your metabolism, resulting in fatigue, constipation and weight gain. If your thyroid is overactive, you may have frequent or heavy periods. Now the pituitary has cut back its production of TSH and the level will be low. Other symptoms include those of a revved-up metabolism: weight loss, nervousness, insomnia, rapid heartbeat, heat intolerance and heavy sweating. The treatment is to correct thyroid function, either by taking a thyroid hormone supplement or by suppressing thyroid hormone production.

I would be remiss if I didn't remind you that *the* most common cause of a delayed period in our twenties is pregnancy. So even though you used contraception or only had intercourse when you thought you weren't fertile, a pregnancy test is in order.

HOW CAN I GET RELIEF FROM MY PMS SYMPTOMS?

What you can do to feel better the week or two before your period depends on how and why you feel bad. PMS symptoms include emotional upset (hypersensitivity, depression, irritability, sadness, anger, mood swings, anxiety and tension). We can also become less sociable, more forgetful and have difficulty concentrating. Some investigators report that we can even become more confused. Any confusion I have stems from reviewing the medical literature on this topic, which at some point attributes every symptom known to woman to PMS. This is usually followed by still other literature refuting the first group of data. But don't let anyone tell you that PMS affects your comprehension and general mental sharpness. These have been tested and found to remain intact.

Fortunately (for this report, but not for you) the investigators do agree on a list of physical complaints associated with PMS. These include bloating, body aches, breast tenderness, headaches, fatigue, food cravings, hot flashes, sleep disturbance, bowel changes and poor coordination. Like a majority of women, you will probably recognize some of these symptoms (you don't need all of them to qualify for a diagnosis). Indeed, 75% to 80% of women have some degree of PMS, and for 30% to 40%, it is moderate to severe.

PMS is produced by a complex interaction between our changing levels of estrogen and progesterone, our "feel-good" endorphins, chemicals in our brain and pain-mediating prostaglandins. It appears that it's the *change* in estrogen and progesterone levels, and not the levels themselves, that leads to symptoms. (Until recently, doctors thought that estrogen was the "good gal" and had little to do with PMS. The rise of progesterone during the second half of the menstrual cycle got all the blame. It's not that simple. If both estrogen and progesterone are eliminated with a medication that causes hormonal shutdown, PMS goes away. But if either hormone is added back, symptoms return.) There's no blood test for PMS—levels of estrogen and progesterone in every part of the cycle are the same for women who have PMS as for those who do not.

Now to the reassuring part—the reason you asked this question in the first place. There is help.

Diet: Low blood sugar and PMS symptoms appear to be linked, so consume meals that are roughly 60% carbohydrate, 20% protein and 20% fat. Frequent small meals are especially helpful at keeping blood sugar levels even. (There is actually a carbohydrate-rich beverage called Escape that's touted to help PMS-related mood and appetite changes by increasing brain serotonin levels.) Although there's no evidence that excess salt causes PMS, limiting your sodium intake may help relieve bloating. Try limiting caffeine as well. It can increase anxiety, tension, irritability and breast pain, making any symptoms you're already feeling worse.

Exercise: Increasing aerobic exercise may reduce some physical symptoms, possibly by increasing your output of endorphins, natural feel-good chemicals. Strength training does not seem to have the same effect.

Supplements: One recent study found that women who took 1,200 milligrams of calcium carbonate daily (in the form of a Tums antacid) had roughly double the decrease in PMS symptoms as women who took a placebo. This gives me a chance to double my recommendation that you take your calcium every day. We then have a long list of supplements, including vitamins E and B_6, as well as evening primrose oil, that have not been given the medical seal of approval because carefully controlled studies have not shown them to be more effective than a placebo. But tradition and patients' testimonials have tempered my skepticism, and my advice is that if you want to try these, make sure that you don't overdose (600 milligrams of vitamin B_6 daily has been shown to cause nerve problems).

Medication: There is no single, overall, "fix PMS" medication, unless we include therapy with Lupron or Synarel, drugs that shut down the ovaries and render us chemically menopausal. In very rare instances where nothing else helps, this has been used. (But then, of course, you develop all the symptoms of menopause—unless you add back hormones, some of which will reinstitute PMS.) The more reasonable therapies are geared to your symptoms.

Over-the-counter nonsteroidal anti-inflammatory drugs (NSAIDs) such as ibuprofen, naproxen and aspirin, and prescription ones like Ponstel, Cataflam and Anaprox DS can help physical symptoms, including cramps, headache, achiness and breast pain. Nonprescription diuretics may relieve that bloated feeling and are often packaged with a pain reliever (Pamprin, Midol PMS Formula and Premsyn PMS). Stronger prescription diuretics are controversial because they can upset the body's balance of sodium and potassium and are habit-forming. However, one type, spironolactone, is less so and may decrease moodiness as well as water retention. Warning: It can also decrease your libido. Parlodel, usually prescribed to suppress lactation after childbirth, may be helpful for severe breast pain.

Birth control pills can ease a wide variety of symptoms because they essentially suppress your ovaries' production of estrogen and progesterone and give you a controlled amount of these hormones. But even this amount may be enough to instigate (and certainly not alleviate) PMS problems in susceptible women. Theoretically, the lower a pill's progestin activity, the less likely it is to trigger symptoms, so try Mircette, Ortho-Cept, Desogen, Ortho-Cyclen, Ovcon, Modicon, Alesse or Levlite. If the week off of the Pill each month causes PMS misery, you can take up to three months' worth of active pills without time off for a pill-free or placebo week.

Antidepressants work wonders when PMS affects your mood and causes depression. Those that are selective serotonin reuptake inhibitors (SSRIs) are especially useful (see page 65). St. John's wort, an herbal product that does not require a prescription, has been shown in German studies to have an effect similar to the SSRIs without many of the side effects.

If your mood is more anxious than depressed, an anti-anxiety medication such as Xanax may be in order. You don't need to take it all the time—just when your symptoms tend to arise.

WHY AM I SPOTTING?

Light bleeding between periods isn't just annoying, it triggers panic for many women. The most common concern is "Is it cancer?" I'd like to say certainly not, but the one thing we know about medicine is that nothing is ever 100% certain. So you'll have to settle for "It's highly unlikely that your spotting is due to a serious condition."

Let's consider the possible sources of blood from the bottom up: Irritation of the vulva or vagina can cause minimal bleeding and a pinkish discharge. If that discoloration on your panties is accompanied by itching or burning, you need to be checked and treated for infection.

The cervix is our next step. It can also be irritated and spot or bleed, especially after intercourse or tampon use. This type of inflammation is frequently due to the exposure of sensitive cervical cells to a bombardment of bacteria present in the vagina. (Believe it or not, the vagina contains more bacteria than the rectum—but less than the mouth.) Spotting may be the only symptom of this inflammation, which is called *cervicitis*. The diagnosis requires an examination with a speculum. Sometimes a doctor will perform a culture to check for abnormal bacteria, including sexually transmitted ones such as chlamydia and gonorrhea. If the wrong bacteria are present from an STD, you need antibiotics in pill form. Other non-STD infections can sometimes be treated with antibiotic creams. If the culture is normal and cervical irritation and spotting persist, some doctors will perform cryotherapy, freezing the cervix to destroy the inflamed cells and allow healthy new ones to grow. None of this should be done until the results of your Pap smear give reassurance that there are no precancerous changes in your cervix. On very rare occasions, spotting is due to cervical cancer.

Benign growths (polyps) coming from the glands lining the cervical canal, or endocervix, can also cause spotting. These are easily removed during your examination. Similar polyps can also grow in the lining of the uterus. These are harder to detect and may require a vaginal ultrasound. Unfortunately, if these polyps are large enough to warrant removal, a surgical procedure such as a D&C or hysteroscopy may be necessary. If the polyps are small, they can often be managed with birth control pills, which can prevent an abnormal buildup of the endometrium. Although it's unusual to have fibroids or endometriosis in your twenties, these conditions can also cause spotting. For more information, see pages 91 and 127.

Finally, if your hormones are off, there may be an uneven buildup or shedding of the endometrium, and spotting can occur. This too can be successfully treated with a hormonal override in the form of birth control pills.

IS THERE ANYTHING NEW I SHOULD KNOW ABOUT SEX?

Yes. It's about time you really understood your sexual response. After all, in your teens your chief concern was "Should I or shouldn't I?" By now you've made up your mind (you should and you will) and you'd like to get the most pleasure you can out of it.

Sexual response occurs in stages. First you want sex—or to put it more medically, your libido is activated. This occurs thanks to a complex interplay between environmental factors such as romantic love or erotica, your brain and hormones secreted by your adrenal glands and ovaries. The principal hormone of desire is testosterone, which increases your sensitivity to physical stimulation and fosters your fantasies. At this age you should be producing it in ample amounts.

The next stage is arousal, which is accompanied by a wonderful sense of warmth, pleasure and an eagerness and readiness to have intercourse. Blood vessels in the lower genitalia expand, allowing increased circulation to the labia, vagina and clitoris, which results in swelling. At the same time, clear fluid, or plasma, is pushed from these vessels to lubricate the vagina. Vasocongestion also occurs in other erogenous zones, such as the nipples and areolae, and may even spread through small blood vessels at the surface of the skin, triggering a total-body flush.

If all goes well, you now get to the peak of your sexual pleasure, orgasm. This phenomenal event is associated with rhythmic contractions of muscles around and in the vagina and reproductive organs, as well as an increase in breathing and heart rate. The response is not limited to the genitals. Apparently an "orgasm center" exists in the brain: Spikes of activity have been recorded in this area during this phase of our sexual response.

All's well that ends well, and the final stage occurs when the body returns to its resting nonaroused but contented state. Your muscles relax and the swelling in the clitoris, vagina and labia abates. This cool-down may be accompanied by fine perspiration. (Multiorgasmic women are capable of being restimulated back to orgasm before completing this resolution phase. Unfortunately, most men need a longer recovery period after orgasm and ejaculation.)

Slightly more than half of twentysomething women report having frequent orgasms as a result of sex with a partner. Still others say they sometimes or rarely experience orgasm. But more than 10% say they never do. Orgasm is a learned response, and your chance of having one increases with practice, self-knowledge and heightened comfort with your body, not to mention your partner's patience and caring. So don't despair if you're not striking gold every time you have sex. Only 30% to 50% of women experience orgasm through straightforward intercourse. Others may need additional clitoral stimulation. The good news is that as you get older, you're more likely to have frequent orgasms.

WHEN CAN I THROW AWAY THE CONDOMS?

I assume you're asking this question because you are in a dependably monogamous relationship, maybe even married. Hopefully you and your partner underwent HIV testing at the beginning of your time together and have been using condoms for at least six months. Provided you now repeat the HIV test and you're both negative, you may be ready to share your lives—and your microbes. Indeed, you might even be ready to share sperm and get pregnant. And share you will—all the sexually transmitted viruses or bacteria that may silently be present in either one of you.

You can both be checked by a doctor for some of these organisms, such as chlamydia, gonorrhea, syphilis and hepatitis B and C, and if you're both negative, you no longer have to worry about becoming infected with them, as long as you remain monogamous.

When it comes to other viruses, there is no surefire test. The sexually transmitted human papillomavirus (HPV) is usually signaled by suspicious changes in your Pap smear, and its presence can be confirmed with special viral testing. Your partner has no equivalent to the Pap smear and may carry this highly contagious virus without knowing it. Since one or another form of HPV—which is actually a family of at least 25 different viruses—is now present in up to 70% of sexually active adults, there's a good chance that at least one of you is silently housing HPV. So at some point, if you're going to stay together, the two of you must decide if it's worth exposing the uninfected partner (assuming he or she is really uninfected) in order for the two of you to enjoy unprotected sex.

The message is similar for herpes. Contrary to common belief, we can have this infection and not know it. Only 10% of people who carry the virus ever see lesions, and lesions aren't necessary in order for the virus to be transmitted. The only test that can uncover a hidden case of herpes is a blood test that checks for antibodies to the genital herpes virus (Herpes 2), but it is expensive and not widely available. If you have unprotected sex and develop herpes, you may get painful sores that can recur, and it may be necessary for you to take an antiviral medication (Famvir or Valtrex). So in making a decision to forgo condoms, know that you're taking that chance. I don't mean to sound cavalier (unfortunately a very male term), but the only time a new herpes infection can be dangerous to a healthy woman is when she is pregnant. So if you've never developed a herpes lesion, pregnancy may be a time to reinstitute condom use with your partner.

I'VE NEVER BEEN TESTED FOR HIV. SHOULD I BE?

If you've had only one partner, he's monogamous and he's tested negative twice in six months' time, you're probably okay. But that description fits very few women. So realistically, yes—you should be tested at least once in your current relationship, after you've been together (and only with each other and protected) for six months. But preferably you'll start the relationship with a test. You obviously have to be more test-diligent if you have had partners who were bisexual, IV drug users or promiscuous, or if this description fits you. And you should be tested if you've ever had any other sexually transmitted disease. All this becomes even more important if you plan to get pregnant.

HOW CAN I TELL IF A POTENTIAL PARTNER HAS A SEXUALLY TRANSMITTED DISEASE?

Unfortunately, you can't. Let's start with the myth that a man can only give you herpes if he has a lesion on his genitals. Only 10% of people with this virus actually develop lesions, and many aren't even aware that they have them. The herpes virus lives sequestered in the nerve root and can replicate and rise to the surface, where it's shed and spreads silently. On any given day, 1% of those who carry the virus are shedding it. This may not seem like a large number, but it is when you consider the fact that 45 million people in this country are infected.

Speaking of viruses, HPV can be just as stealthy, with only 1% of infected individuals developing visible genital warts. They are—you should excuse the expression—just the tip of the viral iceberg. So even though your partner looks fine, if he is shedding this virus you have a 40% to 90% chance of getting infected when you don't use condoms.

Gonorrhea and chlamydia can on occasion cause burning during urination or mild discharge in a man, but generally there's nothing you can see. Unless you approach your partner with a culture swab and wait three days to get the results, there's no way you'll know if he's capable of infecting you.

AIDS, of course, gives no penile signs. Neither does hepatitis. That leaves syphilis, which, in its early stages can cause painless ulcers to develop on the penis.

HOW CAN I TELL IF I HAVE ONE?

You're likely to have more symptoms than a man, but don't count on them to make a self-diagnosis. Vaginal discharge can accompany chlamydia and gonorrhea, while trichomonas, a sexually transmitted parasite, has a distinctive greenish, frothy and foul-smelling discharge. Both chlamydia and gonorrhea can also cause pelvic inflammatory disease (PID), with symptoms that include spotting, pelvic pain, pain with intercourse, fever and burning and frequency of urination.

An initial herpes infection in a woman, like a man, can be silent, and you can shed the virus without ever knowing you have the disease. However, you can also be extremely symptomatic and develop one or more cold-sore-type lesions that look like little ulcers with a yellow or white secretion on top. These can appear on any part of your genitalia, including the buttocks, labia, clitoris and vagina. With initial infection, you may experience flulike symptoms such as fever, general achiness and swollen glands. Voiding can be painful as the urine comes in contact with the lesion. Many women are aware of a tingling or itching prior to a recurrence of a herpes lesion.

HPV can cause visible genital warts in 1% of infected women. There are four types of warts: *condyloma acuminata* are small growths that resemble cauliflower; others can be smooth, red and dome-shaped; some resemble warts on other parts of the body, while the fourth type is flat or slightly raised and pink.

One of the first signs of infection with HIV, the virus that causes AIDS, in women can be recurrent yeast infections that don't respond to the usual therapy.

If you have any of these symptoms, your doctor should test you not just for one STD but for all of them. (The risky penis is an equal-opportunity STD transmitter.)

WHY AM I GETTING ACNE SINCE I STARTED TAKING THE PILL?

Not all birth control pills are created equal as far as your skin is concerned. Combined pills (those with both estrogen and progesterone) all contain the same type of estrogen, ethanyl estradiol, in amounts ranging from 20 to 50 micrograms. The estrogen in these pills will prevent some of the production of your body's own male hormones, which promote oil secretion in the skin and increase development of acne. Additionally, the estrogen encourages the liver to make a protein that binds up male hormone and deactivates it.

Pills differ, however, in their progestin. Until a few years ago, most of the progestins used in the Pill were chemically similar to testosterone and therefore could promote acne. So if you notice you're breaking out, it may be due to the type of progestin your pill contains. The newer progestins, norgestimate and desogestrel, do not have the same androgenic activity as the old ones, and it makes sense to switch to a brand that contains one of them. Ortho Tri-Cyclen has actually been approved by the FDA to treat acne; others that contain a skin-friendly progestin include Desogen, Ortho-Cept and Demulen. The latter is made with ethynodiol diacetate, which also has little male hormonelike activity.

WILL THE PILL CAUSE ME TO GAIN WEIGHT?

I wish I could tell you the only reason you'll gain weight is if you overeat and underexercise. But in some women, there seems to be a link between weight gain and Pill use. Extra pounds (or even half-pounds) that appear just a month or so after you start taking the Pill are most likely due to fluid retention, and you can blame them on either the estrogen or the progestin in the Pill. The solution is to go on a lower-dose estrogen-plus-progestin pill such as Loestrin ½₀, Alesse, Levlite or Mircette. If you start to gain weight after several months of therapy, it's probably due to the estrogen in the Pill, which can do for your body what puberty did: increase fat deposits, especially in the hips, thighs and breasts. Don't despair. Have your doctor switch you to a pill with just 20 micrograms of estrogen—one of those listed above. There's one more aspect of weight-gain that can be fine-tuned: appetite. If after a few months of Pill use you're hungry all the time, you could be on one of the many pills with a male-hormone-like progestin (examples include Lo Ovral and Ortho-Novum). As with acne, the solution is to try changing to a pill with a less androgenic progestin (Ortho-Cyclen, Ortho Tri-Cyclen, Ortho-Cept, Desogen or Mircette). Overall, once you've found the right Pill, you, like a majority of other Pill users, should not gain more than half a pound—which is probably what you would gain premenstrually even if you were not on the Pill.

ALL THE BIRTH CONTROL PILLS I'VE TRIED CAUSE SIDE EFFECTS. WHAT CAN I DO?

In order to help you overcome Pill problems, I have to go over the disheartening list of the most common things that can go wrong as a result of Pill use. But I'll add a disclaimer first: The majority of women taking the current generation of low-hormone pills won't experience any of these problems.

Nausea: It's the estrogen component of the Pill that's to blame, so it makes sense to use a pill with the lowest estrogen possible. These are your 20-microgram pills. Also try taking the Pill with or after dinner (that way you'll sleep through any nausea and not notice it). If this doesn't help, consider switching to a progestin-only "mini-Pill," such as Micronor, Nor-Q D or Ovrette.

Breast tenderness: This side effect can be due to the Pill's estrogen, but on occasion may also come from its progestin. Once more, switch to a very low estrogen formulation or a progestin-only pill.

Headaches: These may occur either while you're on the active pill or, more frequently, when you go off the Pill or on to the placebo in order to get your period. First let's consider the former. Headaches, especially in women who tend to get migraines (vascular headaches), may be associated with the estrogen in the Pill, and there's a chance they might diminish if you use a very low dose 20-microgram estrogen Pill. Warning: Some older studies have found that women who suffer migraines and take the Pill may be more likely to have a stroke. This data was obtained years ago when only high-dose estrogen pills were used, but this caution still exists on all pill labels.

A nonvascular or pressure-type headache may occur as a result of fluid retention and is probably due to the progestin in the Pill. In this case, you want to try using a low progesterone-activity pill such as Ovcon, Modicon or Levlen.

If your headache occurs only when you're on the placebo pills or have stopped taking the active pills, it's due to a sudden fall of estrogen. (This is similar to what happens in women who get menstrual migraines during their regular cycle.) The best way to treat this is to use a low-estrogen pill (there's less of a fall) or to make the fall gradual. A new pill called Mircette does just that. It contains only 20 micrograms of estrogen, and this amount is lowered for two pills (on day 22 and 23); placebo pills are used only on days 24 through 28. If this doesn't help or you experience breakthrough bleeding while on Mircette, there is another secret way to combat your headaches: Any pill can be used continuously without "breaking" for a period for up to three cycles at a time. So if you have a 21-day package of pills, start a new pack as soon as you finish the old one. If your brand contains 28 pills, 7 of which are placebo, don't take the placebo. Instead, switch to a new pack after 21 days. The math is simple: Instead of having 12 periods and 12 headaches a year, you'll now have only 4. Some of my patients protest that this form of pill-taking isn't "natural." But I remind them that the only reason we bleed on the Pill is that we are taking away the active hormones that keep the uterine lining built up. There is no real advantage to doing this monthly, it's just a question of habit.

One last possible remedy: If a fall in estrogen even for a few days or a few times a year is going to result in migraine misery, you can ask your doctor for a low-dose estrogen patch such as Climara (0.025 mg), to be used during the five or seven days it's needed. Finally, I would be remiss if I didn't advise you that if you experience more frequent or intense headaches while on any of the combined pills, you should consider switching to another method of contraception. Or you can try eliminating the estrogen factor by taking a progestin-only pill (Micronor, Nor-Q D or Ovrette).

Spotting: The most common cause of spotting is you, the Pill user. Forgetting to take a pill or not taking it at the same time every day can lead to a drop in hormone levels that causes the uterine lining to begin to slough, and you spot. So if your motto is "Out out, damn spot," you have to "in, in" daily, timely pill-taking. This is especially important if you are on a very low dose pill formulation. For some women, these pills just don't provide enough estrogen or progestin to keep the endometrial lining built up. So if you're taking it right and you're still spotting after two to three months (initial spotting often goes away), you may need an oral contraceptive that contains either more estrogen or more progestin.

A hint to help you and your doctor decide which hormone needs to be raised: If the spotting occurs at the beginning of your cycle, it is probably due to low estrogen or a low estrogen-progestin ratio. The solution may be to increase the amount of estrogen in your pill from 20 to 35 micrograms, or to use a pill with a lower dose of progestin, such as Ovcon, Nordette, Lo Ovral, Modicon or Brevicon. If the spotting occurs toward the middle of your cycle, it may help to gradually increase the dose of estrogen. The Pill that does this is Estrostep, which begins with 20 micrograms of estrogen and slowly increases to 35 micrograms. Spotting that consistently occurs in the second half of your cycle may be relieved by increasing progestin at that time of the month. Pills that do this gradually are called triphasics and include Ortho-Novum 7/7/7, Tri-Levlen, Tri-Cyclen, Tri-Norinyl and Triphasil.

As a short-term solution for spotting (you've been doing fine on the Pill and all of a sudden you're staining), use an extra pack of pills and double up on your dosage for several days, until the spotting stops. Then return to the usual single daily pills.

Breakthrough bleeding: This is more than spotting—it's periodlike bleeding while you're on the active Pill. The things that cause spotting can also result in bleeding, so read the section above. If you smoke and take the Pill (which you should not do, especially after age 35), you are more likely to experience bleeding because the chemicals in cigarettes deactivate and lower the estrogen in the Pill. The solution is not to take a stronger pill but to stop smoking. In nonsmokers it may, in rare cases, be necessary to go from a pill that contains 35 micrograms of estrogen to one that has 50 micrograms. Before I prescribe this for my patients (and I rarely do), I perform a vaginal ultrasound to ensure that there is nothing abnormal in the uterus that might explain the bleeding, such as polyps, fibroids or endometriosis.

No periods: It's not uncommon to skip periods when you take a low-dose pill with 35 or especially just 20 micrograms of estrogen. For many women, this is not a side effect but a blessing, although the tampon manufacturers might not agree. The chief response when this happens, of course, is "Oh my God, am I pregnant?!" Don't freak. If you did not miss any pills or diminish their effectiveness by taking antibiotics (certain antibiotics render oral contraception less effective), you should be fine and in a nongestational state. For reassurance, you might want to perform a pregnancy test. If it's negative, keep taking the Pill. I have many patients who only spot when they're supposed to get a period or who don't bleed at all, and once I reassure them that it's okay, it ceases to be an issue. However, if you'd rather get a period (I personally don't know why . . .), you can switch to a higher-estrogen pill for a month or two to prime the lining of the uterus and trigger a period, after which you might be able to go back to the lower-dose pill and have regular cycles.

Acne: For solutions to Pill-use-related acne, see page 37.

Weight gain: To get the skinny on the Pill and weight gain, see page 38.

Mood changes: Some women find that they have PMS-like symptoms or their existing PMS worsens when they take the Pill. There's an argument among scientists as to whether this is due to the estrogen or the progestin component. So you have to try changing one or the other or both to see what helps. First, try lowering the estrogen component to 20 micrograms. If that doesn't work, switch from a male-hormone-like progestin to one of the newer progestins found in Ortho-Cept, Desogen, Mircette or Ortho-Cyclen. I would suggest avoiding a triphasic pill, which increases the progestin in the second half of the cycle—exactly the time of the month when PMS occurs. If all else fails, you may have to stop the Pill.

I HEAR THAT BIRTH CONTROL PILLS ARE BAD FOR YOU. TRUE OR FALSE?

False. And I'm so glad you asked! There are few medications used by so many women that can have such a positive impact on our lives. The Pill is one. It protects you from unwanted and ectopic (tubal) pregnancies, decreases cramps, prevents heavy menstrual bleeding and the resulting anemia, regulates your cycle and helps prevent ovarian cysts, endometriosis, pelvic inflammatory disease and even ovarian and uterine cancer. I'll take a moment to discuss the latter because they are so important. Just three to six months of Pill use during your reproductive life can reduce your future risk of ovarian cancer by 40%, and the longer you take the Pill, the more protection you get. Seven years or more confers a 60% to 80% reduction in risk. The numbers are similar for uterine cancer, and the risk of colon cancer may also be decreased.

But there's more: The Pill can reduce your chance of getting benign breast lumps (and does not seem to increase breast cancer risk, except perhaps in women who used high-dose pills at a very early age). It may also control fibroid growth, help build your bones and decrease development and progression of rheumatoid arthritis.

WHAT DO I DO IF I MISS A PILL?

Take the missed pill as soon as you remember it, even if it means taking two pills the next day. If you miss two days, you can still catch up by doubling the doses until you're back on schedule, but you should use another method of contraception for the rest of the cycle. If you really mess up and forget to take the Pill for three or more days—and especially if you start to bleed—you should stop taking the Pill and start a new pack seven days later. (Use a backup contraceptive in the interim.) Once you do this, you're immediately covered for contraception.

HOW MANY YEARS CAN I STAY ON THE PILL?

If you wish, you can keep taking the Pill until menopause, as long as you don't smoke or have other contraindications for its use (see page 70). There is *no* medical reason to "take a break" from the Pill. The only thing that can happen when you do this is that you can "break into" pregnancy.

HOW LONG DO I HAVE TO BE OFF THE PILL BEFORE I CAN GET PREGNANT?

The Pill is out of your system as soon as you stop taking it. That's why you bleed during your placebo (or pill-free) week. There does not appear to be any increase in rates of miscarriage or birth defects for women who get pregnant immediately after stopping the Pill. In some cases, however, the Pill may have been masking menstrual or hormonal abnormalities, and so when you stop it your periods could be irregular or absent. This is not the Pill's fault—it was doing the right thing all along, but your body wasn't and is now letting you know. Eighty percent of women who discontinue oral contraceptives and try to conceive will get pregnant within a year. This is the same fertility rate as that of women who stop using other forms of contraception.

HOW WILL I KNOW IF I'M FERTILE?

You can't know until you've tried to get pregnant (or done so inadvertently). However, there can be clues to diminished fertility. If your periods are very irregular (earlier than every 21 days or later than every 45 days), you're probably ovulating inconsistently or not at all. And ovulation is essential to conception. Lack of ovulation can generally be rectified with fertility pills or shots, but this should only be done when you're actively trying to get pregnant.

If you've been diagnosed with pelvic inflammatory disease (PID) in the past, especially more than once, or if you have had a sexually transmitted disease that was not treated on a timely basis, you may have developed scar tissue that blocks the fallopian tubes. This could prevent sperm from reaching the egg.

Endometriosis usually develops in women who postpone childbearing (see page 91), but can also occur in your twenties. Its chief symptom is excruciating menstrual pain that is not relieved with over-the-counter painkillers or birth control pills. In this disorder, endometrial-like cells seed onto the fallopian tubes or ovaries, where they can bleed or secrete substances that block fertilization.

After scaring you with this long list of what can go wrong, let me reassure you: If your periods are regular, your cramps are manageable and you've had no known infections, relax, stop worrying and when it's time, just go about trying to conceive.

WHAT SHOULD I DO IF I'M TRYING TO GET PREGNANT?

Before you let that sperm get to your egg, make sure you've started taking a multivitamin that contains at least 400 micrograms of folic acid. This B vitamin can greatly diminish your risk of having a baby with a neural tube defect, such as spina bifida.

Next, take stock of your body. Is it a place where you would want a pregnancy to grow? If you're smoking, stop. If you're using recreational drugs, detox. And if you're consuming more than one alcoholic drink per day, cut back or quit. (You certainly should give it up the minute you know you're pregnant.) Whether you have to completely forgo caffeine depends on whether you listen to the Canadian or the American researchers. The former say caffeine has a mild adverse effect on fertility and increases miscarriage rates. The latter say either "no it doesn't" or "we're not sure." I tell my patients who are trying to conceive that if they need that one cup of coffee to get going, they can have it. But once they're pregnant, they have to consider whether they would put caffeine in a baby's bottle. Putting it in their body does the same thing.

If you have any chronic diseases such as diabetes, high blood pressure or epilepsy, make sure you discuss your plans to conceive with your doctor and take steps to control your condition with the right medication before you get pregnant.

Once you have a clean bill of health, the next step is to time the encounter of sperm and egg to coincide with your ovulation—otherwise they'll never meet at all. The egg is released into the fallopian tube, where fertilization occurs, 14 days before your period. It's hard to count backward, so count forward from the start of your last period instead. If you have 28-day cycles, you ovulate 14 days after the start of your period; if your cycles last 30 days, you ovulate 16 days after the beginning of your period; and if you have a 21-day cycle, your ovulation may be as early as day 7—even while you're still spotting from your last period. If your cycles are less than 21 days or more than 45 days, there's a chance you're not ovulating, and you should talk to your doctor.

Another way to determine when you ovulate is to check your basal body temperature with a special thermometer sold in any drugstore. Take your temperature when you awaken every morning, before your first cup of coffee—even before you get out of bed. It will go up half a degree at the time of ovulation because of the progesterone that your ovary produces. This elevation should continue for the next two weeks, until you get your period. (If you're pregnant, your temperature will stay up.) If you're thermometrically challenged, you can use an over-the-counter home ovulation test kit, which checks for peaks of luteinizing hormone, which is secreted just prior to ovulation. Lack of a result with this test kit might indicate that you're not ovulating at all. This can be checked by your doctor with blood tests.

Because sperm can live quite happily in cervical mucus for up to a week, it is not necessary to have intercourse the instant your egg is released from the ovary. That means you can begin having sex up to six days before ovulation. The highest rate of conception will be during ovulation, but sometimes if you hold off in order to get to the exact date, you actually miss it. So I generally tell my patients to start trying on day 10 and repeat the effort on days 12, 14 or 16, depending on the length of their cycle. This should get the timing right. Sex after ovulation won't help you conceive, but it might be fun.

WHAT'S MY RISK OF HAVING A MISCARRIAGE?

If you've never had a known miscarriage, you have a 15% to 20% chance of miscarrying once you find out you're pregnant. But the true rate of miscarriage is even higher—up to 57%—because so many fertilized eggs don't implant in the uterus properly and are spontaneously aborted long before a woman ever realizes that she's conceived. The bleeding that signals the end of such an early attempt at pregnancy may be mistaken for an ordinary period. Of the miscarriages that women actually are aware of, 80% occur during the first 12 weeks of pregnancy. The risk of miscarriage increases if you've had a prior miscarriage (see page 84).

The primary cause of early pregnancy failure is faulty chromosomes. A fetus with a genetic makeup that would prevent it from developing or that would cause a severe malformation does not continue to grow and instead is expelled from the body. This is nature's way of protecting you. But don't assume that because you miscarry, either you or your partner are passing on bad chromosomes. These units of our genetic makeup are usually normal, but they must meet, combine and replicate perfectly—an extremely complicated process which, when you consider what can go wrong, is amazing when it goes right. But it *does* go right pretty often, and 80% to 90% of women who have had a single spontaneous abortion (the medical term for a miscarriage) will deliver a baby with their next pregnancy.

WHY DO I GET SO MANY BLADDER INFECTIONS?

Probably because you're sexually active. But relax—you're in good company: Twenty-five to thirty-five percent of women ages 20 to 40 have had a UTI (urinary tract infection). Normally, urine is sterile. But once bacteria get up into the bladder and stick to its walls, they busily multiply in their new environment and cause irritation and inflammation. This leads to the classic symptoms of cystitis: urgency (you constantly feel like you have to go), frequency (you *do* go) and/or dysuria (it burns like crazy when you go). Because an inflammatory response can cause bleeding, some women see blood in their urine.

Why does sex encourage this? If you think about how you're constructed down there, it all makes sense: The urethra (a short channel leading from the bladder out of the body) is near the opening of the vagina. When you have intercourse, bacteria from the genital area are pushed to the entrance of the urethra and ascend from there. These bacteria—usually *E. coli*—originate in the bowel, where they are perfectly harmless and part of your normal flora. They cause symptoms only when they get into the wrong place, adhere and multiply. A new partner, who brings his own bacteria into the bedroom, or an increase in sexual activity are more likely to start this microbial onslaught. That's why it's known as "honeymoon cystitis."

Some women's bladders produce a protein that encourages bacteria to attach, and they are more likely to suffer from recurrent infections. This can be genetic. To add insult to intercourse, our method of contraception can also promote infection. The chief culprits are diaphragms, which press on the urethra and bladder, interrupting normal urine flow, and spermicides (with or without the diaphragm), which change the pH of the vagina and alter normal flora.

And speaking of flora . . . The vagina has a very sensitive ecosystem, and if anything interferes with this, the wrong bacteria can overgrow and reach the urethra and bladder. Sometimes after we've taken a broad-spectrum antibiotic for anything from a sore throat to an infected toe, we, diabolically, end up with a bladder infection, since certain antibiotics can upset the natural balance of bacteria that inhabit the vagina. This may allow other bacteria to grow and spread into the urethra and bladder.

Given all these possible causes, it's not surprising that 40% of women who have one episode of cystitis will have another one within the next year. But you can lessen your bladder woes if you do the following:

Empty your bladder before and after intercourse to help to flush bacteria from the urethra.

Drink six to eight glasses of water a day to dilute any bacteria present in the bladder and stop them from adhering to the bladder wall.

Change your contraceptive method if you're using a diaphragm.

Consume cranberry juice (even the diet kind is fine). This juice has been found to prevent bacteria from clinging to the bladder wall.

Ask your doctor about antibiotics. You should consider taking a low-dose antibiotic (such as Macrodantin, Bactrim or Trimpex) every day if you routinely develop cystitis after sex, or if you've had three episodes of infection in the last year. If you've had just two infections in the past year and they occurred after sex, it might suffice to take an antibiotic only after intercourse. Another option would be to have the antibiotic on hand (or, more precisely, in your medicine cabinet) so that you can take it for one to three days when you feel the first symptoms of an infection coming on.

I BURN AND ITCH. IS THIS YEAST?

Most of us think "yeast" if we itch, and we're probably right. The majority of sexually active women will at some point experience that burning, itching feeling. This is most often due to yeast but can also be caused by a bacterial infection. Let's concentrate on yeast for the moment. Aside from itching and burning, its other signs include redness (erythema) of the vulva that can spread to the inner thighs and around the anus. Painful fissures may appear in the skin around the opening of the vagina, especially in the posterior part where the labia (lips) meet, or between the inner and outer lips. Sometimes the skin is so irritated that the burning increases during urination, but this is not a bladder infection. Only 50%

of the time is there a characteristic white, "cottage-cheesy"-looking discharge.

Yeast may be present in small amounts without any symptoms in 15% of women. It can appear, overgrow and cause symptoms when friendly vaginal bacteria called *lactobacilli*, which normally control yeast, are suppressed by a course of antibiotics or a change in vaginal pH. This can occur as a result of douching or use of spermicides, bubble baths, bath oils, scented soaps or toilet paper or tampons, especially the deodorant kind. Lack of aeration (the result of wearing panty hose or undergarments made of tightly woven synthetic fabrics) or constant exposure to moisture (e.g., a wet bathing suit or sweaty gym clothes) can further facilitate the growth of yeast.

Receiving oral sex twice or more in two weeks' time may be enough to upset the pH (not to mention your mother). And taking oral contraceptives can double your risk of yeast infection. Even if none of these risk factors is present, you can have a genetic tendency to develop yeast infections. The high blood sugar associated with diabetes translates into a change in vaginal glycogen that can in turn raise pH and allow yeast to multiply. Even in the absence of diabetes, both glycogen levels and pH can increase as a result of hormonal fluctuations. This is why some women develop yeast infections before each period. Anything that impairs cells' ability to fight off infection can leave you vulnerable to a yeast infection. This includes the use of corticosteroid medications and infection with HIV.

If all signs point to the fact that you have a yeast infection, you can self-medicate, provided that you had the same symptoms and were diagnosed by your doctor with yeast in the past. Choose an over-the-counter antifungal cream or suppository such as Monistat, Gyne-Lotrimin, Mycelex, Femstat or Vagistat. Antifungals are available in one-, three- and seven-dose packages. If this is a recurrent infection, you're better off using a seven-day regimen. A confusing plethora of feminine anti-itch creams is often found on drugstore shelves alongside bona fide yeast medicines. Don't be deceived: They may help symptoms, but they won't cure yeast. Stronger medications are still the purview of your physician and require a prescription. These include Terazol, Mycostatin, Nilstat and Mycolog. The latter contains a steroid cream that fights swelling. Many of us don't want to be bothered with messy creams or suppositories, especially if we're in the group of women who get these infections repeatedly. That's why single-dose pills such as Nizoral and Diflucan are particularly popular with my patients (and myself). Note that Diflucan can occasionally cause nausea and headaches. And a word about prevention: If you're taking an antibiotic, make an effort to restore the body's normal balance of healthy bacteria as quickly as possible. Yogurt containing live lactobacillus acidophilus cultures, or even acidophilus capsules, may help. Women have tried everything, including placing yogurt (the plain kind) in the vagina. The lactobacilli in this nutritious dairy product is not the same as that present in your vagina, so this probably won't work.

If you've self-medicated your suspected yeast infection and you're still miserable, or if this is the first time you've developed these symptoms, get thee to thy doctor. She will check your vaginal pH and, if necessary, perform a microscopic examination of a sample of your vaginal fluid (a "wet mount") to help distinguish between a yeast and a bacterial infection. Your doctor may also perform a culture, especially if she suspects a sexually transmitted disease.

OKAY, SO IT'S NOT YEAST. WHAT IS IT?

After yeast, bacterial vaginosis (BV) is the most common type of vaginal infection you can have, and indeed up to 25% of women get it. BV is caused by several types of anaerobic bacteria (those that thrive in the absence of oxygen), including gardnerella vaginalis and genital mycoplasm. These can massively multiply and replace healthy lactobacilli. This is particularly likely to happen if you've been taking antibiotics or have had a new sex partner (especially multiple sexual partners). Smoking, having an IUD or being infected with the sexually transmitted trichomonas protozoa are also implicated in infection. For unknown reasons, BV is more common among African-American women. Men can harbor the bacteria in their urethra, under the foreskin or possibly in the prostate gland, and can transmit it to you, but you can get this infection without having had sex (it's found even in children). Half of the women with BV have no symptoms. The major complaint of those who do is a malodorous, fishy or sharp-smelling discharge. The discharge is milky white and its odor often increases after intercourse, menstruation or douching. Since itching is not common with BV, you may be able to distinguish this from a yeast infection on your own.

But even if you are able to self-diagnose, you can't self-medicate. Your doctor can make the final diagnosis by checking to see if your vaginal pH is raised and by performing a wet mount from vaginal secretions. Once she confirms the diagnosis, she'll prescribe the appropriate medication, which can be either a five-day course of the vaginal creams clindamycin or Metrogel (metronidazole), or Flagyl, an oral form of metronidazole that can eradicate BV and will take care of any accompanying trichomonas as well. If you have this type of infection, it's important that you be treated, not just because of unpleasant symptoms, but because BV raises your risk of pelvic inflammatory disease and can lead to complications after pelvic surgery and during pregnancy. Treatment of the male partner has not been shown to reduce recurrence, so although he may have had something to do with your infection, he gets away without needing therapy.

Unfortunately, I'm not able to cease and desist in my vivid descriptions of the sources of itching and burning. There is one more important cause: trichomonas. This unicellular protozoa is sexually transmitted and can lead to a most unpleasant profuse, frothy, yellowish-green discharge, complete with itching and a fishy odor. To make matters worse, it can affect the urethra and bladder, causing painful urination.

The diagnosis is easily made by your physician, who will use a microscope to view the wet mount, in which a characteristic tadpolelike organism is swimming around waving its tail. You and your partner should be treated with metronidazole (even if he doesn't have symptoms).

Less common causes of vaginitis include bacteria such as group A and B streptococcus, which can be diagnosed by your doctor with a culture and treated with either clindamycin cream or amoxicillin tablets or a similar antibiotic. Strep is a bacteria that can colonize the vaginal tract of some women. As long as you're not pregnant, it need only be treated if it causes symptoms. Unfortunately, even with therapy, it often comes back to rehabitate this abode.

Finally, you can itch even in the absence of an infection because of a local skin reaction to douches, scents, soap, laundry detergent, bath products and even the over-the-counter medications you wrongly used to treat what you thought was a yeast infection. The solution here is to stay away from anything that promises you "feminine freshness" because all it might do is cause feminine itching.

SHOULD I DOUCHE?

The vagina is a self-cleansing organ. It is constantly bathed in mucus from the cervix and moisture from the vaginal walls. This clears debris that remains after your period, as well as cells that slough off the wall of the vagina as it is constantly being resurfaced.

The vagina should be acidic, and anything you do in an attempt to "sweeten" or "freshen" it will also ruin its pH balance and allow the wrong microbes to grow—namely, yeast and pathologic bacteria. So obviously, there is no need to routinely douche. Moreover, douching has been shown to increase your risk for pelvic inflammatory disease, perhaps by pushing harmful organisms, some of which could be sexually transmitted, up into your cervix and uterus.

On rare occasions, your doctor may suggest that you use a medicated betadine douche to clear certain types of bacterial infection, either before culture results can be obtained and an antibiotic prescribed, or if you're unable to tolerate the appropriate antibiotic. Some women find that an occasional vinegar douche wards off yeast infections by helping to maintain the acidity of the vagina. I have patients who use a vinegar douche just before their period, when they're most vulnerable to yeast. Myriad items are currently marketed in this country to ensure that you don't smell "down there," the premise being that your odor will compromise personal relationships or be a source of public embarrassment. This advertising is not only misleading but harmful. There is no medical need to douche, spray or dab any of these products in the genital area. In fact, use of talcum powder for feminine "freshening" may increase your risk of ovarian cancer!

HOW RELIABLE IS THE PAP SMEAR?

We've been taught to believe in God, our country and the need to have a routine Pap smear. When you put your legs in those stirrups and have that speculum inserted, you know you're doing it for a noble purpose: to ensure that you don't get cervical cancer. And indeed, the Pap smear has lowered the cervical cancer death rate by 70% in the last 50 years. Why not 100%? Because not every woman is as diligent about testing as I hope you are (80% of women who die of cervical cancer have not had a Pap in the last five years). But there's another reason: The Pap isn't perfect. Depending on what lab is used and the technique of those who handle the slides, up to 20% may be read as normal when they actually are not. These are called "false negative" results. The opposite can also happen, and a lab can report an abnormality when none is present (a "false positive"). Technical error and human mistakes can be made at any point in the process, from the brushing of your cervix to the official reporting of your results.

Let's follow the course of your Pap smear so you can understand how misdiagnosis occurs.

In the doctor's office: You're not always examined at the perfect Pap time. You may be spotting, have an infection or have had sex within the last 24 hours. Up to 40% of the time, the accuracy of Paps is compromised by blood, mucus or inflammation. Sometimes, especially if you haven't had a baby, your cervical canal may be so tightly closed that a doctor can't gain access to get the necessary cells. It can also be hard for the physician to see the entire cervix, especially if you've not been sexually active or you're very overweight. But once there, she collects a cell sample from your cervix with a tiny brush (it looks like an eyebrow brush) that is twirled in the cervical canal. She also uses a small wooden spatula to scrape cells from the outside of the cervix. About 20% of the cells are smeared onto a glass slide, but the other 80% can adhere to the brush and spatula and be thrown away. If by chance the discarded cells are abnormal, no one will ever know.

At the lab: The slide now has to be stained and analyzed microscopically by a cytotechnologist. She must search for abnormal cells among hundreds of thousands of normal ones, and repeat this process up to a hundred times a day. Our demand for accuracy is overwhelming and impossible. Mistakes will be made no matter how well she does her job.

Back at the doctor's office: The third opportunity to make a mistake is in the reporting of Pap results. Your doctor's office may never get a report from the lab, and may not have a method for tracking tests and alerting the doctor to missing results. It's also possible for results to be filed away before the doctor sees them or you are notified. Finally, your address or phone number can be incorrectly entered in a chart or computer, and notification can go astray. No news isn't always good news. That's why you should always check with your doctor's office to get your Pap results.

Attempts are being made to address the problems of sampling and diagnostic errors. Newer, pricier—and perhaps more accurate—ways of reading your Pap are now available, but long-term data has yet to show that they save significantly more lives than diligent use of traditional methods. One system developed to address this Pap smear problem is ThinPrep. Instead of preparing a smear of cells, the practitioner who performs your test will dunk the brush in fluid so that all the cells from your cervix are collected and sent to the lab. There, the solution is filtered to remove blood, mucus and other debris. Only then is a thin, even layer of cervical cells deposited onto a slide, which is stained and examined by the cytotechnologist. This method has been shown to improve the detection of precancerous cells by 65%. Some of the abnormalities revealed, however, are so minor that it's possible they would go away if left untreated.

ThinPrep is still open to human error on the part of the cytotechnologist. In an effort to reduce this, other techniques such as PapNet and AutoPap have been developed. These use computers to screen each slide's hundreds of thousands of cells in order to select those that look particularly suspicious for closer examination by the cytotechnologist.

These new technologies can add $30 to $60 to your bill. Their cost-effectiveness has been analyzed and the current thought is that frequent Pap smears are more of a lifesaver than less frequent ones using these high-tech methods. But if you want greater peace of mind when your doctor inserts that speculum (and you or your insurer are willing to pay for it), you might request one of these new tests.

I KNOW I'M SUPPOSED TO DO A BREAST SELF-EXAM EVERY MONTH. HOW DO I DO IT?

Having breasts does not instill an innate knowledge of how to examine them, so let's go through it step by step. The best time to examine your breasts is immediately after your period, before increased progesterone production makes them more tender and lumpy—so check them when they're on their best behavior. First of all, stand in front of a mirror and take a good look at your breasts. Start with your hands on your waist. Check for any asymmetrical bulge or depression, difference in texture or any other change in appearance. Be especially alert for any changes in the nipples' appearance.

Next, bend over, keeping your hands at your waist, and look for any asymmetry in the contour of your breasts as they hang. Then raise both arms (see diagram on page 54) and check for any swelling or dimpling in this position, especially under the arms.

Lie down with a pillow under your right shoulder and your right hand behind your head. Then, with your left hand, start at the nipple of your right breast and make tiny massaging circular motions using the pads of your middle three fingers. As you're massaging, slowly move your hand in gradually larger concentric circles until you've covered the entire breast and reached its edge, high in your armpit. The pressure should be firm

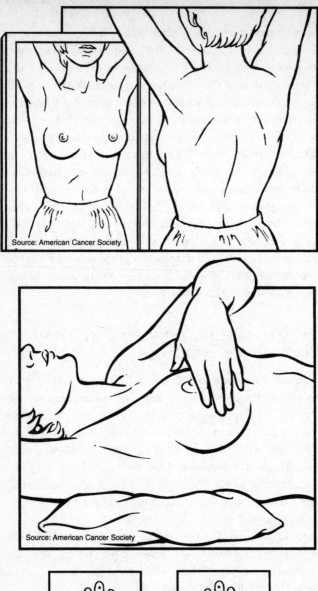

Source: American Cancer Society

Source: American Cancer Society

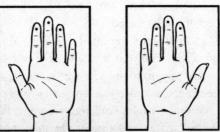

Source: American Cancer Society

but not too hard—you're not trying to palpate your ribs. You're feeling for any unusual lumps or areas of tenderness. I'm often asked what a lump feels like. I use a vegetable analogy that we can all relate to: Think frozen peas, not mushy lima beans. After you've covered the whole breast, feel the nipple for any change in size, shape or consistency, then squeeze it to see if any fluid or blood comes out. Now repeat this entire process using your right hand to examine your left breast while your left hand is behind your head. Initially this all may seem (and feel) very strange. But relax: You can get to know your breasts better than anyone, including your physician. With practice, you'll feel secure that you're not just feeling around; you're checking for—and noticing—any changes that might be important.

WHAT TESTS SHOULD I HAVE?

These are the examinations, tests and procedures I recommend to my patients in their twenties.

Examination/test/procedure	How often
Blood pressure	Every two years
Pelvic exam and Pap smear	Annually; Pap at doctor's discretion after three negative tests
STD testing	At your/your doctor's discretion
Clinical (physician) breast exam	Annually
Breast self-exam	Monthly
Immunizations	Tetanus booster every 10 years
Cholesterol test	Nonfasting total cholesterol and HDL check every five years
Eye exam	Once during this decade or if vision changes
Skin exam by dermatologist	Every two years
Skin self-exam	Annually

WHAT CAN GO WRONG AT MY AGE?

Thyroid Problems

Once our hormones come into play and we reach childbearing age, our thyroid also comes under duress and may malfunction. Women are seven times more likely than men to have thyroid disorders, which include underactive thyroid (hypothyroidism), overactive thyroid (hyperthyroidism), benign nodules on or enlargement of the thyroid (goiter) as well as cancer.

The thyroid is a butterfly-shaped gland at the base of the Adam's apple. It secretes a hormone that influences the growth and development of all our tissues, regulates the oxygen consumption of all our cells and controls all our energy expenditure. "All" is the key word here. The reason you're now susceptible to thyroid problems is that hormonal swings accompanying puberty, your periods and pregnancy may initiate autoimmune responses that can attack and destroy thyroid tissue.

What happens if your thyroid isn't working properly? The most common result is hypothyroidism, which affects 11 million American women. The good news for you is that most of these women are over age 50. But that doesn't mean you're immune, so you should know the symptoms: fatigue, weakness, intolerance to cold, constipation, unexplained weight gain, brittle nails, muscle cramps, difficulty concentrating, menstrual irregularities, lack of ovulation, infertility, increased PMS and nightmares (this list is a nightmare). The tremendous drop in estrogen and progesterone that occurs postpartum can trigger a (usually temporary) form of hypothyroidism in up to 16% of women.

You don't need all of these symptoms in order to qualify for the diagnosis: one or two are sufficient. If you suspect you have an underactive thyroid gland (and given the long list of symptoms, at some point in our lives we'll probably all suspect it), it's easy to find out with a blood test for thyroid stimulating hormone (TSH). This isn't a test of your thyroid hormone levels; it's actually more sensitive because it measures the hormone put out by the pituitary to instruct the thyroid on how to do its job. TSH may change before thyroid hormone levels do, going up when the thyroid is just slightly underactive because it is trying to get the gland to work harder. The therapy is to replace the missing thyroid hormone. The drug most commonly prescribed is Synthroid.

An overactive thyroid gland affects 2 million women, mostly those between ages 20 and 40 (so beware). Symptoms include fatigue, insomnia, tremors, nervousness, diarrhea, rapid heartbeat, palpitations, shortness of breath, hot flashes, intolerance to heat, sweating, frequent or heavy periods, infertility, weight loss or, for some, weight gain caused by increased appetite. If you have undiagnosed hyperthyroidism and become pregnant, you risk premature delivery. One type of hyperthyroidism is Graves' disease, which, in addition to the above symptoms, also causes the eyeballs to be pushed forward and bulge, a condition called exophthalmos. The initial diagnosis of hyperthyroidism is made by a blood test revealing a low TSH level. Treatment involves calming down your overachieving gland with antithyroid medications such as propylthiouracil or methimazole. Or, more commonly, radioactive iodine is given to destroy overactive cells in the gland. Eighty percent of women given this therapy will develop an underactive thyroid and then have to take thyroid hormone supplements for the rest of their lives. There is also a surgical solution, removal of part of the thyroid, which is sometimes recommended if an overactive gland is accompanied by swelling or nodules (goiter).

Multiple Sclerosis

Women are twice as likely as men to develop MS. It's possible that fluctuating estrogen and progesterone levels in our late teens, after childbirth and during menopause interact with underlying genetic or environmental factors to precipitate the disease. Immune cells attack the myelin lining of nerves, causing inflammation and degeneration of the lining (demyelinization). This initially leads to weakness and fatigue with exertion, lack of dexterity, a feeling of numbness, dizziness and blurred vision and possible visual loss. If the disease progresses (and the good news is, the younger we are when we get it, the less rapidly this tends to happen), memory loss, impaired judgment and problems swallowing, walking and controlling the bladder and bowels can develop.

Unfortunately there's no one sign or test that will give a definitive diagnosis of MS. CT scans and an MRI of the brain and spinal cord can show scarring or plaques, while a spinal tap can reveal substances that help confirm the diagnosis. Therapy consists of corticosteroid drugs as well as a medication called beta interferon, both of which suppress the immune systems. A new class of drugs called immune-system-modulator therapies (Betaseron, Avonex and Copaxone) has shown exciting results, and the latest recommendation is that even if the disease is mild and does not appear to be progressing, it should be treated early and aggressively with one of these medications in order to improve future outcome.

MY TOP 10 LIST FOR STAYING HEALTHY IN YOUR TWENTIES

1. Don't smoke.
2. Now that you can legally drink, don't do so in excess or when you'll be driving.
3. Use seat belts.
4. Limit your number of sexual partners and practice safe sex.
5. Don't forget to exercise—even if your body and weight seem fine.
6. Take a multivitamin that contains 400 micrograms of folic acid and consume 1,200 milligrams of calcium per day in the form of dairy products, calcium-fortified foods or supplements.
7. Eat a balanced diet.
8. Build a network of friends and colleagues to serve as your unofficial mental health support system.
9. Establish a relationship with a family or primary care physician.
10. Make sure you have adequate health insurance.

YOUR THIRTIES

YOU'RE STILL PRETTY invincible during this decade, but there are nuances of physical changes, some of which you have no control over, others for which you must take total responsibility. Let's go from the outside in.

From a dermatological point of view, your skin peaked in your twenties—it had the most collagen, moisture, elasticity and thickness it will ever have. Depending upon your childhood and adolescent propensity for sun worship, you may start to see significant collagen loss and even wrinkles at this age. Sun damage can decrease the formation of certain types of vital collagen by as much as 50%. Smoking has an even greater impact, especially when it comes to crinkling around the lips and eyes. It takes 20 years for sun damage to evolve into skin cancer. So guess what? This is the decade when you start to pay for all those childhood sunburns.

Beneath your skin, fat cells may be increasing in size, prompting unwelcome flab and sag, especially if you've given birth. What we stand to gain in pregnancy—aside from our kids—is a future risk of obesity. If you don't lose your extra pregnancy pounds in the first six months after having a baby, they're especially likely to become permanent and prophetic, translating into an even greater increase in poundage after a second baby is born. The longer fat is on your body, the more likely it is to linger. Whether or not you have a childbearing excuse, you can no longer eat with abandon or you may be forced to abandon your slim-fitting jeans.

What about your reproductive system? Although your cycles should remain the same as in your twenties there is a silent change taking place in your ovaries. Your supply of good eggs is dwindling, and that biological clock is ticking. Remember: You started puberty with about 400,000 eggs. (You were born with one million, but most die off gradually in a natural process called *atresia*.) With each month that you've ovulated and released an egg since puberty, atresia has continued and at least a thousand more have died. Simple math allows you to deduce that if you've gone through more than 200 cycles, you've lost at least 200,000 eggs, probably more. In addition, the healthiest eggs went first. Those that remain are not necessarily "Grade A," and the passage of time may cause them to expire.

Our eggs exist in a state of semireadiness, with the chromosome pairs divided and awaiting ovulation and fertilization in order to pair up and double. This condition makes them very vulnerable, and by the time we reach the age of 35, half of our remaining eggs have damaged chromosomes. These defective eggs either can't be fertilized or, if fertilized, can't develop into a normal pregnancy and may result in a miscarriage. But don't completely panic: the other half of the remaining eggs may be just fine and, if fertilized, will usually result in a good pregnancy and a healthy baby.

Because of your ebb in egg power, you may experience a concomitant change in hormone levels, especially in your late thirties. Your control panel for ovarian hormonal production, which includes your hypothalamus, pituitary and ovaries, may be slightly on the fritz, which causes occasional drops in estrogen levels or spurts of estrogen without adequate progesterone production. This may lead to an increase in PMS and occasional irregular periods.

The good news is that for most of us, our internal organs don't show signs that they're aware of our birthdays during our thirties, although wear and tear is silently taking place. So take heart—but also take care of your heart (not to mention your bones, muscles and lungs). Your body will thank you later.

WHY DO I GET A HEADACHE WHENEVER I HAVE MY PERIOD?

I'm sure that by now you've figured out this is hormonally related—and it is. When estrogen levels fall prior to your period, more than your uterus goes into withdrawal. Levels of brain neurotransmitters such as serotonin change, as do the sensitivity of the receptors that pick up the messages these brain chemicals send. This in turn causes adjacent blood vessels to dilate, sensitizes nerve endings and creates muscle spasm. A migraine is born. Estrogen fluctuation also reduces the brain's feel-good endorphins and ensures that you *really* feel the pain.

Meanwhile, back at the uterus, there's another factor contributing to your headache: Prostaglandin levels rise during your period, causing uterine contractions and menstrual cramps. These very same prostaglandins then sensitize pain receptors in your brain and promote spasm of some blood vessels and dilation of others. So, unfairly, if you suffer from severe cramps, you may also be a victim of severe menstrual headaches.

A quarter of all women get migraines, and almost three-fourths of them find that these headaches are linked to their cycle. I'm sure the last thing you want is to be reminded of what a migraine feels like, but a description will at least validate your use of the term "menstrual migraine." The pain is intense and throbbing and often occurs on one side of the head, but it can strike on both sides. It's usually accompanied by nausea and sometimes vomiting. Movement makes it worse. Aside from childbirth, many women feel this is the worst pain they have ever experienced.

A migraine alert, called a *prodrome*, often takes place 12 to 24 hours before an attack. Symptoms include fatigue, euphoria or depression, hunger and sensitivity to light, sound and/or smell. But that's not enough. In 20% of women, the headache is also preceded by an "aura," which develops 20 minutes to an hour before pain strikes. You may see colored or flashing lights, develop temporary blind spots in your vision or feel numbness, tingling or temporary paralysis on one side of your body. Your speech can even be affected. Some women get this aura without a subsequent headache. But if these neurological symptoms occur for the very first time, don't assume it's just aura. You need to be checked to make sure you are not experiencing a potentially dangerous spasm of blood vessels feeding the brain called a *transient ischemic attack*.

There is self-help and medical help for menstrual migraines. First, try lifestyle changes. These headaches are often triggered by certain foods, so look for a pattern in what you eat or drink prior to developing the pain. Prime suspects are aged cheeses, alcohol (especially red wine), caffeine, cocoa, ice cream, monosodium glutamate (MSG, a food additive), sourdough bread, yeast and yogurt. And it's not just what you eat, but when. Missing meals can lead to a headache, as can sleep deprivation. The motto is: Be kind to yourself before and during your period.

Now to drugs. You can start therapy on your own by taking over-the-counter antiprostaglandin medications. If you're wondering what an anti-prostaglandin medication is, it's the pills you're probably taking anyway for cramps—you just need to start them earlier (seven days before you expect your period) and take enough to prevent prostaglandin production in the first place. Try two tablets of OTC naproxen (Aleve) twice a day, or two tablets of ibuprofen (Advil) two or three times a day. If you don't gear up this way and your head begins to hurt, it may not be too late to abort a mild to moderate headache with aspirin (with or without caffeine) or acet-aminophen. When this doesn't work, it's time for the hard stuff: pre-scription drugs developed specifically to treat migraines. Sumatriptan (Imitrex), available as a shot, pill or nasal spray, blocks receptors and inhibits the release of brain chemicals that cause inflammation and blood vessel dilation. It won't prevent a migraine, but it is designed to be taken when one starts. Once one of these drugs wears off, you may develop a "rebound" migraine. Another pill called Amerge may treat or prevent this second migraine. If all else fails and you're unable to tolerate any more pain, your doctor may prescribe narcotics such as Demerol or Stadol NS nasal spray.

In detailing all these painkillers, I really haven't addressed the hor-monal issues. After all, they are what set the whole headache process off. Because menstrual migraines are triggered by falling estrogen levels, one way to treat them is to prevent the fall. This can be done with estrogen supplementation, in the form of a patch (the type used for hormone replacement therapy) or a skin gel. Either is applied for seven days, start-ing two days before you generally get your migraine. (Don't worry; this isn't enough estrogen to stop you from getting your period.) If you're already on the Pill, you can still add the patch or gel during your Pill-free or placebo week. Or you can follow the advice I've given on dosage and Pill scheduling on page 39.

I should add that if you're being treated for general migraines with med-ications such as beta-blockers or calcium channel blockers and your headaches get worse around the time of your period, it may help to step up the dosage of these drugs a week before your period.

Your period may be a pain in your pelvis—but it doesn't have to be a pain in your head.

AM I DEPRESSED, OR IS THIS PMS? AND
WHAT CAN I DO ABOUT IT?

Your depression is PMS-related if it occurs only one to two weeks before your period and abates within four days after you begin to menstruate. From that point until the middle of your next cycle, you should feel no more depressed than the rest of the population. To qualify for a PMS diagnosis, this pattern has to be repeated over successive cycles. Eighty percent of us get some of the complaints associated with PMS (more than 150 have been described!), and more than a quarter of the time, depression is one of the overwhelming issues. If, however, between ovulation and the fourth day of your period you are so depressed that you simply can't cope with work, family or even just getting out of bed, then the diagnosis is more serious. It's called premenstrual dysphoric disorder (PMDD), and it affects 3% to 8% of us.

If you feel like you're PMSing all the time, neither diagnosis applies. You more likely have clinical depression, which is present all month long but can get worse one to two weeks before your period. This condition affects your mood (you feel sad, empty, worried, irritable); thoughts (you can't concentrate or feel guilty or even suicidal); behavior (you're agitated or withdrawn); and body (you suffer insomnia or sleep a lot, feel fatigued, have appetite changes, lose or gain weight or experience a decreased libido). You needn't have every single one of these depressing symptoms to qualify for a diagnosis.

One-fifth of us will develop clinical depression at some point in our lives. It occurs most frequently in women 25 to 44 years old. So, congratulations: You're right in the middle of the time in your life when the incidence of this condition peaks. And when we consider all the reasons for depression, it's amazing that 80% of us get by without being diagnosed. First (as always) are our hormones. They not only affect levels of the brain neurotransmitter serotonin, but they also change the sensitivity of receptors in our brain to this feel-good substance. Then there's the fact that we feel best when our estrogen levels peak and worse when they drop. This is one explanation for premenstrual depression. It's also a major reason for postpartum depression. (At no other time in our lives do estrogen levels plummet so drastically; indeed, half of all new moms will have some degree of baby "blues," and 10% will become clinically depressed.) There's an interrelationship here: Women who have postpartum depression or significant PMS are also more likely than others to develop clinical depression, and half of women who have one episode of clinical depression will eventually experience another. The extreme vulnerability of their neurotransmitters may be the connecting factor. Another interesting neurotransmitter phenomenon: Women produce roughly half as much serotonin as men. This may contribute to the fact that we're twice as likely to develop clinical depression.

Even though I'm a gynecologist and look for hormonal reasons for almost everything that happens in our bodies, it would irresponsible of me not to consider the psychosocial reasons women become depressed. First, there's our parents. Girls are reared to be physically, emotionally and socially pleasing to others, a source of unreasonable pressure from the get-go. Then we're told in subtle and not-so-subtle ways that the ambition and assertiveness we need to advance in life aren't gender-appropriate. And on top of that, we must be nurturing—to others, but not to ourselves. The burden and conflict of parenting and caring for our mates and aging parents falls on us. Meanwhile, we have to earn a living and, yes, may want to pursue a career. Fortunately, most of us can juggle these many roles—that is, until we lose control and become overwhelmed. This is when we become depressed. We also have to consider the uniquely female factors that can lead to depression. Forty-eight percent of women have unwanted pregnancies, while 10% experience infertility. One-third of women have been sexually abused in the past, and between 25% and 50% are sexually or physically abused by a partner. My only conclusion is that women are phenomenally resilient.

Women are also at higher risk for developing another form of depression: seasonal affective disorder (SAD), which tends to strike during the dark winter months and has been linked with sensitivity to changes in melatonin, a sleep-related hormone that is produced only in the dark. SAD's symptoms—depression combined with increased sleeping, overeating, carbohydrate cravings, weight gain and fatigue—affect 10% of those of us who live in middle to northern U.S. latitudes. An additional 25% get a milder case of the winter blues.

Now that you are better able to delineate your true diagnosis (or you're just depressed as a result of reading the above), let me tell you what's available in the way of therapy.

PMS/PMDD: Nonmedical therapies such as cutting back on caffeine, increasing carbohydrate intake, taking calcium and other supplements and exercising may help with general PMS symptoms. If depression remains or is severe enough to be diagnosed as premenstrual dysphoric disorder (PMDD), you may need a prescription antidepressant such as Prozac, Zoloft, Paxil, Luvox or Celexa. These selective serotonin reuptake inhibitors (SSRIs) work by increasing effective serotonin levels in your brain. You can either take continuous low doses of one of these medications and increase the dosage when you're symptomatic, or take the medicine only when you need it—one to two weeks before you get your period. If anxiety is a major part of your PMS or PMDD, an antianxiety medication such as Xanax, taken when symptoms strike, is also very effective.

Clinical depression: Although we live in an era of "take a pill and get better," we can't decide which pill to take, nor can we promise "better" without exploring underlying psychological issues and stresses leading to depression. So consider this my official endorsement of psychotherapy. Just talking to the right mental health professional will help 60% of women with mild to moderate depression get better, the same percentage as will be helped by drug therapy alone. But when you combine the two treatments, the results are even more impressive, especially for women with moderate to severe depression.

There are scores of antidepressant drugs available, and in one way or another they all affect serotonin levels. So on to a quick course in psychopharmacology. The newest mood regulators on the block are the SSRIs (see above). Another, older class of medications is the cyclic antidepressants. They're divided into tricyclics (which have three rings in their chemical makeup) and heterocyclics (which have more). The tricyclics include Elavil, Anafranil, Norpramin, Tofranil and Sinequan. Heterocyclics include Wellbutrin, Desyrel and Ludiomil. A third class of antidepressants, MAO inhibitors, has nothing to do with a former Chinese ruler. MAO is a brain enzyme that breaks down serotonin. This group includes Marplan, Nardil and Parnate. All these medications have complex actions and interactions, so if you don't get relief or experience side effects from them you might want to consult a psychopharmacologist for the right drug or drugs for you.

SAD: Even though SAD is tied to changes in brain chemicals, people who have it don't seem to respond as well to antidepressants as those with clinical depression. The best form of therapy is daily doses of very bright fluorescent light, which blocks release of melatonin. The light is about 12 times brighter than ordinary room light, and while you don't need a prescription to get a light box, you should consult a doctor, who will help you decide whether to use it in the morning or at night and for how long. Most women will feel better within four weeks after using the light for half an hour every morning. When this alone doesn't help, doctors often recommend adding antidepressants.

MY BREASTS HURT. WHAT COULD BE WRONG?

Probably nothing. Almost half of women have breast pain, most of them during the second half of their menstrual cycle. That's because your breasts undergo changes during the phases of your menstrual cycle that are analogous to those that take place in the uterine lining. In the first half of the cycle, the lobules at the tips of the mammary glands are small and widely spaced. During the second phase, when progesterone is dominant, they undergo more cell division and multiply, and the surrounding tissues swell. This is when you feel tenderness or pain. Shortly after you get your period, the swelling disappears.

There is a link between the degree of discomfort and something called fibrocystic breast disease, but in this case the term "disease" is a misnomer. It can't be called a disease if 50% of all women between the ages of 20 and 50 have it! So let's forget the word "disease" and substitute the term "change." Fibrocystic changes are simply enhanced or exaggerated reactions by your breast tissue to the cyclic ups and downs of your hormones. The pain usually occurs in both breasts and is often accompanied by an increased feeling of lumpiness. Your breasts may also feel fuller, and the veins appear more prominent or engorged.

In your age group these changes are not an overwhelming indication that you harbor any hidden cancer (although you may feel that there is no way of telling what's going on in there with all that pain and lumpiness). Nor do they signal that you are destined to develop breast cancer. If you want the technical details: When biopsied, 70% of fibrocystic changes are classified as nonproliferative, meaning they show no overactive cell growth and engender no risk for cancer. Twenty-six percent show proliferative changes indicating that there is cell growth, but none of the cells are abnormal. This too does not increase risk. Only in 4% of biopsies do proliferative changes occur together with atypical cells, and in these rare instances there can be a fivefold increase in your future risk (and we're talking years down the line) of developing breast cancer.

Now on to breast pain control. It's awful if you can't sleep on your stomach or even get hugged! My first suggestion is to get professionally fitted for a really good supportive bra, not a pretty little lacy thing but one that covers most of the breasts and lifts them without squeezing the sides or the lower portion too much. Then on to some lifestyle changes: Stop drinking or significantly decrease your intake of coffee, tea and caffeinated soda. Decaffeinating your body can decrease pain and lumpiness by nearly 70%. While you're changing your diet, consider reducing the amount of fat you consume. Doctors see less breast tenderness in women who eat a low-fat diet or who are vegetarians. Another stop order: To stop pain (and in this case ultimately cancer), don't smoke. Most doctors will also tell you to take 400 IUs of vitamin E, but I have to confess that there are no good clinical trials that officially show that vitamin E works, perhaps because the women who were studied didn't use this supplement long enough. My clinical experience leads me to feel that it is helpful, and at least it won't hurt.

Another therapy you can self-prescribe is a painkiller, probably the same one you would use to help ease cramps: Tylenol, Advil or Aleve. If this is not enough, you may need a prescription from your doctor. Diuretics can help reduce breast swelling and tenderness. Birth control pills, especially those with low estrogen and/or low progestin activity, may decrease fibrocystic changes and discomfort. But it may be months before you feel the difference. There is an antiestrogen medication called Danazol that is also quite effective in reducing pain. This has mild male-hormone-like activity and should never be used if you are going to get pregnant. It can alter your periods or cause your skin to become oily or develop acne. Some of these side effects can be reduced if small doses of danazol are used, just 100 mg daily. In extreme cases doctors are also prescribing tamoxifen, a selective estrogen or SERM (see page 164) that is currently used to treat postmenopausal women who are at high risk for breast cancer. This drug may, however, increase the risk of endometrial cancer and change your cycles, and we don't know how long you can safely stay on it. If all else fails and your pain is horrendous, it's possible to shut down the ovarian hormone production that's contributing to this cyclical breast pain with GnRH analogs such as Lupron shots or Synarel nasal spray. Therapy beyond six months, however, can lead to bone loss, so this is a temporary solution.

All of the above does not apply if you suddenly develop localized pain, especially in just one breast, that is unusual and not associated with your period. First check to see if the area that hurts is red, swollen or has a thickening or lump. (Please note that you won't know if it feels different unless you are used to touching your breasts, so here is where I insert a plea for monthly self breast exams . . . see page 53.) If there is redness or if the area feels hot, it's possible you have an infection or mastitis. (You may also feel a lump in your underarm.) Most of us associate this with breast-feeding, but it can (rarely) occur when you are not lactating, especially if you have had an infection in the same area in the past that could have resulted in a blocked duct. In this case, you should see your doctor imme-diately. She will prescribe antibiotics and then should reexamine you three weeks later to make sure the pain and mass have disappeared. If you experience pain in one area of your breast but there is no redness, you can wait a few weeks or at least until after your next period to see if it dissipates. But make sure you check carefully for a lump or any changes in consis-tency. The adage that if it hurts it's not cancer is *not* true. Women may have pain as a presenting symptom of cancer as often as 10% of the time. So, once more, if the pain or lumpiness persists for two or more months, see your doctor. At this point it's advisable to get a mammogram and an ultrasound to see if there are any suspicious changes, and if there are, a biopsy is required. If noninvasive testing still shows nothing, but your doc-tor feels something, a biopsy may also be appropriate.

HOW DO I KNOW WHAT CONTRACEPTIVE IS RIGHT FOR ME?

The reply hinges on whether you want to have any (or any more) babies in the future—in other words, whether you want reversible or irreversible contraception. By the time they reach age 30, half of women say they don't want more children. Knowing they'll need protection for the next 20 years, they opt for the easiest course: doing it once and getting it over with. This may be why sterilization is the number one contraceptive choice in your age group, elected by more than one-third of women. So let's begin with this procedure.

Sterilization

When I say "sterilization" here, I'm talking not about hysterectomy, but about tubal ligation. There are several ways this can be performed, but all involve obstructing the fallopian tubes so that sperm cannot gain access to and fertilize an egg. Many women elect to undergo this procedure during a scheduled C-section or immediately after vaginal delivery. In the latter, a small incision (called a mini-lap) is made under the belly button. Because the uterus is still very large, the tubes are easily exposed and can be cut and sutured while you're still under the epidural used for child-birth, if you've had one. The other option is to wait and have the proce-dure once you've recovered from the delivery and you know that your baby is doing well. Remember: This surgery is considered irreversible, and you want to make sure that your family is complete and healthy.

"Interval" sterilization is usually performed through a laparoscope with a general anesthetic. A special needle is placed under the belly button and the abdomen is inflated with carbon dioxide to move the abdominal wall away from the internal organs. A lighted viewing device called a laparo-scope is then inserted through a hollow tube, allowing the surgeon to view the pelvic organs. Another, smaller incision is made below the pubic hair-line and an instrument is inserted that allows the surgeon to either "burn" or place a permanent clip or band around each tube. Rarely, your surgeon may elect not to use the scope but to make a slightly larger incision in the pubic hairline and go directly into the abdomen. The incisions are so small they can be covered by Band-Aids, hence the somewhat disparaging term "Band-Aid surgery."

Failure rate: In the ideal world, the failure rate of this method would be zero. But it's not, sometimes because a surgeon doesn't achieve complete blockage of the tubes, other times because the ends of a tube grow back together. In the real world, 2 out of every 100 women who use this method get pregnant after 10 years. Because the pregnancy takes place in a dam-aged tube, there is a 20% possibility that it will be ectopic (tubal). So if you have a tubal ligation, miss a period and develop pelvic pain, consult your doctor immediately.

Contraindications: Unless you are absolutely certain that you will *never* again want to conceive, you should not choose sterilization. The only way you can have a baby after this procedure is to undergo in vitro fertilization or, in rare cases, have major abdominal surgery in an effort to reverse the tubal ligation. Surveys have shown that up to half of the women who elect to be sterilized have second thoughts years after the surgery, often because they realize too late that other long-term contraceptive options are available.

Advantages: This method is user-friendly and ever-lasting (you'll never need another contraceptive). But there's a hidden benefit: tubal ligation has been associated with a 33% reduction in your future risk of developing ovarian cancer. No one knows why for sure. Blocking the tubes may also decrease your risk of developing pelvic inflammatory disease, because bad microbes can't gain access to the pelvic cavity. (Of course, sterilization provides no protection from STDs.)

Disadvantages: Tubal ligation is expensive ($1,000 to $3,000) and may not be covered by all health insurance carriers. The laparoscopic procedures require a general anesthetic. On occasion (0.6% of the time), there can be big complications behind those little incisions. The bowel or a blood vessel can be punctured or inadvertently burned, requiring subsequent major surgery. Thankfully, this is rare and is more likely to occur if you've had multiple abdominal surgeries or infections that have caused extensive scarring. There is also a so-called post-tubal-ligation syndrome of irregular periods that occurs chiefly in women who stop taking the Pill when they undergo the surgery. The menstrual problems probably aren't the fault of the surgery—it's more likely that stopping the Pill has unmasked a woman's own natural irregularity. If, however, the surgeon was overenthusiastic in destroying tubal tissue, it's possible that the ovarian blood supply and hormone production were compromised. The final disadvantage is that you have to go through the procedure—not your partner. I should point out that getting him "fixed" is your other sterilization option. It's less expensive, does not require general anesthesia and can be performed in the doctor's office.

Oral Contraceptives

If you're not interested in permanent contraception, a combined estrogen-progestin birth control pill is a good choice, and indeed one in every five women in your age group uses it. The synthetic estrogen in the Pill misleads the brain's hypothalamus and pituitary so that production of hormones that trigger ovulation is shut down. The progestin adds to this effect and also makes mucus in the cervix inhospitable to sperm.

Failure rate: Used perfectly, these pills work 99.9% of the time. But in the real world, where you don't take the Pill at the same time every day, miss it altogether or take antibiotics, which can impair its absorption, the efficacy rate is more like 97%. As you get older, however, your fertility rate decreases, so failure rates (of any contraceptive method) will go down.

Contraindications: You should not take the Pill if you've had any of the following health problems: heart attack; stroke; blood clots in your lungs, eyes or in the deep veins of your legs; breast cancer; uterine cancer; cervical cancer; vaginal cancer or liver tumors. Also avoid oral contraceptives if you have uninvestigated vaginal bleeding or had jaundice during previous pregnancy or use of the Pill. And certainly avoid them if you are over age 35 and you smoke.

That's the official disclaimer. But there are conditions that might make your doctor reluctant to prescribe the Pill, and the two of you will have to weigh the possible advantages against the potential disadvantages. These include uncontrolled high blood pressure and severe migraine headaches with accompanying neurologic symptoms such as numbness or transient paralysis.

Advantages: There are a lot. For a long list, see page 42.

Disadvantages: Currently, the Pill is not covered by many insurers. (The fact that these same insurers cover Viagra has caused a furor, and state legislatures have begun to rectify this embarrassing inequity by passing overdue laws to mandate this coverage.) If you buy pills at your pharmacy, they'll cost $25 to $30 per month, though you can get certain brands at lower prices by buying online or through the Femscript program sponsored by Organon (1-800-511-1314). Another drawback for some women: You have to remember to take the Pill every day at the same time, and even if you take it properly, the Pill may not function right in your body. You can have breakthrough bleeding or stop bleeding, get acne, have headaches, gain weight, develop breast tenderness or find that PMS starts or worsens. Some women also develop melasma, spots of dark skin that appear on the face in response to sun exposure. Others note a decrease in their libido (for further discussion, see page 79). Also beware that the Pill doubles your risk of gallstones, and that birth control pills can change the effectiveness of other medications (or vice versa). If you're taking the following, know that the Pill can sometimes make them more potent or their side effects more severe: anticoagulants, benzodiazepine tranquilizers, beta-blockers, corticosteroids, theophylline or tricyclic antidepressants. The Pill has been found to decrease the effectiveness of salicylates, including aspirin. Whenever you put any combination of drugs into your body, the resulting pharmacologic mishmash may affect how well the Pill inhibits ovulation. Drugs that can impair the Pill's effectiveness include antibiotics and the epilepsy medicines phenobarbital, phenytoin and rifampin. One last word of caution about intermixing: The Pill increases your sensitivity to caffeine.

Finally, my public health pronouncement: The Pill will not protect against STDs, although it may decrease your risk of pelvic inflammatory disease by making the cervical mucus more hostile to invading microbes.

The Mini-Pill

These progestin-only pills (POPs), sold under the brand names Micronor, Nor-Q D and Ovrette, have a strong negative effect on the hypothalamus and pituitary, preventing signals that lead to ovulation. They also make the cervical mucus unwelcoming to sperm and the endometrium inhospitable to a fertilized egg.

Failure rate: Taken at exactly the same time every day, this method protects against pregnancy 99% of the time. But this number falls to just 90% if you miss your dose by even a few hours. This is because the levels of progestin the pill delivers drop after 20 hours.

Contraindications: There are very few. If you're taking hepatic-enzyme-inducing medications such as rifampin, phenobarbital, carbamazepine and phenytoin, which are often given for epilepsy, you should not take POPs.

Advantages: You can take this pill in many situations when you should not take combined estrogen-progestin pills—for example, if you are older than 35 and you smoke (tsk, tsk), or if you have heart disease, congestive heart failure, stroke, migraines with neurologic symptions or an increased risk of clotting problems. You can also use this pill without worry if you are breast-feeding. And if you've experienced estrogen-associated side effects such as nausea, breast tenderness or headaches with combined birth control pills, it's worth trying these instead.

Disadvantages: This method is not for the forgetful. If you are more than three hours late in taking a pill or forget one altogether, you should resume your schedule as soon as possible, but you'll have to use a backup contraceptive for at least 48 hours. If you do get pregnant while taking a POP, there is a 10% chance that it will be a tubal pregnancy. You can also develop menstrual changes that may be worrisome or annoying, such as short cycles, spotting, breakthrough bleeding or no bleeding at all. Some women develop acne, and a very few get ovarian cysts.

Depo-Provera

This is the low-maintenance way of getting hormonal contraception. A shot of long-acting progestin every three months, and you're covered. Depo-Provera stops ovulation but doesn't completely shut down the ovaries, so you produce estrogen levels similar to those you produce during your natural cycle.

Failure rate: With a 99.7% efficacy rate, this is one of the most effective methods you can use.

Contraindications: Women with a history of liver disease or uninvestigated abnormal bleeding should not use Depo.

Advantages: You might welcome the fact that there is a 50% chance of having no periods after a year on Depo-Provera. (This increases to 75% after the second year.) Another plus: You don't have to worry about forgetting a pill or taking another medication, such as an antibiotic, that might interfere with hormone levels. Depo-Provera can also be used if you are on antiseizure medication. Indeed, Depo seems to have a quieting effect on brain seizure activity, so it provides birth control while improving seizure control. The shots have also been associated with an 80% reduction in the risk of endometrial cancer because the uterine lining is subjected to less estrogen and more progesterone. Additionally, Depo-Provera may lower your risk of pelvic inflammatory disease much in the way the Pill does. Unlike the Pill, however, it does not increase your risk of gallstones. Finally, women who smoke after age 35 or who have had a heart attack, stroke or clotting problem can use these shots.

Disadvantages: Depo-Provera has quite a few annoying side effects, but the biggest one is that if you develop them, you're stuck with them for three months, sometimes longer, until the shot wears off. Here's what you may have to contend with: unpredictable bleeding (chiefly during the first few months of use), weight gain (an average of 5 pounds in the first year and 2 to 4 pounds every year after that), headaches, bloating, breast tenderness, depression, dizziness and hair loss. You should also know that once you stop getting the shots, it could take an average of 10 months for fertility to return.

Norplant

Like Depo-Provera, Norplant gives you a long-term, slow release of progestin. But this time it's *really* long: five years. These six matchstick-size rods are implanted just under the surface of the skin in your underarm above the elbow. They prevent ovulation about 50% of the time, but their chief effect is to stop the egg from maturing properly so that it cannot undergo fertilization. "Arming" yourself against pregnancy with Norplant also makes your cervical mucus hostile to sperm.

Failure rate: This method's efficacy ranges from 99% to 99.6%, depending on how many years the rods have been implanted.

Contraindications: See Depo-Provera, above.

Advantages: This is one-stop contraception, good for five years. Like Depo-Provera, it decreases your risk of pelvic inflammatory disease and endometrial cancer.

Disadvantages: One deterrent is the high start-up cost: $500 to $700. But amortized over five years, this isn't too bad. In the first couple of years of use, as many as 80% of women on Norplant have changes in their cycles. These include bouts of prolonged or heavy bleeding, spotting between periods, frequent bleeding or no bleeding at all. Half of the patient requests for early removal of the implants are due to this side effect—and therein lies the rub: The implants can be much more difficult to remove than to insert.

IUD

The most commonly used intrauterine device is the Paraguard, a T-shaped piece of polyethylene wrapped in copper wire. It is inserted so that the top part of the "T" fits across the upper portion of the uterus and the body points down toward the cervix. A single-filament string hangs from the lowest part of the "T" out of the cervix so that the wearer and doctor or nurse can check to make sure that the device hasn't gotten lost. The IUD is truly a contraceptive and not a device that causes early abortion, as many people mistakenly believe. Its copper has a toxic effect on sperm. It also makes the cervical mucus hostile and the fluid in the fallopian tubes unconducive to fertilization. The presence of the IUD in the uterine cavity also increases the activity of white blood cells, which gobble up sperm and release chemicals that destroy the sperm and the egg. A second type of IUD, Progestasert, has no copper but instead slowly releases progestin, which prevents sperm from traveling to and fertilizing the egg.

Failure rate: The Paraguard is 99% effective over 10 years of use, while the Progestasert, which is good for only one year, has a pregnancy prevention rate of 98%.

Contraindications: You're not a candidate for an IUD if you have a history of unexplained bleeding, PID, ectopic pregnancy or uterine infections or if you have uterine abnormalities or fibroids. Allergy to copper disqualifies you from getting a Paraguard. But above all, you should steer clear of an IUD if you're not monogamous or if your partner puts you at risk for an STD.

Advantages: You don't know it's there—and neither does your partner. And the Paraguard is good for 10 years. Because of its progestin, the Progestasert can also reduce heavy periods. Once an IUD is removed, fertility immediately returns to precontraception levels.

Disadvantages: The potential drawbacks start with insertion. Although it's rare (occurring in one in 1,500 women), there is a chance that the IUD could perforate the uterus. This is more likely to happen if your uterus has not been stretched by a previous term pregnancy, or if the doctor performing the procedure is inexperienced. Once the device is in place, the uterus may protest with heavy or prolonged periods, cramping or spotting. It may even contract hard enough to expel the device. This is more likely to happen if you've never had children.

Your doctor (and you) may harbor fears of infection and scarring based on the history of another form of IUD, the Dalkon Shield. This device was popular in the 1970s and, unfortunately, had a multifilament tail that encouraged bacteria to grow and travel to the uterus. Women who had this IUD were at risk for PID, and if the device failed and they conceived, they sometimes died of septic miscarriage. The Dalkon Shield was taken off the market, but the reputation of all IUDs was damaged and has never recovered. There is still a risk of PID with today's IUDs, but it is primarily due to the risk associated with the bacteria your partner carries on his penis and not to the IUD itself. Because bacteria from your vagina can be carried into your uterus with insertion, most doctors will follow this procedure with 72 hours of antibiotics.

In the rare instance that you become pregnant while you have an IUD, you should be checked to make sure the pregnancy is not tubal and have the device taken out immediately in order to prevent the possibility of a miscarriage and systemwide infection, or later premature delivery. Note, however, that the removal may cause a miscarriage.

Finally, there is cost. The initial price for the device and its insertion ranges from $300 to $500. This may seem like a lot, but over 10 years the copper IUD becomes a bargain. The one-year Progestasert will obviously be less cost effective.

Condoms

This great barrier method, the condom, is obviously the one I will promulgate for the prevention of STDs (although nothing's perfect but the perfect partner). Eighteen percent of women in your age group concur and are using condoms as their primary contraceptive method.

Failure rate: With typical use, the condom protects against pregnancy 88% of the time. But you improve upon this number with appropriate "penis dressing" (I don't mean a condiment—I mean putting the condom on the right way) and diligent use of spermicide. (For more information about proper condom technique, see page 13.)

Contraindications: Latex allergy. But you can try using a polyurethane condom, sold in specialty condom shops or by mail order. Less is known about their effectiveness against STDs, however. (Sheepskin condoms are too porous and won't prevent infections.) Your allergy can also be due to the spermicide, so also try eliminating this, although that will eliminate some of the protection. You should suspect an allergy if you or your partner develop irritation, swelling and discharge every time you use a condom.

Advantages: It's the cheapest, most effective STD protection you can buy.

Disadvantages: Stopping to put on the condom can take away from the spontaneity of sex, and you have to wait until your partner's penis is erect to put on the condom. "Fooling around" (specifically, having genital contact) before the condom is on can cause pregnancy and infection. Many couples also claim that they feel less when they use a condom—and bemoan a reduced sensitivity as well as spontaneity.

Diaphragm

Two percent of you are relying on this soft silicone disc that is filled with spermicide and placed in the vagina. The spermicide kills any sperm that attempts to pass up the vagina, through the cervix and into the uterus.

Failure rate: The diaphragm plus spermicide protects against pregnancy 82% of the time.

Contraindications: Being allergic to spermicide or having recurrent bladder infections disqualifies you from using this method.

Advantages: The spermicide used with the diaphragm may kill off bad microbes and somewhat reduce their ability to ascend into your pelvis and cause PID. (But the reduction in risk is never as good as with a condom, nor is this considered protection against STDs.) The diaphragm does allow for slightly more spontaneity and sensation than a condom, however.

Disadvantages: Using a diaphragm with spermicide can increase your risk of getting a bladder infection. On top of that, inserting a diaphragm can be awkward and messy. The diaphragm is not sperm-"tight." It only works if spermicide is applied around the rim of the cup before insertion in order to kill any sperm before they enter the cervix. The device must also be put in place within two hours of intercourse and left there for at least six hours afterward. If you're feeling energetic and decide to go for it again before the six hours are up, don't remove the diaphragm. Instead, you should keep it in place and use a special applicator to insert more spermicide.

Cervical Cap
This "mini-diaphragm" is filled with spermicidal jelly or cream and placed directly on the cervix, where it should fit tightly.

Failure rate: The cervical cap plus spermicide protects against pregnancy 82% of the time.

Contraindications: Being allergic to spermicide or having recurrent bladder infections disqualifies you from using this method.

Advantages: Unlike the diaphragm, it can be left in place for two days at a time, although you'll still have to reapply spermicide to the vagina before each act of intercourse. Because the cervical cap does not press directly on the opening of the bladder, it may carry a lower risk of bladder infections than a diaphragm (although spermicide or any device that remains in the vagina can increase risk for this problem).

Disadvantages: The cap is more difficult to insert than the diaphragm, and its fit must be just right or it may be dislodged. Like the diaphragm, it does not give adequate STD protection.

Spermicides
Some vaginal spermicides are intended to be used alone, without diaphragms, caps or condoms. Sold in the form of suppositories, foams, creams, gels and absorbable films, they melt or spread inside the vagina to form a protective coating inside the vagina or over the cervix. Like other spermicides, they contain nonoxynol-9, which immobilizes and kills sperm.

Failure rate: These products protect against pregnancy 79% of the time.

Contraindications: Being allergic to nonoxynol-9 disqualifies you from using this method.

Advantages: No fitting or training is needed in order to use these products, and the spermicide may kill some viruses and bacteria, perhaps decreasing PID, though it won't provide the STD protection of a condom.

Disadvantages: You may have to allow up to half an hour for the product to melt, spread and coat the vagina. And if you have sex a second time, you have to insert a new dose. This can get messy, and you're not allowed to wash or douche the stuff away for six hours after intercourse.

The Rhythm Method

This method of timed abstinence is dependent on your having a regular cycle and being able to predict when you will ovulate. By the age of 30, you probably know when to expect your period (and thus when you're ovulating, two weeks prior to menstruation), although by your late thirties this may be less predictable.

Failure rate: If you abstain from the beginning of the cycle until after ovulation (at least two weeks), this method is 93% effective. But if you try to fudge it even a little ("I just got my period . . . I can't be *that* fertile . . ."), the success rate drops dramatically.

Contraindications: Not wanting to abstain the first two weeks of your cycle (though you could always use condoms if your libido acts up) or having irregular cycles means you're not a candidate for this method.

Advantages: It's free and 100% natural, no additives, preservatives or artificial flavorings.

Disadvantages: Keeping track of your cycle can be a drag. Anything that upsets your ovulation timing can throw off this pregnancy prevention plan.

These are the responsible forms of contraception used by women in your age group. I'm going to assume you're old enough and wise enough now not to rely solely on withdrawal ("He didn't come inside me . . .") or prayer.

I'M OVER 35. CAN I CONTINUE TAKING THE PILL?

If you don't smoke, yes. Once upon a time, long, long ago (okay, 15 years ago), when our pills were more potent and our doctors more scared of side effects, women were told in no uncertain terms that once they reached the age of 35, they were too old to take the Pill. But that was then, and the Pill of today is much lower in estrogen and does not come with age limitations. As a matter of fact, the Pill will help even out any irregularities in your body's production of estrogen and progesterone, and will give you all the benefits it did when you were younger.

WILL THE PILL CAUSE A STROKE OR A HEART ATTACK?

The Pill won't put you at higher than average risk for a stroke unless you smoke or have underlying high blood pressure or diabetes (all of which can increase stroke risk on their own). This is provided that you're on a low-dose pill that has less than 50 micrograms of estrogen. See page 39 for more information on higher-dose pills and stroke.

The same goes for heart attacks. In fact, using a third-generation oral contraceptive that contains the progestin desogestrel may cut your risk of heart attack slightly.

A third concern for women who've been watching the news is that European studies cited the new third-generation pills as causing a higher risk than the older type of pills of pulmonary embolism (blood clots in the vessels of the lungs) and other problems with clot formation (thromboembolism). But the reports cried "clot" too quickly, and more recent analysis of all data on this subject indicates that the women who developed clots were actually at greater than average risk for them before they were ever put on the Pill. However, *any* birth control pill can increase your risk of nonfatal clot formation. Out of 100,000 healthy, nonpregnant women who do not take the Pill, 4 will develop thromboembolism each year. Among 100,000 who take any type of birth control pill, 10 to 15 will have this problem. But you have to consider this in its reproductive context: 50 out of every 100,000 women who become pregnant experience thromboembolism.

EVER SINCE I STARTED ON THE PILL, I'VE BEEN LESS LUSTY. IS THERE A CONNECTION?

There could be. Your libido is hormonally driven by your testosterone, and in order for this hormone to have its sexy effect, it has to be unbound—that is, not attached to a protein called sex hormone binding globulin (SHBG). When you take birth control pills, they not only prevent ovulation, they also prevent some of the secretion of testosterone from your ovaries. Moreover, the Pill increases SHBG levels, so more of whatever testosterone is produced is bound up and rendered impotent. The Pill may have caused you to be functionally testosterone-deficient.

If your libido problem started with Pill use, you might want to try switching to a pill that is triphasic (providing gradually increasing doses of progestin over the menstrual cycle). These have been found to have a less profound effect on sex drive. If there's still no improvement, consider another form of birth control. After all, you're using contraception so you can have sex in the first place.

WE'VE BEEN TRYING TO GET PREGNANT, BUT IT SEEMS TO BE TAKING A WHILE. WHAT SHOULD WE DO?

This depends on what you mean by "a while." Eighty percent of all women who try to get pregnant for one year will succeed. But if you're over 35 you may be worrying about your biological clock, and waiting a year to get an official diagnosis of infertility seems too long. So my advice is to track your basal body temperature or use a home ovulation test kit to see if you appear to be ovulating, and to time intercourse to peak fertility (see page 44). If nothing happens after six to nine months, you might want to start preliminary infertility testing if you're 35 or older. If you're under 35, you can wait a year.

A basic infertility workup begins with hormonal tests. Your follicle stimulating hormone (FSH) level will be measured on day two or three of your cycle; a high level is a marker for poor-quality or poorly performing eggs (egg problems can appear years before menopause). This test becomes extremely important as you enter your late thirties and early forties. If FSH test results are consistently high, you probably won't be able to conceive with your own eggs and may need to consider donor eggs. Blood progesterone levels will be checked at day 21, when they should peak, to help determine if and how well you're ovulating. Prolactin should be measured if your cycles are irregular or if you secrete fluid from your breasts; elevated levels could indicate a pituitary adenoma (see page 27), which could interfere with ovulation. Irregular cycles also call for a thyroid stimulating hormone (TSH) blood test to check for thyroid problems.

Because sperm's movement is aided and abetted by cervical mucus, this should also be checked at midcycle, when it's most abundant. A postcoital test, done anywhere from 2 to 12 hours after intercourse, checks to see if mucus production is adequate and if sperm are actively swimming in it.

Infertility is not just a woman's thing. Forty percent of the time it is due to male factors. And in another 20% of the cases, the problem is a combination of both male and female factors. That means the cause is purely female just 40% of the time—and that may be a slight exaggeration, because 10% of the time we can't figure out why a couple is infertile. So obviously your partner should have his semen analyzed for sperm count, motility or activity of the sperm and their ability to penetrate an egg as well as antisperm antibodies.

If results of all the above tests are normal, you should be checked for "mechanical" problems that can stop sperm from meeting the egg or prevent implantation and normal growth of an embryo. These include scarring of the fallopian tubes from endometriosis, previous infection or surgery; uterine malformation; or growths such as fibroids and cervical abnormalities. Hysterosalpingography (HSG) is an X-ray in which dye is injected into the uterine cavity to show whether the cavity is normal and the tubes are free of blockages. If the results of this test are questionable or abnormal, the next step is a laparoscopy to view the pelvis and establish whether there is scar tissue or endometriosis blocking the tubes. Fibroids, scarring or malformations inside the uterus can be seen first with vaginal ultrasound or HSG and further assessed with hysteroscopy, in which a telescope placed through the cervix shows the uterine lining. Laparoscopy performed through an abdominal incision will confirm a diagnosis. If scarring, endometriosis, tumors or other abnormalities are found, your doctor may be able to use these procedures to correct these problems.

This is a very short answer to what I know is a very complicated and emotionally charged issue. The first thing you have to do is establish what, if anything, is wrong and then proceed with appropriate therapy. Remember, despite all of these tests, doctors can't figure out what's preventing a couple from conceiving 10% to 20% of the time. But they can still use fertility techniques to help them get pregnant.

WHAT TREATMENTS CAN WE EXPECT TO GET AT A FERTILITY CLINIC?

When a woman's ovulations are deemed inadequate or infertility is unexplained, ovulation induction or enhancement is the treatment of choice. The easiest (but not necessarily most effective) method is an oral fertility drug called clomiphene citrate (Clomid or Serophene). This tricks your pituitary into "thinking" there's no estrogen in sight, causing this gland in your brain to work harder and produce more FSH, which in turn stimulates the ovary and causes follicles to develop in preparation for ovulation. In any given cycle, 6% of women with unexplained infertility who use this drug will become pregnant, but this isn't terribly impressive given that 4% of them would become pregnant with no therapy at all. To slightly better the odds, clomiphene citrate is often combined with a shot of human chorionic gonadotropin (HCG) to enhance release of the stimulated egg or eggs. This is usually followed by intrauterine insemination, in which sperm are separated from semen, placed in a special solution and inserted directly into the uterine cavity. (I like to think of this as "Federal Expressing" the sperm.) When these methods are combined, the average per-cycle pregnancy rate minimally rises to 6.7%.

If all this doesn't work, the bigger guns are called in: shots that contain FSH. You have to administer the shots to yourself daily in specially tailored amounts determined by (sometimes daily) blood tests for estrogen and ultrasound exams. Once egg-containing follicles in your ovaries are adequately developed, HCG is given to prompt the eggs' release. (In an attempt to better the chances of success, superovulation, or development of multiple follicles, is common and even necessary. But if too many eggs develop and HCG is administered, you risk a multiple pregnancy. Twins are acceptable, but when more than three embryos develop, pregnancy complications are likely. So you and your doctor should be prepared to discontinue therapy before you get your HCG if an ultrasound examination shows too many developing "ready to go" follicles.) Intrauterine insemination is generally performed 36 to 40 hours after the HCG shot. Some reproductive endocrinologists will make sure that your own ovarian hormone production is shut down with a drug such as Lupron before beginning this process. This ensures that you start at ground zero. The overall per-cycle success rate for this technique is 18%, which means that 18 out of 100 women who try this method for one month will become pregnant. But almost a quarter of those pregnancies will not continue to term; still others will be multiple. In couples with unexplained infertility, this technique is three times likelier to result in pregnancy as insemination alone, and twice as likely as treatment with superovulation, intracervical insemination (just putting the sperm in the cervix) or intrauterine insemination alone.

If this superovulation-plus-insemination technique doesn't work or your fallopian tubes are blocked or the clinic wants to quickly get the best results they have to offer, in vitro fertilization (IVF) is used. Pregnancy rates can be as high as 45%, depending on your age and the clinic where you are treated. Here, after ovulation induction as described above, eggs are harvested by aspirating the stimulated follicles. The word "harvested" means that a needle is inserted through the vagina and used to puncture the swollen egg-containing follicle. The eggs are then mixed with your partner's sperm (or donor sperm, if necessary) and incubated for several days. Meanwhile, you are given progesterone to help prepare the uterine lining for implantation. Fertilization and initial cell division can be checked, and if they appear successful, the fertilized egg is placed in the uterine cavity. Once a pregnancy "takes," HCG levels are checked and an ultrasound will be done to evaluate whether the embryo (or embryos) is in the right place and is viable. Because this technique is so expensive and invasive, many women and their reproductive endocrinologists want to go for the gold, and a large number of fertilized eggs will be placed in the uterus in hopes that at least one or maybe two will implant and grow. Unfortunately, this may result in multiple pregnancies that threaten miscarriage, fetal loss, prematurity and even the mother's own health. To help reduce this risk, some clinics observe the dividing fertilized eggs slightly longer before implanting them. This allows doctors to select the best, most mature, fertilized eggs (now called blastocysts) and implant a smaller number. Reports have shown that at least in younger women, two eggs may be just as successful in creating at least a single viable pregnancy as four or five and are less likely to result in multiple pregnancy.

Even a woman who doesn't have ovaries or viable eggs can undergo an IVF using donor eggs. The average per-cycle pregnancy rate for this procedure is 22.5%, but it can rise to 35% to 45% at some fertility clinics, depending on the quality of their lab and the age and health of the patients they treat.

Provided your tubes aren't blocked, some clinics will attempt to put a fertilized egg into the fallopian tube and let it travel to the uterus under its own power. This is called *gamete intrafallopian transfer* (GIFT). GIFT has an average per-cycle pregnancy rate of 27%, but may be slightly more successful in some clinics; however, unlike IVF, GIFT requires a laparoscopy. It's also more expensive, and most reproductive specialists now feel there's little advantage in resorting to this over IVF.

There are also techniques that micromanipulate the fertilization of the egg by sperm. These include intracytoplasmic sperm injection (ICSI), in which the sperm is injected directly into the egg. This also allows a viable sperm to be selected and used in cases where sperm count is very low. ICSI is now routinely used in many labs because reproductive technologists believe that fertilization is generally improved with this technique. This may result in a slight increase in genetic abnormalities in the developing embryo in some instances when the man's natural sperm count is very low.

There are more developments, combinations and permutations in the world of infertility treatment even as I write. A nucleus that contains all the genetic material from an "old" egg can be transferred into the cytoplasm or "shell" of a younger person's donor egg, and implanted in the older mother. This makes it possible for her genetic material to be passed on to her offspring. Methods have been developed to freeze young, healthy eggs or egg-producing ovarian tissue and store them for later use in IVF. Although this is still experimental, it could be valuable to young women who will lose future ovarian function due to cancer therapy.

Going through all this can be one of the most stressful and expensive experiences of your life, and success is not guaranteed. Before you begin infertility treatment, do your homework. Find out what options are offered for your particular problem and what the cost and success rates are in the clinic you're planning on using. The key is to ask not just for pregnancy rates but for the clinic's "take-home baby" rate—the percentage of clients whose pregnancies end in delivery of a baby. An infertility support group such as Resolve (617-623-0744 or www.resolve.org) can help you with up-to-date information on therapies and clinics and can help you cope with your emotional stress. (This section has not dealt with the tremendous sense of frustration and anguish that accompanies each "failed" cycle. An apt description used by one of my patients is that "infertility is like a cancer of the soul").

I'VE HAD TWO MISCARRIAGES. WHAT SHOULD I DO?

Once you've had two or three miscarriages—and especially if you've had no living births—your chance of having another miscarriage is 25%. (The normal chance of having a miscarriage is 15%.) A fourth miscarriage would push your risk to 40%.

Successful implantation and development of a pregnancy requires a good housing unit (the uterus), proper hormonal support and a willingness on the part of your system not to reject the fetus as a foreign body. From the fetal side, the right amount of chromosomal material compatible with development is needed. Finally, the pregnancy requires a sterile, nontoxic environment in which to grow.

Ten to fifty percent of women who experience recurrent pregnancy loss (RPL) have some type of anatomic problem. This can sometimes take the form of a uterine malformation. If only one half of a woman's uterus develops, it's called a unicornate uterus and may have only one fallopian tube. When the two halves develop but don't meet, there can be two uteri (uterus didelphys); if the two halves partially meet, the result is a bicornate uterus. Another possibility is that the uterus can have a normal exterior contour, but that a wall, or septum, is present between the two halves. All of these malformations can prevent normal implantation and development of a pregnancy and result in first or second trimester miscarriage. In addition to these or in combination with them, the cervix may be short or weak (incompetent cervix) so that it dilates under the pressure of a pregnancy, causing a second-trimester miscarriage. The lining of the uterus may also be a factor. A fibroid projecting into the uterine lining or scarring of the lining (Asherman's syndrome) resulting from a previous dilation and curettage, the scraping of the uterine lining, may leave the uterus unable to support a pregnancy.

Fifteen to sixty percent of RPLs are hormonally related. There may be too little progesterone to maintain the lining of the uterus. This is called a luteal phase insufficiency, and may be due to inadequate FSH or LH production, or to an abnormal ratio between the two. (This occurs in women with polycystic ovarian syndrome.) Hormones from other glands such as the thyroid can also affect these levels. Finally, women with poorly controlled insulin-dependent diabetes may have a two- to threefold increased risk of miscarriage.

We know an overactive immune system can be important in rejecting a pregnancy, and this is more likely to occur in women who, for some unknown reason, produce antibodies against their own tissues (autoantibodies). This explains why autoimmune conditions such as lupus are associated with an increased risk of pregnancy loss. The autoimmune antibodies that are most frequently linked to pregnancy problems and miscarriage are the antiphospholipids, which can be present even in perfectly healthy women with no history of an autoimmune disease. These antibodies are found in 10% of women with RPL. They cause clots to form in vessels feeding the placenta, which can then no longer nourish the pregnancy, so it aborts.

Not only do we not need the wrong antibodies, but we also need the right ones. The mother's body must make special antirejection antibodies in her placenta so that the fetus is not considered a foreign invader and rejected. In certain immunologic conditions, the mother's immune system is too similar to that of the father, and the antirejection antibodies are not properly formed.

Although 60% of first trimester miscarriages are caused by chromosomal abnormalities, most of these are spontaneous and have nothing to do with either your or your partner's own genetic makeup. If you are experiencing RPLs, the chance that either of you is passing on a chromosomal malformation to the fetus is only 3% to 6%.

Infections compromise the sterile surroundings needed for growth and development of the pregnancy. Some studies have shown an association between RPL and two types of bacterial infection that can be silently present: mycoplasm and ureaplasm. Herpes virus has also been shown to triple the rate of miscarriage.

Exposure to toxins by you or your partner can also "poison" a pregnancy and result in its expulsion. Smoking "just" 10 cigarettes a day increases your risk of miscarriage, as does drinking two or more alcoholic drinks a day. (Your mate should avoid overconsuming alcohol too—paternal alcoholism has been associated with RPL.) Drinking more than three cups of coffee a day (or consuming the caffeine equivalent of 300 milligrams) may put you at higher risk, and the more you drink, the greater your risk.

Having given you this long and complicated list of what can lead to a miscarriage, let me reassure you: With the exception of RPLs caused by smoking and alcohol abuse, these miscarriages are almost never caused by what you personally do. There is no evidence that moderate exercise will prompt a miscarriage, although it's traditionally advised that women stop exercising in the first trimester of pregnancy if they have experienced RPL or if they are bleeding. Likewise, working does not increase your risk. However, holding a job that requires you to work long hours and/or stand for long periods of time may increase your chance of a premature delivery. Happily, having sex—even experiencing orgasm—has not been shown to put you at risk for miscarriage. Nor is there any evidence that exposure to computer video display terminals increases risk.

There's no consensus among experts as to how many miscarriages constitute the need for a complete medical workup, although many consider three the minimum number. But because miscarriage is so deeply troubling to couples and you may not want to take the chance of enduring a third (or fourth) pregnancy loss, it's not unreasonable to ask your doctor to perform a basic diagnostic workup after two miscarriages if you have not successfully given birth in the past. Before you put yourself through the physical and financial hardship of testing, though, consider this: Even after three miscarriages, patients who receive no therapy for RPL can deliver a healthy infant 50% of the time.

The diagnostic workup for RPL should include the following:

- Pelvic ultrasound after ovulation, to assess the thickness of the endometrium and rule out fibroids.
- Hysterosalpingography to rule out uterine malformations (see above).
- Endometrial biopsy and/or measurement of blood progesterone on day 21 of your cycle to check for a luteal phase defect.
- Thyroid stimulating hormone test.
- Autoantibody testing.
- Cervical cultures to look for bacterial infections.
- Chromosomal testing (karyotyping) of both parents and, when available, of the abortus. (This test is very expensive and there is only a 3% to 6% chance that it will be positive. And even if it is, you can still have a normal pregnancy. My recommendation is that you undergo karyotyping only as a last resort.)

If the suspected cause of your RPL is determined with testing, you can consider therapy. The highest rate of success will be with surgical procedures to correct uterine malformations or remove fibroids. Luteal phase deficiency can be treated with progesterone in the second half of the cycle, or with drugs that improve ovulation from the get-go. In the rare instance that thyroid function is abnormal, it should be corrected. If you have RPL associated with positive antiphospholipid autoantibody disorders, therapy with heparin, aspirin or corticosteroids in a subsequent pregnancy may help. If your antigens are too similar to your partner's, there is a therapy called mixed leukocyte immunization, in which his white blood cells are injected into you. This therapy is very controversial and there can be immune complications, so make sure it is done through a specialized center.

Women who test positive for mycoplasm or ureaplasm should be treated with erythromycin or tetracycline, although no one can guarantee that this will make a difference. Finally, if karyotyping reveals chromosomal abnormalities, you can keep trying to get pregnant and make sure that early chorionic villus testing is performed to check for genetic defects. Or you can consider use of donor eggs or sperm. In the future, it may be possible to correct the chromosomal abnormality in the fertilized egg before implantation.

Once you become pregnant again, there are several tests that can reassure you that the embryo is viable. Blood tests for HCG, human chorionic gonadotropin, the hormone produced by placental cells during pregnancy, should show that levels are doubling every 48 hours in the first 10 weeks of pregnancy. By seven weeks, ultrasound should reveal a normal-size gestational sac and fetus, with a heartbeat of 110 beats per minute or more.

WHAT CAN GO WRONG IF I GET PREGNANT AFTER AGE 35?

Pregnancy involves two beings, you and (ultimately) the baby, so we have to examine each one separately. Let's start with you. I'm assuming you're generally healthy, but there are a few things you'll want to watch out for. After 35, you are at increased risk for miscarriage, especially in the first trimester, because of a 50% decrease in your number of chromosomally perfect eggs. And if the eggs do allow for a pregnancy, you'll want to ensure that there are no chromosomal abnormalities in the developing fetus. This is where genetic testing may be considered the most important aspect of your over-35 pregnancy. The chance of a genetic problem is slim. Your risk of delivering a baby with a significant chromosomal abnormality rises from 0.26% at age 30 to 0.56% at age 35 (It continues to rise, hitting 1.5% percent at age 40 and 5.4% at age 45.) If we look only at Down's syndrome, your risk at 35 is 0.3%; at 40 it's 1%. At 45 it rises to 3% and at 49, it's reached 9.1%. There is an even higher rate of abnormal chromosomes if we test in the first two trimesters of pregnancy, but about one-third of these pregnancies will be lost at later dates or are stillborn. The bottom line is that after the age of 35, these numbers are high enough that having genetic testing is worthwhile.

There are two ways we can detect chromosomal abnormalities: amniocentesis and chorionic villus sampling (CVS).

Amniocentesis: This is performed between 14 and 20 weeks of pregnancy, when there is abundant amniotic fluid surrounding the fetus. Using ultrasound guidance, your doctor will insert a needle through the lower abdomen into the uterus and aspirate fluid. The cells in this fluid are then separated and cultured so that they multiply for about 10 days. (This is the reason you have to go through that tense waiting period before results are available.) Once adequate cells have been grown from the fluid, they are stained and their chromosomes are measured and counted. The most common chromosomal abnormality is Down's syndrome, or trisomy 21 (in other words, there are three of this chromosome instead of a matched pair), but other extra or missing chromosomes associated with severe developmental abnormalities or even inability to survive can also be found. Additionally, genetic problems can be diagnosed by studying the cells' enzymes and DNA. These include more than 70 hereditary disorders including sickle cell anemia, thalassemia, cystic fibrosis and Tay-Sachs. The fluid that's obtained can also be tested for high levels of alpha fetoprotein, which is associated with neural tube defects, abdominal wall defects and certain gastrointestinal problems. The latter test used to be one of the reasons that amniocentesis was preferred over CVS, but now maternal blood testing is almost as accurate and is routinely performed on women of all ages. The current advantage of amnio is that it is easy to perform and has a slightly lower rate of miscarriage associated with it than CVS—about 0.5% versus 1% to 2%. The disadvantage is that the results are not available until late in the second trimester. Emotionally—not to mention technically—it is much more difficult to terminate an abnormal pregnancy at this point.

Chorionic villus sampling: This is done between 10 and 12 weeks of pregnancy. Under ultrasound guidance, a thin tube is placed through the cervix or through a small puncture site in the lower abdomen, and tissue from the edge of the placenta is aspirated. Because this contains large amounts of fetal cells, it can be immediately stained and the chromosomes examined. Some of the cells are also cultured to confirm that the initial assessment is correct. Like amnio, CVS allows enzyme and DNA testing for hereditary disorders. Its advantage is that you can miss only two periods and yet be reassured that there is no detectable genetic problem. And if there is, you can choose to terminate with a simple, first trimester abortion performed in a doctor's office. In the likelier case that everything's fine, you can rejoice in your condition and begin the process of bonding. (If you choose to learn the sex of your baby, you can even starting decorating the bedroom in pink or blue.) The risk of fetal loss in most clinics is twice as high as with amnio, and these numbers might scare you off if you've tried to conceive for a long time. Bleeding, spotting and cramping can occur in 1 in 10 women. Rarely, if the cells obtained during CVS are questionable, you may have to have an amniocentesis to confirm the first finding.

Because not all abnormalities are caused by changes that can be detected in chromosomes, a normal CVS or amnio does not guarantee a completely healthy baby. And so it is also advisable for you to have a special ultrasound at 20 weeks to carefully scrutinize the anatomy of the fetus and rule out developmental abnormalities in the brain, heart, major vessels, abdomen and limbs. Many anatomic problems can be detected, and finding them gives you the option of discontinuing the pregnancy or arranging possible surgical correction in utero or immediately after delivery. This type of testing is now performed fairly routinely on women of all ages.

In addition to possible chromosomal abnormalities, you face certain hazards during labor and delivery. Once you're 35, you're almost twice as likely as a younger woman to get gestational diabetes (the type that develops during pregnancy). This is associated with an increased risk of high blood pressure and large babies, and subsequent cesarean section. The majority of women who get gestational diabetes are at significant risk for developing true diabetes later in life. (So if you have or had gestational diabetes make sure you get a fasting blood glucose test once a year from here on in).

You're also more likely to develop pregnancy-induced high blood pressure. This may require bed rest, hospitalization, medication to lower your blood pressure and vigilant monitoring of the baby's well-being. There is also a higher risk of bleeding complications from separation of the placenta, and again, a higher risk for C-section.

Now on to the hard part: labor. If you haven't had a previous delivery, you now have the dubious distinction of being called (in the less than P.C. terms of obstetrical textbooks) an "elderly primipara." Whether or not you agree you *are* more likely to have prolonged or dysfunctional labor and require contraction stimulation with intravenous doses of the hormone oxytocin. This doesn't always work, and the baby's head may fail to come down and/or the cervix may not dilate. This may ultimately cause you to need a cesarean section. Even if your doctor does not need to perform a C-section, forceps or a vacuum may be needed to help get the baby out.

Fetal distress is more common after age 35 because with age (this is all relative again), the arteries that supply blood to the placenta become less expandable, and during contractions may provide insufficient oxygen to the baby. This is called diminished fetal reserve, and if it happens, your doctor may have to rescue the baby with an emergency C-section.

Then there's the psychological issue: You've waited a long time to have this baby, perhaps you even underwent fertility treatments in order to conceive. You and your doctor don't want to take any chances. So the decision to opt for a C-section is made more readily.

If you've had several children in the past (now you're called an "elderly multipara"), and especially if you've had C-sections, you're at greater risk for placenta previa, which means that the placenta has developed in the wrong part of the uterus and covers the cervical opening. This can cause significant bleeding in the last few months of pregnancy as the cervix begins to thin and dilate, and can result in a need for early delivery with cesarean section.

Now let's look at what happens to the other being, the baby. Once you've safely gotten through the first trimester, you will probably have a viable, healthy baby. But you'll need closer surveillance than younger women, since your greater risk of diminished placental blood supply can cause growth retardation and low birth weight. Conditions that are especially likely to lead to this include high blood pressure, diabetes and other types of chronic illness, as well as smoking.

You're probably not at significantly increased risk of having a premature baby just because you're over the age of 35. But being over 35 means you're more likely to have had a previous D&C (which can lead to an incompetent cervix), fibroids, multiple pregnancies as a result of infertility therapy or high blood pressure. All of these can promote premature delivery.

Pregnancy after age 35, like pregnancy at any age, requires that you take care of your body and get appropriate prenatal care. This includes eating a healthful diet, taking prenatal vitamins, making sure that you get adequate calcium (1,200 milligrams per day) and avoiding smoking, drinking alcohol or taking medications not deemed safe in pregnancy.

I HAVE REALLY BAD CRAMPS. HOW CAN I TELL IF IT'S ENDOMETRIOSIS?

It's not easy to tell. Ten percent of women have been found to have some degree of endometriosis during their reproductive lives. How do you know if you're one of the 1 in 10? If your cramps don't get significantly better with over-the-counter pain medicines or birth control pills, then they could be due to endometriosis. You're certainly in the right age group, especially if you haven't had a baby. Unfairly, endometriosis is a disease that may be associated with a willing or unwilling postponement of childbearing.

This insidious disease originates in abnormally located endometrial cells that grow and respond to your hormones. One theory is that the cells get misplaced by something called retrograde menstruation. Normally when you have your period, cells from the lining of the uterus slough off and go down the cervix and out of the vagina. With retrograde menstruation, some cells go up through the tubes and seed onto the ovaries and pelvis, where they implant.

Another mode of displacement for these wayward endometrial cells is thought to be through blood or lymphatic vessels, which can allow cells to wander as far as the lungs or even the skin. And finally, multipotential cells may be present almost anywhere in the pelvis or even abdomen, and may convert to hormonally stimulated endometrial-like cells and grow.

In most situations, these cells will be cleaned up by intricate immune system processes. But if this control fails, the cells take root and begin to respond to your own hormones by growing or multiplying and causing local reactions such as scarring and bleeding cysts (endometrioma). All this may be diminished by (or even regress during) pregnancy.

The most prominent symptom of this endometrial cellular invasion is severe pain with your period, because that's when the cells react and bleed. The degree of disease has very little to do with the intensity of the pain, and indeed pain can occur and be quite horrendous even if the disease is mild. You may also hurt at other times, such as midcycle with ovulation or premenstrually. You may even spot between periods. Women with endometriosis sometimes feel deep pelvic pain with intercourse as well as during bowel movements, particularly when menstruating. If endometrial implants are present on the bowel, they can cause diarrhea or constipation during menstruation.

Unfortunately, your gynecologist cannot always tell if you have endometriosis by doing a simple pelvic exam. And if implants are less than one-quarter of an inch in diameter, they can't be seen on a pelvic ultrasound, nor can scar tissue. So the absence of any findings on a pelvic exam or ultrasound doesn't guarantee you don't have the disease. The only way to be sure is to undergo laparoscopy, at which time your physician can look for round, beige or red implants of abnormal endometrial cells. Even then, some of the implants may not be easily distinguished by the naked or laparoscopically aided eye. Nonetheless, 26% of women with pelvic pain turn out to have endometriosis when they are carefully examined laparoscopically.

In some women with endometriosis, the disease progresses, with the formation of fairly large blood-filled ovarian cysts. These endometriomas can be felt during your pelvic exam and certainly will be visible during an ultrasound. Laparoscopy can help confirm that this cyst is benign and allows its removal.

Endometrial cells and the glands that they are a part of can even implant deep into the wall of the uterus (the myometrium) and, once there, can also create severe pain with your period. This is called *adeno-*

myosis and is often associated with heavy bleeding. Adenomyosis may begin to develop through the next two decades of your life. By the age of 50, half of all women have some degree of this endometrial invasion. Again, diagnosis can be difficult. Your doctor may tell you that your uterus is a little "boggy" (or soft) and enlarged. An ultrasound might show small cystic areas in the wall of the uterus. Neither laparoscopy nor D&C will help in confirming that you have adenomyosis. The only way to be sure, unfortunately, is to remove the uterus. And clearly the goal is to treat the problem in you rather than take the uterus out to make the diagnosis.

Before you resort to surgery to check out your cramps, it's important to consider what other conditions might be causing them. It may be that you haven't developed any disease at all, but that you're extremely sensitive to prostaglandins. However, for most women, nonsteroidal anti-inflammatory drugs or birth control pills will bring relief. Another possibility is that you have a chronic pelvic infection or pelvic scarring from a previous infection. In this case, every time you have your period or even ovulate and prostaglandins are produced, the scar tissue is irritated and cramps become severe. To complicate matters, any disorder in the pelvis can also be made worse during your period and result in pain or cramping. That includes fibroids, irritable bowel syndrome or inflammatory bowel disease.

So now I've given you all the possibilities, but you still have your cramps. What should you do? I'll assume that you've already taken OTC painkillers and they've failed. You need a thorough pelvic exam. During this checkup, a rectal exam should also be performed to see if there are any nodules or if there is severe tenderness behind the uterus. This could indicate implants on the uterosacral ligament, which supports the uterus. If a pelvic exam shows nothing, you can either be persistent and ask your physician for a pelvic ultrasound, or you can try treating the problem with birth control pills (provided you're not trying to become pregnant). If the pain does disappear, you may never have a firm diagnosis. But know that the Pill may help prevent development and progression of endometriosis, so you should simply stay on the Pill until you want to get pregnant, in which case your contraceptive will be doing double duty as a stand-off therapy for endometriosis.

If the Pill doesn't help, it's certainly time to get that pelvic ultrasound to see whether there are ovarian cysts that appear to contain blood. If they do not diminish in size even after you take birth control pills, then laparoscopy is warranted. This procedure is also called for if you have severe, disabling pain that prevents you from continuing your normal activities for several days each month, despite attempts at conservative therapy.

Not only will laparoscopy allow your doctor to make a diagnosis, but at the time of surgery she can vaporize or burn the endometrial implants, excise them and remove endometriomas or any pelvic scarring that has occurred as a result of this disease. A presacral neurectomy, in which nerve fibers running from the back of the pelvis are severed, can also be performed via the laparoscope to help control disabling pain. All these forms of surgical treatment may not be adequate for pain control. Nor are they always permanent. The tendency for cells to reimplant will always be there. In fact, up to half of patients who've had surgery develop a recurrence within nine years. For some women, the only definitive cure for this disease is a radical one: removal of the uterus and both ovaries. Obviously this is truly a last resort in your age group, particularly if you still want to have children. So even if you've gone through laparoscopic surgery, you will probably need to continue with some kind of drug therapy if you aren't planning on becoming pregnant in the near future. If your disease was severe or your doctor feels she hasn't removed all the implants, total ovarian suppression with GnRH analogs, which essentially render you temporarily menopausal, will help control aberrant cells that may have been missed during surgery. The most commonly used analogs are Lupron, given as a monthly shot, or Synarel nasal spray (a puff a day). These medications are generally used for only six months at a time because they can lead to bone loss and subsequent development of osteoporosis. They also cause menopausal symptoms of hot flashes or sleep disturbances. If this occurs, talk to your physician about taking the mini-pill (such as Micronor) or a very low dose birth control pill during therapy. Alternatives to GnRH analogs, which also cause shrinkage of the endometriotic implants, include Danazol, a malelike hormone that suppresses ovulation, or Depo-Provera, which induces a pseudopregnancy state and ultimately robs the implants of their natural ovarian hormone supply. If you're not planning to get pregnant when you finish your therapy, it would be wise to take a birth control pill to diminish the chance that endometriosis will recur.

Although I want to be reassuring about the success of these treatments, there are valid concerns about this disease's effects on your future fertility. More than one-third of women with endometriosis are infertile. (Doctors don't know whether to blame the disease for the infertility or the infertility for the disease. It's possible that these women developed endometriosis because they didn't have protective pregnancies.) In any event, endometriosis can cause mechanical problems (the fallopian tubes may be blocked by scar tissue or endometrial implants) as well as chemical ones (the implants produce substances that compromise the tubes' ability to pick up the egg and move it along, and that also impair sperm's ability to fertilize the egg). Infertility therapy is similar to that for pain: Get rid of the implants, free the area of scar tissue and remove any ovarian cysts. If this is not effective, you may need to resort to high-tech in vitro fertilization procedures. Although half of women treated with GnRH agonists alone will go on to become pregnant, the chance of conceiving is slightly greater if medication is combined with surgery.

Now back to your pain. If your doctor thinks your cramps are due to adenomyosis, you should be able to control it with birth control pills. On rare occasions, if this therapy doesn't work by itself, a GnRH analog can be combined with the Pill for better results.

If your doctor diagnoses chronic pelvic inflammatory disease, the first line of therapy is still the Pill. This will prevent the monthly ovarian trauma of ovulation and decrease the chance of reinfection or irritation of local scar tissue. The ovaries—and hence the pelvis—should remain quiet, calm and comfortable. In some cases, if flare-ups of infection occur during menstruation, it may be necessary to add on an antibiotic during your period.

When a previous infection has caused pelvic scarring, the Pill may not provide relief, and surgery may be required to remove the scars and free the pelvic organs so they don't hurt. This is usually done through the laparoscope. A word of warning: Any surgery can itself lead to scarring, and there's no guarantee that if the scars are removed they won't re-form. On rare occasions, a tube, ovary or even the uterus may need to be removed because of recurrent scarring and pain.

The treatment of fibroids is dependent on the severity of pain, bleeding or size (see page 144).

I HAVE PELVIC PAIN, BUT IT DOESN'T REALLY FEEL LIKE CRAMPS. WHAT COULD IT BE?

In order to help you, I have to get a more specific description of your problem. Is the pain constant, or does it come and go? Is it so severe that you can't continue your normal activities? Is it accompanied by nausea or vomiting? Does eating make it worse? Is it worse when you need to have a bowel movement or while you're having one? What happens during intercourse? Do you have any burning or frequency of urination, or does the pain increase when you void? How long has the pain lasted? Did it come on suddenly? Is it associated with weight loss, lack of appetite or fatigue? Do you have any coexisting problems such as frequent headaches, sleep disorders, depression, mood disorders or diffuse tender points all over the body?

After I ask you these questions, I must also remind you that there's more to your pelvis than your uterus, tubes and ovaries. It contains the large and small intestine, the bladder and the ureters leading into it from the kidneys, as well as all the nerves that enervate these organs. The abdominal wall muscles, pelvic bones and lower spine are there as well. If there's anything wrong with any of these, pelvic pain can result. So let's examine your symptoms and see which diagnosis fits best.

Severe, Unremitting Pain Chiefly on One Side of the Pelvis

This is not something you should try to self-diagnose (a) because you're in too much pain to think clearly and (b) because lack of a proper diagnosis can be serious, even fatal.

If your period is late or you have had a positive pregnancy test: You may have a ruptured tubal (ectopic) pregnancy, so see your physician immediately. Your doctor will perform a blood test for the pregnancy hormone HCG and, if this is positive, do a vaginal ultrasound to look for the absence of a viable pregnancy in the uterus and presence of a swelling or mass in the tube or ovary. Roughly 1 in 250 pregnancies is ectopic. You're especially at risk if you've had previous STDs, pelvic inflammatory disease, pelvic surgery or tubal ligation. Treatment doesn't necessarily require surgery. Methotrexate, a form of chemotherapy, can be given to cause regression and reabsorption of the tubal pregnancy if it's not too advanced and there is no heartbeat. If you're not a candidate for methotrexate or the drug fails, laparoscopic surgery needs to be performed to remove the pregnancy and, sometimes, the entire tube.

If your periods are regular, and the pain comes on suddenly: You may have either a ruptured ovarian cyst, a twisted ovarian cyst or fallopian tube or a degenerating fibroid. Every ovulation is really a rupture of a very small ovarian cyst (i.e., the follicle that's developed around the egg in the first two weeks of your cycle). Sometimes, more than the usual amount of fluid accumulates in the follicle, and its rupture with egg release can cause significant pain. This of course should correspond to the time of ovulation—in other words, the middle of your cycle. Although this pain can be fairly severe, it will usually subside within a few hours and, at most, will leave you with a sense of achiness until your next period.

Subsequent to ovulation, the follicle becomes a corpus luteum. This too entails some cystic risk. The corpus luteum can bleed into itself and form a hemorrhagic cyst. This can cause pain in the second half of the cycle, especially if it ruptures. At no time in our cycle are we immune from cysts or the pain they can produce. The fact that these cysts resolve after your period means they are functional cysts and should not be a health concern. But if they occur repeatedly, it's probably worthwhile (or, more precisely, pain-while) to inhibit ovulation and cyst formation with birth control pills.

Nonfunctional cysts, which do not disappear from cycle to cycle, include those resulting from endometriosis, those caused by an infection and benign ovarian growths. Rarely, these too can rupture. The diagnosis is usually made with ultrasound. Nonfunctional cysts can trigger inflammation of the lining of the abdominal cavity, causing pain to persist for up to several days. This irritation can also cause nausea, vomiting, bloating and even abdominal hardening and diffuse tenderness. Laparoscopy may be necessary if pain and other symptoms persist. However, your doctor may want to simply keep you under observation if there are no signs of internal bleeding, because the fluid will slowly be reabsorbed by the body.

Just when you thought we were done with cysts, the plot takes another twist: Ovarian cysts or the ovaries and tubes themselves can twist and, in doing so, shut off their own blood supply and undergo tissue death. This "torsion" is very painful and will often be accompanied by an elevated white blood cell count, fever and signs of an "acute" abdomen (the abdomen swells, gets hard and is supersensitive to the slightest touch; nausea, vomiting and constipation can also ensue). These symptoms do not go away—if anything, they get worse. This is a medical emergency that requires surgery.

If the pain starts around the belly button and spreads to the right side and is accompanied by nausea, vomiting and/or fever: You may have appendicitis. This pain gets progressively worse and, once more, is a medical emergency requiring surgical intervention. If the condition is caught early, the appendix can be removed through a laparoscope.

Central Pelvic Pain with a Previously Diagnosed Fibroid

If your doctor has told you that you have fibroids and you develop pain that is constant or increasing in intensity, it's possible that your fibroid tumor is undergoing "red degeneration." This is not a political affiliation. Rather, the fibroid is outgrowing its own blood supply and is deprived of oxygen and undergoing tissue death (it's sort of like a heart attack in the uterus, except that it's not fatal). Ultrasound may show that the fibroid has fluid in its center, and blood tests may reveal internal bleeding. If the amount of tissue death is not too great, your doctor might suggest you take aspirin and wait to see if the pain diminishes (this is legitimate therapy and not a medical copout). If it doesn't or if tissue death is extensive, surgery to remove the fibroid (and in some cases the entire uterus) may be necessary.

Intermittent Pain and Bloating That Gets Worse After Eating or Before/During Bowel Movements, Often Accompanied by a Change in Bowel Habits

This may be due to irritable bowel syndrome (IBS), which strikes one-sixth of women, or it could be the result of inflammatory bowel disease. In the former, muscles of the bowel malfunction, causing spasm or abnormal expansion. This leads to pain, constipation or diarrhea and bloating. If the symptoms become more severe or persistent over time, it's possible that either an infection or ulcerative colitis is present. Your doctor should do a stool culture and test for blood in the stool. You may need a colonoscopy, in which a thin flexible scope is used to view the entire colon, or the viewing can be done with colon X-rays. Therapy is determined based on findings during the examination. If your symptoms are not severe or testing doesn't turn up infection or inflammatory bowel disease, the diagnosis will probably be one of exclusion: IBS.

There are many things you can do on your own to relieve the symptoms of IBS: Eat small and more frequent meals, and eat slowly and chew thoroughly. Another recommendation that I personally cannot follow: Don't talk while you're eating. You should also gradually increase your intake of fiber to 25 to 30 grams per day, and drink eight glasses of water a day. Moderate exercise helps improve the intestinal muscle tone. Limit your consumption of alcohol and caffeine: Both can affect the motor function of the bowel. And don't chew gum or suck on candy, which will stimulate gastric and intestinal activity.

If you're having a lot of cramping and diarrhea, avoid raw fruits and vegetables, with the exception of bananas (eat cooked fruits and vegetables instead). Also try eliminating dairy products for a while to see if your symptoms improve. Finally, remove wheat and rye products from your diet. If this helps, slowly reintroduce them to see which foods cause sensitivity.

And now, the most difficult Rx: Ease the stress in your life—it not only cramps your style, it cramps your intestines.

Pain Accompanied by Frequency, Urgency or Pain During Urination and/or Lower Back Pain and Fever

You've probably already guessed that this is due to a urinary tract infection. However, some women experience pain without concomitant bladder symptoms. Since a urinary tract infection can only be diagnosed with a urinalysis and, if necessary, a culture, make sure filling a specimen cup is part of your workup for pelvic pain. Pyelonephritis, a kidney infection, can present very suddenly without prior bladder-related symptoms. This should be suspected if you suddenly develop a fever and severe pain radiating from your pelvis to one or both sides of your back. If this occurs, see a doctor immediately; you may need intravenous antibiotics.

Spasmodic Pelvic Pain That Radiates to One Side of the Back, Sometimes Accompanied by Visible Blood in the Urine

When kidney stones (nephrolithiases) travel down the ureter or block this passageway, the pain can be worse than labor and delivery. It should quickly get you into the doctor's office or, more likely, the emergency room. The diagnosis is made by checking your urine for blood. An ultrasound, CT scan or intravenous pyelogram (IVP), in which dye is injected into your veins and followed as it's excreted through the renal system, will be performed. These tests will show the number, size and position of the stone(s). Hopefully, while all this is being done, you'll be given adequate pain medication (morphine). Then a decision can be made as to whether to let you pass the stone on your own or go in to retrieve it with a "basket" procedure or crush it with lithotripsy, in which the stone is bombarded with sound waves. Once you've had a stone, you're not going to want one again. Your doctor will do 24-hour urine testing for calcium excretion and special blood tests and will analyze the stone, when it's available. Based on these test results, you may be told to limit your calcium ingestion, and you will certainly be told to drink lots of fluids. However, you don't want to substitute one disease (renal stones) for another (osteoporosis). Ask your physician about using calcium citrate as a supplement; this is considered to be more stone-safe than other calciums.

Constant Achiness with Periodic Flare-Ups of More Intense Pelvic Discomfort, Combined with Pain at Other Sites in the Body as Well as Generalized Fatigue

This sounds like the pelvic symptoms that are sometimes associated with fibromyalgia, an autoimmune disorder that primarily affects women. This syndrome strikes soft tissues, resulting in widespread pain throughout your body. To qualify for diagnosis, you must feel pain in multiple tender points. Usually there is chronic (greater than six months) achiness and pain in the muscles, bones or joints. This can often be accompanied by stiffness, especially in the morning. (The diagnosis of this disorder is very difficult and frustrating; virtually all standard laboratory tests and X-rays are completely normal.) This condition is almost always found together with a sleep disorder. With fibromyalgia, there is also an exaggerated response to almost any stimulus. Forty percent of women with fibromyalgia have painful periods, while 12% have irritable bladder and 10% have vulvar pain. If together with your pelvic pain you have the more generalized symptoms noted above as well as sleep problems, a consultation with a rheumatologist is in order, and your pain should be treated in the context of this syndrome. This includes medications to improve sleep, lifestyle changes such as exercising and reducing stress, as well as the judicious use of painkillers, muscle relaxants and antidepressants, particularly tricyclics.

Unexplainable Moderate to Severe Pelvic Pain That Often Worsens During Intercourse

Don't feel guilty or crazy if your doctor can't explain your pain. More than half of women who suffer pelvic pain have no discernible cause. "Discern," for many doctors, is limited to what they see below the belly button. There are women in whom the only physical finding is an expansion or dilation of the pelvic veins, a condition known as *pelvic congestion syndrome*. Some physicians question the term, or even the existence, of this so-called syndrome. Traditionally, it was treated with hysterectomy, but up to half of women who have had this drastic therapy continue to experience pain. Another possible explanation for pain is the development of abnormalities in or increased sensitivity of nerves that conduct sensation from the pelvis. This is found more frequently in women who have been sexually abused. Indeed, 48% of women undergoing laparoscopy for chronic pelvic pain report sexual trauma as adults, and 63% report childhood sexual abuse! I don't like to use the expression "It's all in your head," but neural stimulation emanating from your brain can trigger pain. Our nerves conduct impulses in both directions, from the brain to the pelvic organs, and vice versa. When extreme stress or emotional pain is translated into nerve stimulation downward, it can be conducted back in the other direction as physical pain. This is called *somatization*. You're not making it up; your physical discomfort truly is there. So, in treating your pelvic pain, your doctor should not be dismissive of what she can't easily diagnose. *All* of you should be considered. This includes psychological issues such as underlying depression and post-traumatic stress from previous abuse, or current relationship trauma. Your pain may not go away without the right psychological intervention. At the same time, you should also get help with pain control, learn relaxation techniques and, if warranted, be given a prescription for antianxiety, antidepressive, or antipsychotic medications. Seeing is not necessary for believing and treating your pelvic woes.

I HAVE VULVAR PAIN, BUT MY DOCTOR CAN'T TELL ME WHY; CAN YOU?

Sometimes we doctors are unable to tell you why you have a particular condition, but we won't admit defeat without the proper medical terminology. The official catch-all term for vulvar pain is *vulvodynia*, from the Greek word *odynia*, meaning pain. The pain can be anywhere in the vulva but most frequently occurs in the lower portion near the entrance of the vagina (the vestibulum). You may experience extreme sensitivity to touch or pressure or even have a constant feeling of burning, stinging, irritation or rawness, which is made worse by any contact, even with underwear. In their need to classify, doctors have divided this pain disorder into primary (it begins with a woman's first tampon use or sexual experience) or secondary (it began long after these initial vulvar "insults"). Then, to further complicate the issue, vulvodynia is subdivided into two more categories: organic, or having a known cause, and idiopathic, which, despite its similarity to idiotic, refers only to being without a known cause.

If you've already seen several doctors, I have to assume they have ruled out identifiable causes for your vulvar pain and have treated you accordingly. But just in case, here's a list of the organic causes of vulvodynia and what can be done to treat them.

Infections

Yeast infection: Sometimes the predominant symptoms of yeast infection may be pain rather than itching. This infection, which causes redness, swelling and cracking of the vulvar skin, should be treated with either local or oral antiyeast medication (see page 47).

Genital herpes: Infection with this virus is chronic. Herpes lives in the nerve root and can multiply and rise to the surface. Sometimes it causes the typical cold sore–like lesion; at other times, it simply irritates the nerve without a visible skin eruption. Pain with or without a lesion may be associated with the onset of your period. Continuous viral suppressive therapy with either Valtrex or Famvir will help prevent recurrence of pain or lesions, as well as decrease viral shedding so you are also less likely to infect your partner.

Human papillomavirus: HPV infection is dreadfully common and is found in up to 70% of sexually active young adults. But we're not sure how often small lesions that are invisible to the unaided eye actually cause vulvodynia. In order to diagnose vulvar or vaginal HPV, a vinegar solution should be applied to the area and colposcopic examination done to see a characteristic whitening. Even then, an actual biopsy is necessary to confirm this diagnosis. Many physicians feel there is no pain benefit in treating these widespread microscopic lesions, and that the therapy may be worse than the disease. Most of the topical medications, which include trichlorocetic acid, the antiwart ointment podophyllum, the chemotherapy cream 5-FU, as well as laser vaporization, often result in diffuse irritation and pain and, worse yet, will not eradicate the actual virus. There may be a somewhat better result with vulvar injections of the antiviral medication Interferon, but this drug can cause significant flulike symptoms. Aldara 5% cream, which is used to treat warts, is far less irritating and clears visible external warts in over 70% of women after 16 weeks of use, but whether this is helpful for widespread microscopic HPV is not established.

Trichomonas: Aside from a greenish, foul discharge, infection from this sexually transmitted parasite can cause considerable vulvar pain. It is treated with oral metronidazole (Flagyl).

Infection of a Bartholin's gland: These glands are present on the lower inner portion of both sides of the vulva at the entrance to the vagina and secrete a viscous lubricating fluid during sexual stimulation. If a gland opening is blocked, it can swell and form a Bartholin's cyst or become infected and become a Bartholin's abscess. The latter causes one of the labia to become extremely red, swollen and painful; it may even break open and exude pus. If this should occur, therapy requires having the abscess drained and taking oral antibiotics. If the gland remains blocked and a cyst or abscess should recur, a new route for the gland's secretions can be surgically created by opening the cyst and suturing its walls to the outer labial skin, a process that has been aptly named *marsupialization*. If this small procedure doesn't work, the entire cyst wall and gland can be removed with a Bartholin's cystectomy. This usually requires general anesthesia, can entail blood loss and, unfortunately, may result in scarring.

Trauma

Sexual assault not only causes the physical trauma of lacerations, infections and, rarely, scarring of the vulva and vagina, but it can also result in a horrendous psychic trauma that affects the pain pathways from the entire pelvis, as well as the vagina and vulva (see page 100). Previous sexual abuse may also lead to *vaginismus*, the involuntary spasm of the outer musculature of the vagina. If you experience pain or vaginismus with attempted intercourse or even tampon use, consider exploring your sexual past with the appropriate psychotherapist. You may also need to begin a program of gradual desensitization by inserting tampons, fingers or special dilators into the vagina until you can finally attempt intercourse.

Systemic Diseases

Vulvar pain has been associated with autoimmune diseases, including systemic lupus erythematosus (SLE), which often occurs during our childbearing years. In this disorder, autoantibodies may attack small blood vessels and nerves in any organ (see page 113), and the vulva and vagina may be affected. In these situations, the vulvodynia is treated with lubricants and estrogen cream, as well as NSAID painkillers or, if the disease warrants, steroids or immunosuppressive therapy.

Another autoimmune disease, Sjögren's syndrome, is characterized by a white cell attack on glands and mucous membranes throughout the body, including the vagina. It is unlikely that this disease will cause pain in your thirties. Its peak occurrence is in women in their fifties.

Unfortunately, vulvodynia also occurs more frequently in women who have other chronic "down there" diseases such as Crohn's disease and irritable bowel syndrome.

Irritants

Nearly everything you apply to the vulva can irritate it and cause pain. The long list of possible culprits includes soaps (especially those containing deodorants or perfumes), sprays, douches, antiseptics and creams and suppositories you use to treat yeast or vaginal infections. These vulvar insults don't even have to be applied directly. Laundry soaps or the softener used to fluff your underwear can cause vulvar irritation. Then there is a group of caustic substances your doctor may have applied to treat HPV and warts such as tricholorocetic acid, 5-FU and podophyllum, as well as laser therapy, which can cause ongoing pain.

Other Conditions

These include the skin reactions we associate with the other parts of our bodies such as contact dermatitis, eczema and psoriasis. There is one condition, however, that is unique to the vulva; it's called *lichen sclerosis*. It can occur at any age, although it seems to be more common after menopause. The vulva loses its normal fat and becomes thin and atrophic. The overlying skin turns shiny and may develop fissures, and the top folds of the labia fuse together over the clitoris. This condition can cause itching, pain with intercourse or burning. Your doctor should biopsy the affected area to make a diagnosis. In the past, the treatment of choice for lichen sclerosis was testosterone ointment (that's how we found out that topical testosterone can increase sexual desire), but less erotically, the current, more effective, therapy is a potent steroid cream of 0.05% clobetasol.

There is one particular type of idiopathic vulvodynia that has driven many women to go from doctor to doctor in hope of a diagnosis and cure. This frustrating disorder can cause generalized vulvar pain or pain that's confined to the lower portion of the entrance to the vagina (vulvar vestibulitis). It appears more frequently in women in their twenties and thirties, but can be seen as early as the teens, and as late as menopause. Touch or pressure during sex, or touching with only a Q-tip during an exam, can elicit extreme burning or a stinging pain that may be similar to what it would feel like if an open wound were rubbed. Yet there is no visible lesion, and at most a doctor sees mild redness. You may also feel burning or throbbing while sitting or walking. Rarely symptoms are constant. No expert can tell exactly what has caused your condition, but studies have shown that it is often linked to previous infections and/or the treatment of these infections with antibiotics, antibiotic creams, cryosurgery or laser surgery.

The issue becomes not why you hurt, but how you can get relief. Unfortunately, there is no rapid surefire cure. Improvement of your symptoms may take weeks or months and although on occasion they can go away on their own, it's more likely that you'll have to try various forms of medical or even surgical therapies. Pain management with the antidepressant amitriptyline (Elavil) can help, not because you are depressed, but because this medication inhibits the reuptake of the neurotransmitter norepinephrine and will block pain fibers that enervate the vulva. You should start with a dose of 10 to 25 milligrams at night and slowly increase to 100 milligrams. If this is not sufficiently effective, your doctor may try long-term topical antifungal therapy, Vitamin A and D ointment, 1% hydrocortisone ointment (not the cream, which contains alcohol and will burn) or a numbing lidocaine gel. Some women are helped by a low-oxalate diet (oxalates, found in foods such as tea, chocolate and spinach, can be excreted in urine and may cause vulvar burning), together with up to 2,000 milligrams of calcium citrate supplementation daily. Transcutaneous electrical nerve stimulation (TENS) can be helpful, as it is with other pain disorders. This therapy uses mild electric pulses to bombard and confuse the pain signals of the vulvar nerves. Biofeedback and/or physical therapy are especially helpful if the pain occurs together with vaginismus. In general, women with vestibulitis have been shown to have increased resting muscle tone in the vulva and a decrease in contraction tone. They can use a biofeedback machine to "grade" nerve and muscle tension and practice voluntary relaxation of that tension. A physical therapist can also show you specific exercises to correct muscle tone imbalance.

If all of these medical techniques fail, surgery to remove the sensitive tissue in the vestibule can be performed and is successful for 60% to 80% of women who use it as a last resort.

Vulvodynia is a condition that requires a lot of trial, error and coping. You may get depressed, but don't give up. And don't forget that along the way, you, like many other chronic pain sufferers, may need appropriate emotional and psychological support.

IS IT NORMAL TO LEAK URINE DURING EXERCISE OR SEX?

If you've ever taken an aerobics class, you'll undoubtedly have noticed the rush to the bathroom when the instructor announces the imminent onset of jumping jacks or any other form of unnatural jarring to the lower pelvis. Unfortunately, the only thing that prevents women from having urinary loss is a short, one-inch-long urethra, which, at rest, should be at an angle and elevated above the bladder. The minute this angle is lost, the urethra loses much of its ability to block the flow of urine from the bladder. The urethra's blocking action is supported by two other mechanisms: an internal sphincter muscle and external pelvic muscles and tissues. When you exercise, pounding can place pressure on the bladder. This pushes the urethra down and changes its angle. It may also cause the bladder to contract—and, voilà, urine flows in an uninhibited fashion. This is termed stress incontinence, and the same mechanism can cause urine loss during coughing, sneezing, laughing, lifting, pushing or, in severe cases, just standing up. Abdominal muscle contraction during sex will also strain the bladder, and the mechanics of intercourse result in further pressure on the bladder that changes the urethra's angle.

We all know that childbirth and age loosen pelvic and bladder support. But you don't have to have gone through this trauma in order to suffer from stress incontinence. Up to 38% of women who have not given birth have some degree of urethral malfunction. There may be a genetic component when it comes to sphincter strength: If your mother had stress incontinence, you're three times more likely than usual to have it too. And, of course, if you have had a baby, especially with a fairly difficult vaginal delivery requiring hours of pushing, your bladder, as well as your other pelvic organs, may weaken and even drop so that it protrudes from the vaginal opening. This protrusion is called a cystocele, and it will leave you even more prone to stress incontinence and bladder infections.

Before you decide to depend on the absorbency of Depends to get you through your aerobics class, try some simple self-help bladder strategies. Don't let your bladder overdistend—this in itself puts a strain on the urethral angle. That means voiding frequently during the day and waiting no more than 20 minutes after you first sense that you need to go to get to a bathroom. Always empty your bladder before intercourse or exercise class (whichever comes more frequently!). You need your six to eight glasses of water a day, but you might want to consume it after the act rather than before. Inserting a tampon before exercise will help elevate the bladder angle and may allow you to get through your class without a bathroom break.

Exercising the muscles that help strengthen and support the bladder may also help. Kegel exercises involve contracting the muscles around the opening of the vagina. In order to isolate these muscles, try putting your finger in your vagina and squeezing as though you were trying to stop the flow of urine. Then, after removing your finger, contract these same muscles for 10 seconds and relax them for 10 seconds. Repeat this 15 times and try to do this three times a day. You know you're in peak form if you can work up to a "set" of 25 "reps" three times a day. Be sure you are not using your abdominal, leg or buttock muscles instead of your pelvic muscles. You can check this by putting your hand on your abdomen; if it's moving during this exercise, you're cheating. When you do Kegels in a sitting position, you should remain motionless. Unlike your aerobics class, which brought on the symptoms in the first place, you can do Kegel exercises without donning spandex or going to the gym. Although you may not want to confess to the traffic cop (or your boss) that you're doing your Kegels, you can even perform them while driving or sitting at your desk.

If these techniques don't keep you dry, you should seek medical help. Don't become one of the 80% of women who feel that this form of incontinence is part of the normal adversities of being female and never consult a doctor about it. Your physician will check for pelvic prolapse, in which the uterus, bladder and even rectum drop from their normal positions because they lack adequate support. Special techniques can be used to assess the urethral angle, the integrity of the bladder and the tone of the urethral sphincter. (This usually requires cystoscopy, in which a small scope is placed through the urethra.) Measurements of pressure in the bladder and urethra and their relationship will also be checked.

Because the underlying problem in women with stress incontinence is lack of support, help should usually be mechanical, not pharmaceutical. Your doctor may first try to help you strengthen your pelvic floor muscles by having you use specially designed cones of progressively heavier weight during Kegel exercises. If that is insufficient, she may prescribe a diaphragmlike device to support the bladder or a cap or plug to block the urethra. If the urethral angle has been severely compromised by childbirth, bladder neck suspension surgery may be necessary to reestablish a working angle. This can be performed vaginally, laparoscopically or abdominally, depending on the severity of the damage.

IT ALWAYS BURNS WHEN I URINATE, AND MY DOCTOR SAYS I DON'T HAVE AN INFECTION. WHAT COULD IT BE?

If your symptoms are present but your urine doesn't test positive for signs of infection, you may have interstitial cystitis (IC). This causes urinary frequency, urgency and pain that can be so severe that you may be unable to sleep, go to work or care for your family. The pain often gets worse during your period and is exacerbated by sexual intercourse. Unfortunately, because the symptoms are so similar to those of a simple bladder infection, you've probably received several rounds of antibiotics before this diagnosis is even considered.

Thankfully, this condition is not common—less than 1% of women develop it, and doctors are still puzzled regarding its cause. Infection may set off IC in the first place, but once the condition takes hold, bacteria are not found and antibiotics don't help. There may be autoimmune factors at work (the same antinuclear antibodies that have been linked with lupus have been tied to IC); however, symptoms do not consistently respond to immunosuppressant drugs. Mast cells, which release histamine in allergic reactions, are present in the bladder wall of a significant number of sufferers. Perhaps these cells are activated by changing female sex hormone levels; this could explain why symptoms sometimes worsen during your period. Alterations in a component of the protective coating of the bladder (glycosaminoglycan, or GAG) may also be a factor. This would permit urine to penetrate the bladder wall, causing irritation and injury.

In order to make a diagnosis of IC, your doctor will look inside the bladder with a cystoscopy and then fill it with water to look for a pale surface with small ulcers and hemorrhages as well as diminished bladder capacity. In up to 25% of patients, the mere filling of the bladder will provide temporary relief of pain that may last for several months. Your physician may also perform a biopsy to document inflammation. If IC is diagnosed, treatment revolves around alleviating the symptoms. Antihistamines may decrease mast cell activity, tricyclic antidepressants can be used to block pain signals and Elmiron, a synthetic GAG, will help coat and protect the bladder lining. The latter can take 12 to 16 weeks before it begins to produce symptom relief. Dimethyl sulfoxide (DMSO), an older therapy, can be injected directly into the bladder to coat its surface. It is sometimes combined with heparin, which can help keep urine from penetrating the bladder walls. This procedure often needs to be repeated several times before relief is obtained. When all else fails or if IC is part of a chronic pelvic pain syndrome, you may want to consider adding transcutaneous electric nerve stimulation (TENS), self-administered imperceptible electric shocks that desensitize nerve responses. Some patients also get relief from acupuncture. Surgery is truly a last resort. It consists of burning or lasering bladder ulcers or, on rare occasions, removing the bladder and diverting urine into a pouch constructed from the bowel.

MY PAP SMEAR IS ABNORMAL. WHAT'S MY NEXT MOVE?

Don't panic. At least one out of every 10 Pap smears shows some type of abnormality. Most of the time it's due to changes associated with inflammation or is what doctors call a "low-grade" lesion that will clear up on its own. But that's not to say it's safe to ignore it. So let's go over the terminology of your Pap results in order to determine what needs to be done.

Your Pap smear is written in the "secret" language of the Bethesda system, which classifies cervical cells according to their well-being. The Pap report card says it as follows:

1. **Adequacy of the specimen.** If adequate cells are not present, you need to repeat your Pap.
2. **General categorization.** This either says "within normal limits" or shows "benign cellular changes" (which can occur during or after an infection) or "epithelial cell abnormality" (this is the report's way of saying something's wrong, and the wrong is then detailed under "descriptive diagnoses").
3. **Descriptive diagnoses.**
   BENIGN CELLULAR CHANGES. There is either an infection or "reactive" changes. The latter can result from a previous infection, trauma, lack of estrogen or the presence of an IUD.
   EPITHELIAL CELL ABNORMALITIES. These are the cells on the surface of the cervix. Changes can occur in the *squamous cells*. They are as follows:
   Atypical squamous cells of undetermined significance (ASCUS). This means the cytopathologist is not sure what's going on, but the cells are not quite normal.
   Low-grade squamous intraepithelial lesion (LSIL). These are mildly abnormal cells, also called "mild dysplasia" or cervical intraepithalial neoplasia (CIN 1), and are usually linked to HPV infections.
   High-grade squamous intraepithelial lesions (HSIL). This is moderate to severe dysplasia, also called CIN 2 and CIN 3, and carcinoma in situ (cancer cells that are confined to the surface of the cervix).
   Squamous cell carcinoma. Cancer cells are present and may have invaded the cervix.

GLANDULAR CELLS. It's also possible that glandular cells from deep in the cervix or the endometrium can be picked up during the Pap smear. These include:

Endometrial cells. These are usually benign, but their presence is recorded on the report because it may signal endometrial precancer in menopausal women who are not taking hormones.

Atypical glandular cells of undetermined significance (ASGUS). Another "we're not sure what this is but there may be something wrong in the glands" found deep in the cervical canal or in the endometrium.

Cervical adenocarcinoma. This is a rare cancer of the glands of the cervix.

Endometrial adenocarcinoma. Cancer cells from high in the endometrium are shed and picked up on the Pap smear.

Extrauterine adenocarcinoma. This is extremely rare and may mean fallopian tube cancer.

OTHER MALIGNANT NEOPLASMS. These are unidentifiable cancer cells and may even come from the ovaries.

4. **Hormonal evaluation**

The cytopathologist can look at vaginal cells and determine whether their condition is appropriate to your age, menstrual cycle and history of hormone use. If there are a lot of bacteria in the vagina, this evaluation can't be made.

This is probably a lot more than you want to know. I'm not expecting you to read or interpret your own Pap smear, but your doctor should tell you if the report shows adequate cells and if the cells are normal or abnormal. If they are abnormal, find out if the cells fall into a low- or high-risk category, and whether cells are present that shouldn't be there. Finally, do the hormone readings match where you are in your cycle?

The Pap is a screening test and won't give definitive answers, so if something is abnormal it needs to be investigated further before you (a) panic or (b) get therapy. Your doctor will tell you which one of the following steps is indicated.

Further Diagnostic Tests

1. **Repeat the Pap smear right away.** The slide broke on the way to the lab, or when it got there there were too few cells or blood that made interpreting the smear impossible.

2. **Repeat the test in two to three months.** This would be the recommendation if an infection was present, making it difficult to read. If you've been getting regular, normal Paps and have no history of STDs, you can wait to repeat the test if your last reading was ASCUS. Two to three months may seem like a long time to wait, but that's how long it takes cells to regenerate after the cervix is scraped, so repeating your Pap immediately might give you falsely reassuring negative results.

3. **Get a colposcopy exam and possibly a biopsy.** If your Pap is ASCUS and you have a history of previous abnormal Paps, an STD, or have tested positive for a high-risk HPV infection, or if the reading is LSIL, HSIL, ASGUS or cervical cancer, your doctor will examine your cervix with a special magnifying scope (colposcope) to identify abnormalities. Then she'll decide if they warrant a biopsy. To perform a biopsy, she'll pinch off a tiny piece of cervical tissue, which will be sent to a pathology lab. At the same time, she will often perform an endocervical curettage (ECC), scraping the cervical canal with a small curette to collect cells from the part of the cervix she can't see. If precancerous changes are confirmed, you'll go on to the next step: treatment.

4. **Endocervical curettage and possible dilation and curettage (D&C).** This should be performed if your Pap showed ASGUS, cervical adenocarcinoma or extrauterine adenocarcinoma, or if unidentified cancer cells are present.

Treatment

There are two basic ways to get rid of cervical abnormalities that are diagnosed after colposcopic biopsy and ECC. One entails destroying, or ablating, the tissue, the other excising it. The latter allows the doctor to send the tissue sample to a pathologist, who can make sure that its borders are clear and that the treatment was adequate.

Ablative Methods

Cryosurgery: Extreme cold destroys cells just like extreme heat. The abnormal cervical tissue is frozen with a special probe that is applied to the cervix. This procedure is done in the doctor's office and takes about six minutes. It requires no anesthetic and causes cramping at most. This is usually reserved for LSIL.

Laser: A laser beam is used to vaporize abnormal tissue. This can be performed in a doctor's office or outpatient facility with local anesthesia and can be used to treat HSIL.

Excisional Methods

Loop electrosurgical excision procedure (LEEP): A small loop powered by a special electric current is used to slice through the cervix and remove the abnormal tissue. A smaller loop can then be used to remove a portion of the endocervical canal. The loop's current is not conducted to surrounding tissue and is designed to minimize pain and bleeding. The LEEP is performed in a doctor's office with local anesthetic. It's appropriate for HSIL and in rare instances will also be used for LSIL.

Surgical conization: A scalpel, laser or cautery needle is used to remove a cone-shaped portion of the outer cervix and cervical canal. Sutures are often required to stop bleeding. This is done in an outpatient facility or hospital OR and usually requires an epidural or general anesthesia. Aside from hysterectomy, this is the strongest weapon your doctor has against cervical cancer. It is used for advanced HSIL and carcinoma in situ. In rare cases, it can also be used for squamous cell carcinoma, to establish whether or how deeply the cancer has invaded the tissue.

Hysterectomy: This, of course, is the maximal excisional treatment there is and is reserved for invasive carcinoma. (Note: Depending on the stage of the cancer, the hysterectomy should be "radical," and radiation or chemotherapy may also be rquired.). A vaginal or simple abdominal hysterectomy can, on occasion, be used as a final therapy for carcinoma in situ or microinvasion if you've completed childbearing and want to make sure there is no chance of recurrence.

An abnormal Pap, even if it shows severe cell changes, does not mean "Oh, my God, I'll need a hysterectomy!" This is not a time to jump to conclusions—it is time to jump to the right tests and therapies.

WHAT TESTS SHOULD I HAVE?

These are the examinations, tests and procedures I recommend for my thirtysomething patients.

Examination/test/procedure	How often
Blood pressure	Every two years
Cholesterol test	Nonfasting total and HDL every five years
Pelvic exam and Pap smear	Annually; Pap at doctor's discretion after three negative tests
STD testing	At your/your doctor's discretion
Clinical (physician) breast exam	Annually
Breast self-exam	Monthly
Immunizations	Tetanus booster every 10 years
Eye exam	Once during this decade or if vision changes
Skin exam by dermatologist	Every two years
Skin self-exam	Annually

WHAT CAN GO WRONG AT MY AGE?

Systemic Lupus Erythematosus (SLE)

This autoimmune disease is one of "our" diseases—it's 10 times more likely to occur in women than in men. Eighty percent of women who get it will develop SLE during the childbearing years. This, like other autoimmune disorders, occurs when our immune system fails to recognize the body's tissues as our own and attacks them as if they were foreign invaders. Of all the autoimmune diseases, lupus attacks the most organs, including the skin, the joints, the blood and blood vessels and the kidneys, as well as, less frequently, the heart, lungs, gastrointestinal tract, brain and pancreas. And that's not all: If the disease is active, and especially if it causes kidney inflammation and high blood pressure, there is an increased risk of miscarriage, premature delivery or stillbirth. SLE can begin with nonspecific symptoms such as episodes of aching joints, fatigue, sore throats, headaches and mood changes or loss of mental sharpness. It may also cause a characteristic butterfly-shaped skin rash across the nose bridge and both cheeks, or a raised, red rash on sun-exposed areas of the body. Some women notice that their hands and feet tend to become blue or white in response to cold temperatures. This is known as Raynaud's phenomenon.

In order to qualify for an official diagnosis of SLE, you need to have at least three of the disease's telltale symptoms: a rash, arthritis, a lowered platelet count (thrombocytopenia), kidney inflammation (nephritis) and the presence of an antinuclear antibody (ANA). The latter attacks the nucleus of our cells; it is present in 90% of women with SLE and is thought to be one of the culprits underlying this disease. Many factors have been blamed for the development of these antibodies, including exposure to sunlight, infection and environmental toxins, as well as changes in a gene or group of genes that hamper normal immune system recognition. Because lupus tends to strike after we've reached peak production of reproductive hormones, SLE may be hormonally aided and abetted. But how estrogen and SLE are connected and whether hormone or antihormone medication can alter the course of this disease are not clear. We do know, however, that high-estrogen birth control pills and pregnancy can make SLE worse.

The younger a woman is when she develops lupus, the poorer her prognosis. Symptoms depend on which tissues are attacked by the errant immune system. If it's the joints, they may become damaged or, rarely, deformed. When the kidneys are affected, they may fail. Central nervous system attack can lead to migraines, fever, high blood pressure and seizures. If large blood vessels in the brain are involved, potentially fatal stroke or brain hemorrhage can result, although, fortunately, this is rare. One-third of women with SLE develop inflammation of the lungs, heart, pancreas or blood vessels leading to the intestines. If platelet counts drop, potentially fatal bleeding may occur.

The above details the worst-case scenario. But the good news is that at least 90% of women with full-blown SLE survive more than 10 years after their diagnosis. This is despite the fact that there is no sure cure for the disease—only therapies can curb the immune system's attack. These include steroids, immunosuppressive drugs and immunomodulating drugs. Unfortunately, these medicines compromise our ability to deal with infections, and long-term use of steroids can lead to osteoporosis. Treatment can often be directed at specific symptoms. Antimalarial drugs are used for skin problems, while clotting disorders can be controlled with anticlotting drugs. Large doses of DHEA, a weak male hormone, have been shown to help some patients, and research is ongoing in an attempt to find better therapies.

Skin Cancer

It can take 20 years or more for malignant melanoma, the most deadly form of skin cancer, to develop. So now that you're in your thirties, you may start paying for the sunburns of your childhood. Skin cancer is one of the most rapidly increasing forms of cancer in women, second only to lung cancer. (Between cigarettes and sun exposure, we've really done a number on our bodies.) One in 75 women will be diagnosed with melanoma during her lifetime, and still others will develop one of the even more common nonmelanoma skin cancers, basal and squamous cell carcinoma. This gives skin cancer the dubious distinction of being the most prevalent form of cancer in the United States.

Melanoma originates in the melanocytes, cells that lie in our outer skin or epidermis. They produce melanin, a pigment that gives us our skin color and also protects us against ultraviolet damage. Abnormal growth of these cells results in a malignancy. Melanomas often arise from atypical, or dysplastic, moles, which are clusters of pigmented cells. We now know that exposure to the sun's UVB and even UVA rays can damage DNA and ultimately increase risk for skin cancer. The younger you were when you were exposed to high doses of UV radiation (in the form of a sunburn or deep tan), the more likely you are to develop melanoma. Three or more outdoor summer jobs as a teen and three or more blistering sunburns before the age of 20 quadruple your risk. Having fair skin, blue eyes, red or blond hair or a tendency to freckle, especially on the upper back, further adds to your risk. If two or more of your family members have developed melanoma, and especially if you have more than 50 moles on your body, your risk of the disease may be as high as one in two.

This is one of the few cancers that doesn't require X-rays, blood tests or other invasive, unpleasant detection methods. All you have to do is look at yourself in a mirror from head to toe. Most of us do this anyway to check on our skin tone and weight changes. The only difference is that you'll need to scrutinize areas that you normally would pay little attention to, such as your scalp and between your fingers and toes. Pay attention to any pigmented mark or mole on your body, and know your ABCDs. The American Academy of Dermatology recommends that you look for the following:

> A = asymmetry
> B = a ragged, blurred or irregular border
> C = color variations within a mole,
>   or moles that are tan, brown,
>   black, red, white or blue
> D = diameter larger than a pencil eraser

I also like to add "G," which stands for either growth of a new lesion or increase in size of an existing lesion, and a second "C" for change. If any mark or lesion changes its size, color, shape or surface (in other words, if it gets bumpy, scaly, crusty, forms an ulcer or bleeds), see a dermatologist. (You should probably start getting professional screenings once a year. The exam should include the skin of the genitals.) The dermatologist will remove any suspicious lesion and send it for biopsy. The good news is that 80% of melanomas are found before they spread to the lymph nodes. But that does not mean that 80% of those of us with the disease will be easily cured. The cure rate depends on the size and depth of the lesion. A thin, early lesion means a 96% chance of five-year survival, while a thicker, more advanced one (greater than 4 millimeters deep) has a five-year survival rate of less than 50%. The 20% of people whose melanoma has spread to the lymph nodes or farther face a diminishing survival rate. This means that the difference between near-certain death and near-certain cure lies in your diligence in self-exam and dermatologic screening.

Two other less malignant but more common forms of skin cancer are basal cell and squamous cell carcinoma. Basal cell cancers arise from the basal (or bottom) cells of our skin. They often begin as translucent or pink, raised nodules that may have fine blood vessels on their surface. As they grow, they can ulcerate and form small sores. Other types can start as red, scaly patches on the arms, legs or torso. These may become crusty or scaly. A third type appears as flat, off-white patches or elevated plaques. As these grow, they may resemble scars. Long-term sun exposure, rather than the acute burns associated with melanoma, is implicated, and could explain why 80% of these cancers develop on the head and neck. I'm speaking from experience here: I developed a basal cell carcinoma on my forehead near my hairline. As a child, I spent my summers on the New Jersey shore, where my mother proudly declared me to be as "brown as an Indian." Like anyone else who has had one basal cell carcinoma, I face a 50% chance of developing another one within five years. We former sun seekers are all dermatologically challenged and need to be monitored.

Squamous cell carcinoma is a cancer of the superficial cells of our outer layer of skin. Eighty percent of these cancers occur on the arms, head and neck. Again, long-term exposure to UV rays is to blame. But tumors can also develop as a result of other skin insults such as chronic inflammation or scarring, radiation or smoking. These cancers begin as reddish, raised nodules with indistinct margins. The nodule may have a cavity or ulcer in the middle and can also look like a warty bump or superficial scabby plaque. The bottom line for all these cancers is that if anything looks new or different, get it checked.

Both types of nonmelanoma skin cancer need to be biopsied in order for a diagnosis to be made, and therapy requires removal or destruction with cautery, laser, freezing, radiation or topical chemotherapy. Once you've been treated, staying out of the sun will help prevent recurrence.

Speaking of prevention: While you can't erase the sun damage done in childhood, it's clear (and pale) that avoiding sun exposure at any age will decrease your chance of developing skin cancer. Most of us associate sun damage with sun*burn,* but we're wrong. There's no such thing as a healthy tan. Any color change in the skin, from mild pink to dark brown, is an indication of a biologic effect from the sun that may be sufficient to instigate the DNA changes and immune suppression that result in cancer. The horrendous increase in the incidence of skin cancers is directly linked to our society's preference for outdoor activities and women's preference for bathing suits, shorts, tank tops and miniskirts. (Not to mention civilization's preference for industries and products that reduce the earth's protective ozone layer.) While I don't bemoan leg exposure (I'm jealous of those who can look great in such fashions), I should point out that one of the prime sites for the increase in skin cancer incidence has been women's legs. So when possible, cover up: Wear a hat, long sleeves and, yes, pants and try to avoid any sun exposure in the peak UV hours between 10:00 A.M. and 3:00 P.M. If you must be outdoors, use a broad-spectrum sunscreen (one that protects against both UVA and UVB rays) with a minimum SPF of 15 and don't forget to put it on your legs, since most of us apply sunscreen too thinly. Since we also tend to sweat, swim and not reapply, this means that we're probably getting only half of the expected SPF coverage listed on the bottle. Slathering on a stronger SPF—as high as 50—may afford slightly greater protection. When you're spending consecutive days in the sun, decrease your time outdoors and increase your SPF on each successive day. Even if you don't plan a sun-exposed outing, incidental exposure when you're driving, walking or going about your normal activities can still cause damage, so wear sunscreen under your makeup.

And now a word about tanning booths: The fact that the UV rays come from an artificial source doesn't make them any safer than those that come from the sun. Most tanning salons use UVA-emitting equipment. It's true that these rays are less likely to cause acute burns, but they actually penetrate farther into the skin than UVB and cause damage that can lead to cancer. If you're tanning for vanity's sake, know that these rays also cause premature aging—you know, that wrinkled, leathery-skin look. Great for a purse, but not for your dermis.

Complications of Smoking

If you picked up cigarettes as a teenager, you now have 15 to 20 years' worth of tar and nicotine under your chest, and you're going to start feeling the effects. Many of us think that seeing is believing, so here's what you're going to see: Lines around your eyes and lips proclaim a "skin age" 10 years older than you really are. Your aging skin also mirrors your bones. Smoking causes osteoporosis by decreasing the laying down of new bone while increasing its breakdown or resorption. Like your skin, your smoked-out bones are at least 10 years older than you are, and by the time you end your next decade you will have 10% less bone mass than women who have not smoked. This translates into a 45% increase in your future risk of hip fracture. Some studies suggest that the numbers are worse and that if you continue to smoke, your risk of bone fracture increases by 250%. Think of a loss of height, curved spine and pins in your hip. In smokers' cases, "little old lady" applies way before they're old.

To continue with what those cigarettes are doing to your body, you have to admit that no matter how much you brush or even bleach your teeth (and fingers), they are becoming a disgusting yellow. You're also going to start to hear a hoarseness in your voice and feel a tickle in your throat that's followed by a hacking cough. You develop frequent colds that often lead to bronchitis or sinus infections. You feel short of breath and may have trouble sleeping. These are the first outward signs of what's going on inside your body—and what's happening there is even more distressing. Let's start with the gynecologic: Nicotine alters the pituitary hormone surges needed for ovulation and hormone production. As a result, the risk of abnormal vaginal bleeding is 67% higher in heavy smokers than in nonsmokers. Your fertility is decreased, not only because of inadequate hormones but also because nicotine may hamper the function of the fallopian tubes and double your risk of having an ectopic pregnancy. If you do get pregnant (in your uterus), your risk of spontaneous miscarriage is more than doubled. While we're on the subject of "down there," let me mention that smoking results in a five-fold increase of the likelihood that infection with the human papillomavirus will result in venereal warts. It also seriously ups your risk of vulvar and vaginal cancer and more than doubles your chance of cervical cancer.

Although heart attack may not seem like a significant threat when you're in your thirties, smoking is responsible for more than half of cardiovascular deaths in younger women. Smokers have four times as great a risk of heart disease as nonsmokers, but that number rises to 9.25 if you started smoking before age 15. The more than 2,500 chemicals present in cigarette smoke diminish the oxygen content of your blood, damage blood vessels, cause platelets to become stickier and increase clotting factors while also increasing bad cholesterol and decreasing good cholesterol. This results in malnourished, damaged blood vessels that will bruise easily, allow clots to form and ultimately get clogged. When this happens in your heart, it's called cardiovascular disease; when it happens in your brain, it's a cerebrovascular accident, or stroke. Doctors are seeing a rise in the incidence of strokes and what we call "prestrokes," or transient ischemic attacks (TIAs), in younger women who smoke, and particularly among those who smoke and take the Pill. Hence our warning that smokers should not continue taking birth control pills after age 35.

Because I feel so strongly about this, I probably should take this "you're thirty and it's time to change" opportunity to mention the other health disasters that can result from smoking, even though it may take another decade before these occur. They include Graves' disease, a form of thyroid disease, and cancer of the mouth, pharynx, larynx, esophagus and stomach as well as the pancreas, kidney, ureter and bladder. Breast cancer rates can be higher in women who smoke, especially if they lack a gene that promotes enzyme reactions that help detoxify the chemicals in cigarette smoke. (Until the tobacco companies pay for this particular gene testing, it's wise to assume you're at risk.) Indeed, one study found that the median age of smokers with breast cancer is eight years younger than that of nonsmokers. If all these facts haven't caused a haze to form in front of your eyes, cataracts will. Up to 20% of cataracts are due to smoking. Moreover, smokers are twice as likely to develop macular degeneration, a virtually untreatable cause of blindness. Smoke not only gets in your eyes—it can blind them.

Now for my antismoking pièce de résistance, lung disease. Whether it's emphysema or lung cancer, the result is the same: a slow, painful death. It takes 20 to 30 years for smoking to begin to kill you. So guess what? If you started smoking at 15, you're getting there. And you have company. Lung cancer (not breast cancer) is now the leading cause of cancer death in women, and smoking is to blame for over 85% of cases. Smoking damages the cells lining the airways and may quickly cause them to become atypical and potentially cancerous. This is not something *any* smoker can get away with: 93% of current smokers have been found to have these damaged airway cells. But once you quit, that number goes down to 6%.

This is probably the lengthiest, most whining wind-up that I've proffered thus far in an effort to effect a change in your behavior. You simply can't get away with it anymore. And if you stop now, I can almost promise you a rose garden in the next two to four years. Just about every increased health risk from heart disease to stroke as well as most cancers will diminish or even be canceled. The damage to the cells in your lungs may still leave you with a 2.2-fold increased risk of lung cancer for the next 15 years (that's how long it may take for the distressed cells to undergo malignant conversion and create a tumor), but this is a huge improvement over the 35-fold increase in risk that would occur if you continued to smoke. Your bone mass will still be low, but at least you won't lose more, and with proper bone care you may be able to build back some of it.

I don't want to underestimate or deprecate the degree of your addiction, or the difficulty in stopping (nicotine is as addictive as heroin), but there is better living through chemistry when it comes to kicking this habit. First pick a quit date and let everyone know. Next, choose your nicotine replacement method. You can get gum or patches over the counter, or your doctor can prescribe a nicotine nasal spray or an inhaler (the latter may make you feel as if you're still smoking). These will all help you overcome many of your symptoms of nicotine withdrawal. And do we have symptoms! Women metabolize nicotine more slowly than men, it stays in our systems longer and we need a lower dose in order to create a nicotine "high." Not surprisingly, it's harder for us to quit. Many women subconsciously use nicotine to self-medicate for depression. Nicotine raises dopamine and serotonin levels. Sudden withdrawal may instigate changes in these brain chemicals that you and your body are unprepared for, resulting in anxiety, irritability, difficulty concentrating, anger, restlessness and problems sleeping. Without nicotine substitution, these symptoms peak two days after you quit smoking and diminish after two weeks. Those may be the hardest two weeks of your life, and it's perfectly legitimate to add the nicotine without the other 2,499 chemicals that you get from cigarette smoke to make quitting easier. Some of my patients are afraid to use the patch because they fear it will give them a heart attack, especially if they sneak a few cigarettes while wearing the patch. *Au contraire*. Studies have shown that transdermal nicotine does not cause a significant increase in heart attacks even in high-risk patients with cardiac disease—smoking, however, does. As a matter of fact, the levels of nicotine in your blood, even when you use a full-dose patch, are likely to be lower and steadier than those of the average smoker, whose levels spike with each cigarette. That said, if you cheat and have even the occasional cigarette, chances are unlikely that you're going to kick the habit.

If you fail with the patch or the gum on your own, it's worth making a second attempt with a different method of nicotine replacement. Also consider joining a smoking cessation self-help group or trying hypnosis. Nicotine replacement is less effective alone than when combined with the antidepressant drug buproprion, marketed under the name Wellbutrin, or with Zyban, an identical stop-smoking medication. (The drug's manufacturer renamed the drug in order to avoid the appellation "antidepressant," which some smokers found too depressing.) Because nicotine acts on the brain chemicals like an antidepressant, it makes sense to substitute it with a medication that does the same thing. After four weeks of combined therapy with Zyban and a nicotine replacement method, two-thirds of smokers quit, versus fewer than half of smokers who tried nicotine replacement alone. And after one year, 22.5% of those on combined therapy were still successful, versus fewer than 10% of those who took a placebo. Aside from the success rates, the good news about Zyban is that it diminishes withdrawal symptoms, and for those of you who are concerned about weight gain, it may decrease some of the carbohydrate cravings associated with quitting. When you use either nicotine replacement, Zyban or a combination of the two, weight gain is minimized; my clinical experience is that weight gain rarely occurs in patients who take Zyban.

If, despite all these pharmaceutical aids, you just can't seem to quit, you may have to face the fact that you have an underlying mental health problem such as major depressive disorder, adult attention deficit/hyperactivity disorder, an anxiety disorder or bulimia, and that these may need to be treated by the appropriate professional in order for you to be able to conquer the ultimate health threat, smoking.

MY TOP 10 LIST FOR STAYING HEALTHY IN YOUR THIRTIES

1. Don't smoke.
2. If you want to have children, start trying now and make sure your body is a healthy venue for a pregnancy.
3. Periodically reevaluate your choice of contraception.
4. Practice safe sex with any new partners and get checked for STDs.
5. Wear your seat belt.
6. Do not hesitate to seek help if you experience increasing PMS or depression.
7. Maintain a steady, healthy weight and return to it after pregnancy.
8. Take a multivitamin that contains 400 micrograms of folic acid and consume 1,200 milligrams of calcium per day, in the form of dairy products, fortified foods or supplements.
9. Make sure you are informed about the results of all your lab tests, and if they are not normal (especially your PAP smear), get appropriate follow-up and/or therapy.
10. Do some form of exercise for half an hour a day on most days.

there is a quantitative and qualitative difference in forties follicles compared with those of the two previous decades. They are fewer in number (remember, for each follicle that committed to producing a releasable egg in the past, thousands more died), and the ones that have remained to do their duty have been kept waiting a long time. In their state of dormant readiness, they have been extremely vulnerable to genetic changes and are now less likely to allow complete viable fertilization or become reliable hormone providers. Incomplete development of those follicles results in surges or deficits in estrogen and inadequate or absent progesterone. The outcome is the decreased fertility, cycle changes and hormonal swings that are part of perimenopause. But before you declare your body a hormone disaster area, relax and remember that the average age for perimenopause is 47, and that for many women, it is a nonevent (and, as I've promised on the cover of this book, I will advise you on how to make sure this transition won't hurt).

Your ovaries are just one pair of glands among many, and we need to expand our endocrinologic horizons in order to understand all the hormonal changes that can occur at this time of your life. Your forties and the decades to come will continue to tax the immune integrity of your thyroid, the mother of all glands and the one that controls your metabolism. Autoimmune attacks on this gland increase with age and cause subsequent development of hypo- or hyperthyroidism. Another gland that may have been overworked over the past three decades, especially if you've gained a lot of weight, is your pancreas. While you've been consuming the wrong food (you know—cheeseburgers, fries, candy . . .) and gaining weight, an energy battle has gamely been fought by your pancreas. It has literally worked its tail off producing sufficient insulin to allow you to process the excess glucose that accompanied your overabundant caloric intake. At some point, the pancreas just can't keep up. Meanwhile, age, hormonal changes and weight have all conspired to make you more likely to develop insulin resistance. Your body is presented with insulin, but ignores it and resists its action, so your blood glucose levels rise. Your pancreas now has to work harder than ever to make more insulin. High insulin levels stimulate fat production in your liver (while also increasing production of low-density lipoprotein or LDL, the bad cholesterol that forms plaque and causes cardiovascular disease). This liver-made fat is then stored in your body and replaces muscle, and a vicious cycle is perpetuated. Fat does not utilize calories and glucose as well as muscle. Levels of unmetabolized glucose continue to rise, and at some point, the exhausted pancreas can no longer effectively cope. Blood glucose levels remain elevated, and you now have Type II or non-insulin-dependent diabetes. We're not sure which came first, obesity, which causes insulin resistance, or high insulin production, which causes obesity. But the entire process can be delayed or even stopped in our forties with weight control and subsequent energy control.

While on the subject of energy intake, let's consider the gastrointestinal tract, which has, most likely, been serving you in good stead for the last 40 years. Its daily wear and lack of tear is phenomenal. The bowel lining constantly resurfaces itself, its cells sloughing off and regenerating every 24 to 72 hours. In your forties, your GI tract may start to protest. You are more likely to develop lactose intolerance, a condition in which you don't produce enough lactase enzymes to break down milk sugar, or lactose. If this sugar isn't "enzymed," it can't be absorbed, so it remains in the intestinal tract, where it causes gas, bloating, cramping and diarrhea. This occurs in 25% of Caucasian and more than 80% of African-American and Asian women. But for most, small amounts of milk products will still be tolerable. (Try up to one glass of milk, or better yet one cup of yogurt, which has its own enzymes to degrade the lactose.) You can also use lactated products so that you get your natural calcium and eat or drink it too.

The muscles that propel your intestinal content down its long, tortuous route may begin to lose their synchronicity of action as you eat (and often bloat) your way through your forties. One-sixth of all women develop irritable bowel syndrome, which can cause diarrhea, constipation or a combination of both, as well as bloating and cramping. Unfortunately, bloating seems somewhat ubiquitous in our forties (between PMS, gut sensitivity and weight gain, most of us begin to wonder where our flat abdomens went). This symptom, together with nausea, pain and general heartburn (an unfortunate term that has led to some serious diagnostic mix-ups), may be the primary symptoms for gallstones, known by many medical students as the (you should excuse the expression) F-disease. "F" stands for fat, fecund and forty. High fat consumption causes a double "F" whammy: cholesterol stones and obesity. Pregnancies caused elevated estrogen levels, which promoted stone development. So gallstones (cholelithiasis) and gallbladder inflammation (cholecystitis) reach a peak incidence of 20% in our forties. Apparently estrogen really does make a difference, since only 8% of men in this same age group develop these stones.

MY PERIODS HAVE BECOME HEAVY AND PAINFUL. WHAT'S GOING ON?

Heavy is a very subjective term that, at least medically, should be quantified. If you're changing your pad or tampon (or both) at least once an hour for 24 hours or more, or you're passing large (silver dollar size) clots every time you go to the bathroom, you qualify as having menorrhagia, or abnormally heavy periods. Pain, of course, is more difficult to measure. But if you're spending your day counting the hours until your next dose of ibuprofen, and even then you feel that your best position is fetal and in bed, your periods are truly painful.

One of the most prevalent causes of both symptoms is *adenomyosis*, in which glands from the endometrium grow into the muscle of the uterus. This may be a variant of endometriosis, in which cells from the uterine lining get "lost" and end up in places such as the fallopian tubes, ovaries and peritoneal lining. In adenomyosis, endometrial cells invade the muscular wall of the uterus and respond to hormonal directives to swell and even bleed. As a result, the uterine muscle cannot do its thing, which is to contract uniformly and close off the vessels running through it to the uterine lining. Once these vessels have been opened during the period, they continue to bleed until they are properly squeezed shut. If something (in this case, aberrant endometrial glands) prevents this viselike action, your period becomes heavy. The swollen tissue also generates pain.

More than half of women in their forties have some degree of adenomyosis. In a way, it's a natural consequence of all those years of hormonal stimulation of the endometrium. Its diagnosis is almost as subjective as its symptoms. Your doctor will probably feel that your uterus is somewhat enlarged, or in certain cases exclaim, "My goodness, your uterus feels like a three-month pregnancy. You couldn't be . . . ?" In gynecologic vernacular, the uterus also feels "boggy," or soft, again referring to what the examiner feels when you're pregnant. Ultrasound may reveal small cystic areas within a thickened uterine wall that correspond to islands of blood-filled endometrial glands. The final diagnosis, unfortunately, can only be made by sectioning the uterine wall and discovering the misplaced endometrial glands. Since this is done by a pathologist, it means that the uterus was removed in order to make the diagnosis—which is a bit extreme, considering that we have therapies that can allow you to keep your uterus intact (and in pelvis).

The treatment is usually medical rather than surgical. Strong—even prescription-strength—painkillers will certainly help with the cramping and often diminish blood flow. Birth control pills will minimize endometrial buildup both in the lining and in the muscle, resulting in lighter, less painful periods. On rare occasions, it might be necessary to treat this disorder aggressively, much as one would a severe case of endometriosis, by stopping hormonal production with a GnRH analog such as Lupron or Synarel. Since the latter should not be done for more than six months because of concerns about bone loss with low estrogen, your doctor may add back hormones in the form of birth control pills or HRT and still be able to control the bleeding and pain.

A surgical procedure can also be considered: a hysteroscopic endometrial ablation, in which the lining of the uterus is heated, or cauterized, making it less likely to shed and result in heavy bleeding. But remember: Adenomyosis occurs in the uterine wall, not in the lining. As a result, ablation does not eliminate the underlying pathology. Although it can diminish heavy periods, some women continue to have severe cramps.

A less common but perhaps more dramatic cause of heavy bleeding with or without cramps is *fibroids*, especially the type that grow into the lining of the uterus (submucosal fibroids). Other forms of these benign tumors, consisting of smooth muscle fibers, can grow either in the wall of the uterus (intramural) or project outside the uterus like Mickey Mouse ears (subserosal). Fibroids occur in about a third of women over the age of 35. Their growth is stimulated by your own hormone production and they may suddenly enlarge in your forties, when your estrogen surges are not always balanced by the appropriate progesterone production. It appears that certain women are more likely to develop these tumors, perhaps because of a genetic tendency to produce a type of growth hormone in their uterus. If your mother or sister had fibroids or if you are African-American, you may fall into this genetically predisposed category.

It's rare that subserosal fibroids cause abnormal bleeding, but both intramural and submucosal fibroids can be culprits. The former does so by interrupting the ability of the uterus to contract and close off blood vessels. These fibroids also seem to instigate abnormal vascular growth, increasing blood flow to the area. Submucosal fibroids totally throw off the mechanisms for constriction of blood vessels and blood flow. They poke into the lining and may have large, abnormal vessels that, when exposed, pour out excessive amounts of blood. Submucosal fibroids are a deep, dark secret. Since they are present in the lining, your doctor can't feel them during an exam unless they are accompanied, as often occurs, by the other forms of fibroid growth in the wall or outside it. Ultrasound will show where the fibroids are located and allow measurement of their size and number. Sometimes, in order to delineate the extent to which a fibroid is projecting into the uterine lining, the ultrasound is combined with infusion of a saline solution into the endometrial cavity. (This is done by inserting a very fine catheter through the cervix.) Inserting a hysteroscope through the cervix and into the uterine cavity can also allow your doctor to make this diagnosis. On rare occasions, a doctor may order an MRI for better assessment, but usually this expensive test is unnecessary.

The basics of fibroid therapy (i.e., do you or don't you need a hysterectomy?) will be covered on page 144. But I want to focus here on the types that most commonly cause heavy bleeding. *Submucosal fibroids* can be treated with an outpatient surgical procedure called *hysteroscopic resection*, which is performed under a general anesthetic or an epidural. A scope the diameter of your index finger is inserted through the cervix and a cautery loop is passed through it, allowing the doctor to "burn" off pieces of the tumor until it is destroyed. After this is done, a rollerball that carries an electric current is used to cauterize the tumor's base and, if desired, the entire lining of the uterus. The latter procedure, called an ablation, will permanently diminish or even stop your menstrual flow by scarring the lining.

An alternative to rollerball ablation is balloon ablation, a newer procedure in which a balloon is inserted into the uterine cavity, inflated until it fills the uterus and then heated for six minutes until the uterine lining is destroyed. This technique involves less cervical dilation than a hysteroscopic surgery and may not require a general anesthetic. In the future, it may become a fairly common office procedure.

If no anatomic cause for your pain and heavy bleeding is found, your complaint is likely to be due to the usual female scapegoat, "your hormones." Don't worry—I'll deal with this at nauseating length in the section on perimenopause (see page 129). The therapy in this case is birth control pills, which will correct your misbehaving ovarian hormone production and regulate and limit your cramps as well as the amount of uterine bleeding. If you can't take the Pill, progestins such as Provera or even natural progesterone such as Prometrium can be used to evenly build up the lining of the uterus during the last 12 days of your cycle. When you stop taking this progestin, the lining should slough evenly, resulting in a normal period. If you cannot or choose not to medicate this problem and you're sure you don't want a future pregnancy, endometrial ablation with one of the methods explained above is also an option.

This assumes that your doctor has already ruled out the last possible causes of heavy bleeding: endometrial cancer or its predecessor, atypical endometrial hyperplasia. Both of these conditions are more common in women who have had long intervals of unopposed estrogen stimulation, or high estrogen levels. This occurs in those who have a history of poly-cystic ovarian syndrome (see page 28) and irregular periods, as well as in women who are obese and/or who have diabetes. Use of tamoxifen to pre-vent breast cancer or its recurrence can, like unopposed estrogen, cause abnormal endometrial changes or even cancer. If you fall into any of these categories or if ultrasound shows a very abnormal thickening of the uter-ine lining, your doctor should make a complete diagnosis based on a tis-sue sample taken from the endometrium. This can be accomplished by inserting a small catheter through the cervix into the uterus and aspirating cells (endometrial sampling) or by scraping the lining (dilation and curet-tage, or D&C).

Sometimes this test shows that the glands are swollen and overly abun-dant, but aside from this crowded condition, there are no abnormal cells. This is termed "simple hyperplasia without atypia." Therapy is geared to replacing the missing progestin (see above) or, on occasion, to using an even more potent progestational agent called Megace to overcompensate for the estrogen-mediated changes. If atypia is found, you still may get by without a hysterectomy. Your doctor can prescribe daily Megace for three months and then do another sampling. Often the worrisome changes will have disappeared. In a few instances, this can even be done, with caution, in early endometrial cancer. But most doctors would suggest a hysterectomy.

IS IT PERIMENOPAUSE, OR AM I JUST HAVING A BAD DAY?

There may be days, or even weeks, when you feel that your hormones have conspired to make you feel subcharged or completely power-depleted. Although that feeling of fatigue and emotional letdown may have been part of your PMS pattern for the past two decades, there is, unfortunately, a tendency for this to worsen and last longer in your forties. Blame can justifiably be placed on the dwindling number and quality of your ovarian follicles, which, in turn, cause an overall decrease in your estrogen and progesterone levels. Researchers have also found that there can be spurts of unopposed estrogen from these less-than-disciplined folli-cles. This hormonal situation becomes even more complicated. We know that estrogen affects the number of receptors to progesterone and vice versa, so that the ratio between these hormones may be more important than their actual level when it comes to activating cellular responses throughout your body, including in your brain. In the latter organ, they alter levels of neurotransmitting substances, which can in turn affect your mood.

Many of these complex interactions are currently under investigation by neuromolecular biologists and are still indecipherable to most of us, so I'll "synapse" to the end result. As your hormones fluctuate more radically in your forties, your brain centers are sensitized and may "feel" that at times there is too little estrogen. So you can get symptoms similar to those of menopause just before or during your period, i.e., hot flashes, mood swings and sleep disturbances. But just because you're more sensitive to these fluctuations doesn't mean you have to assume that your first hot flash, or really bad hormone day, equates with perimenopause or menopause. Some of us are more sensitive than others to this ebb and flow of estrogen. The truly sensitive include the 20% of women in their twenties and thirties who have hot flashes way before they undergo follicular depletion.

In order to officially justify using the term *perimenopause* to explain your symptoms, you are supposed to have these symptoms in combination with irregular cycles. Let's get through the semantics of the word. *Peri* is a term that means "around" and, in this case, also means "before." The term *menopause* connotes a pause of menses (Latin for period, not the misspelled plural of men), and that pause is supposed to last for six months to a year before the condition is correctly defined. During perimenopause, not only are your follicular numbers down, but those that are left may fail to take up the gauntlet of the pituitary imperative of FSH to go forth and develop. As a result, there is diminished or absent estrogen production, causing a late or missing period. This lack of estrogen upsets the hypothalamic brain center, which controls your menstrual cycles. It knows that something is missing (namely, estrogen), and begins to work harder to get the pituitary to produce more FSH, which will finally get those recalcitrant follicles to do their thing.

Once the ovary is literally bathed in a pool of FSH, one of the follicles may respond and begin its belated and belittled course of development and estrogen production. If it has perked up sufficiently, it may even release an egg and go on to produce progesterone. So, in the midst of what seems like a hormonal standstill, you have a perfectly good cycle, and if your hormone levels were to be checked, you would be told they are fine. But, alas, the correction is temporary, and in cycles to come, your ovarian follicles may once more fail to respond, and hormonal testing at that time would show menopausal elevations of FSH (greater than 30 milli-international units per milliliter) and low estrogen or estradiol levels. So, if you want laboratory proof of your perimenopausal condition, you can request that your FSH level be checked, but you may not be able to rely on the results of a single examination. If your follicles are working properly (and remember, timing is important), your FSH should be low in the beginning of a normal cycle, then rise in mid-cycle together with LH just prior to ovulation, so there's no sense in checking it at that time (here you are, ovulating nicely, and the lab report declares your FSH is high or menopausal!). Get the test on day 2 or 3 of your cycle after you begin your period. If it is high but you're still bleeding every few months, you're perimenopausal. If it's low and declared "normal," it doesn't clear you of perimenopause; it simply indicates that in that particular month, your ovaries behaved properly. It might be worthwhile to repeat the test in another cycle. Or, if your symptoms justify it, consider the same therapy you would use for perimenopausal complaints—low-dose birth control pills. These will help regulate your cycle and hormonal "imbalance" at any age.

OKAY, SO IF I AM PERIMENOPAUSAL, HOW LONG WILL THIS LAST, AND DO I NEED TO TREAT IT?

I'll have to answer the first part of this question with the typical medical use of averages: The average duration of the perimenopausal transition is 3.8 years. The average age of natural menopause is 51.3 years, so subtraction tells us that the average age at the beginning of menopause is 47.5. But since there is a menopausal range, from 47 to 53, you can obviously be part of a similar range for the onset of this peritransition, and it can begin when you're as young as 43 or as "old" as 50 or more. To confuse the timing issue, I have to report that 10% of women will abruptly cease to menstruate without going through perimenopause at all, and 1% of women actually become menopausal before age 40. In this latter group, there is often a maternal history of early menopause. These women probably have a genetically determined decrease in their overall supply of follicles. It's also possible that some women who undergo early, unexpected menopause were exposed to viruses that destroyed a portion of their developing follicles while in their mother's uterus or during infancy. So age does not necessarily predict or confirm your perimenopausal status. If you have all of the symptoms, despite the fact that you or your doctor think you're too young, it might be worthwhile to get your FSH level checked.

It's clear that the "about four years of this" prediction can vary, and I can also predict that it can vary more if you're a longtime former smoker or are still smoking. The questionable good news is that perimenopause is shorter for smokers. The regrettable news is that menopause begins an average of 1.8 years earlier in women who smoke. (A preachy aside: Isn't it ironic that so many young girls begin to smoke so that they seem older, and if they continue this lousy habit, they inevitably get their wish? The chemical toxins of tobacco destroy their follicles and age their ovaries.)

Now that you have a sense of how long perimenopause will take, the issue is whether you should do anything about it. So, I'll give you both the "Leave it alone; it's a perfectly natural hormonal transition" and the "Why suffer through it?" arguments.

Let's start with the former. Of course this is natural, and if you are only mildly inconvenienced by a few hot flashes or inconsistent cycles, then just wait it out until you are menopausal, and then you can decide if you want to consider hormone replacement therapy. But there are a few things you should watch out for. (This is the "why suffer?" part.) One is heavy or prolonged bleeding. The poorly responding ovarian follicles of peri-menopause may cause an uneven buildup and shedding of the endometrium. The crucial mechanism in your cyclical bleeding control is that the entire top layer of the uterine lining is evenly built up, first by estrogen, then by progesterone, and then evenly sloughed off when the two hormones simultaneously drop two weeks after ovulation. This should be followed by repair of the "wounded" endometrium, under the guid-ance of the rising estrogen production of newly developing follicles. If this entire process is not complete or perfectly coordinated, the endometrium becomes unevenly or overly built up and then sheds irregularly (more graphically, bits and pieces come off). Bleeding becomes prolonged or heavy. Aside from the inconvenience and cost (you may begin to wish you had stock in a tampon company), you can develop anemia with symptoms of severe fatigue, rapid heartbeats and, yes, the peripatetic hot flashes. Moreover, back at the endometrium, your confused glands may undergo swelling and abnormal convolutions and become hyperplastic. With time, abnormal or atypical cells can appear and multiply, leading to pre-cancerous or cancerous changes. This bleeding pattern should not, there-fore, be dismissed as part of nature's intended transition. It warrants therapy. The first course of action is, of course, to get your bleeding to stop. One way to do this is to take a 10-day course of synthetic progestin (Provera, Cycrin or the generic medroxyprogesterone acetate). If this doesn't work, or if your other symptoms such as hot flashes indicate you are low on estrogen, you may need to take one of the estrogens used in hormone replacement therapy (see page 209), together with progestin or progesterone, to properly build back the endometrium.

I usually opt to perform a vaginal probe ultrasound before initiating this medical therapy just to make sure that endometrial polyps or fibroids projecting into the lining of the uterus are not causing the bleeding, and that the overall buildup is not consistent with a precancerous condition. If your bleeding verges on hemorrhaging (you need to change your pad or tampon every hour or are passing large, dollar-size clots), or if the ultrasound shows a very thickened lining, it may be necessary to perform an office D&C or, minimally, an endometrial sampling. The former will scrape the top layer off and help stop the bleeding. Both will provide diagnosis before beginning medical therapy. If polyps or fibroids show up in the ultrasound, I would recommend hysteroscopy to confirm this finding and help in removing the tissue.

AM I TOO OLD TO BE ON THE PILL?

No. That is, unless you smoke, in which case: Shame on you! You're old enough to know better and, as a smoker, you should have stopped the Pill by the age of 35 because of your substantially increased risk of heart attack and stroke. Your risk will be especially high if you smoke more than 15 cigarettes a day. But the good news is that if you quit smoking, the chance that you will suffer one of these adverse events while using the Pill returns to a safe, normal level. I use the Pill as a carrot when treating fortysomething smokers. Many of them have early, horrendous perimenopausal symptoms, and the Pill is their best hope for relief. So we make a deal: They stop, and I supply them with the Pill. When I use the term "the Pill" here, I am referring to the combined estrogen-progestin version. The progestin-only minipill is not off limits to smokers; however, it may not adequately correct perimenopausal symptoms and can be associated with irregular menstrual bleeding.

In this decade you may be more likely to develop high blood pressure, diabetes and elevated lipids, and although these are not absolute contraindications for use of the Pill, it is preferable to select a type of pill that is low in estrogen, and possibly a version that contains one of the newer forms of progestin. Brand names include Ortho-Cyclen, Ortho Tri-Cyclen, Ortho-Cept, Desogen and Mircette. Your hypertension, diabetes and high cholesterol levels should also be under medical control before you go on the Pill.

Although estrogen-containing oral contraceptives have not been shown to cause gallstones, a common problem among women in their forties, they may accelerate the development of symptoms if you already have stones or a history of gallbladder disease.

As you enter your forties, the issue of breast cancer takes on heightened importance. But relax: The Pill has not been shown to increase the risk of this disease in women between the ages of 35 and 44, and even appears to decrease the risk in women ages 45 to 54. Furthermore, Pill use has not been shown to pose any increased risk for women with a history of benign breast disease or a family history of breast cancer.

There are absolute contraindications for Pill use at any age (see page 70), and you and your doctor should consider these before starting this therapy.

WHAT OTHER FORMS OF BIRTH CONTROL MIGHT BE ESPECIALLY GOOD FOR ME IN MY FORTIES?

The methods that were available to you in your younger years are adequate if not better in this decade—better because your natural fertility rates have diminished. As a result, the vaginal spermicides, diaphragms and condoms that offered less than desirable efficacy rates in your twenties may be all the pregnancy protection you currently need. On the other hand, the rhythm method, or timed abstinence, becomes less reliable. This is because your ovulations are imperfectly timed, particularly toward the end of this decade. Without the right cadence, you can't have rhythm. My contraceptive favorites for women in their forties are:

Birth control pills: At the risk of sounding like an ad, let me say that a pill a day can keep perimenopause, uterine cancer, ovarian cancer, ovarian cysts, anemia and both ectopic and intrauterine pregnancy away. In a less rhyming fashion, it may also help minimize breast lumps and prevent osteoporosis, colon cancer, perhaps even heart disease.

IUDs: Most women in your age group are perfect candidates for this hands-off, long-term form of contraception. One Paraguard (the most commonly used IUD) inserted in your early forties can give you birth control until you're menopausal or for 10 years, whichever comes first. Hopefully, you're in a monogamous relationship and don't have to worry about coming into contact with new microbes. The only drawback to this method is that as you go through perimenopause you may experience irregular and at times heavy periods. If this happens, you might need to take the Pill to regulate your cycles, in which case your IUD will become obsolete and need to be removed.

Tubal ligation: By the age of 44, almost half of all women have already had this procedure, many while in their 30s, when the specter of pregnancy loomed large (and long). Unfortunately, up to 24% of these women may subsequently regret their decision. But you're older now and have a clearer perspective on childbirthing and childrearing, and you're less likely to want to rescind a decision never to enter this realm again. It might be worthwhile to quickly survey your mother's or older sister's menopausal history because it's a good indicator of the age at which you will go through this change. If you're destined for an early menopause, you might want to consider forgoing surgery and using a more temporary method. On the other hand, if your mother or sister didn't go through menopause until her midfifties, 8 to 10 more years of birth control may warrant this surgical "fix" even if you're in your early to midforties.

Another option, which I rarely use for my patients, is Depo-Provera shots. Because half of women who use Depo find that it stops the period, it might be ideal for those who have heavy bleeding. It also will decrease the risk of developing uterine cancer. But irregular bleeding is another possible scenario, and this tends to make fortysomething women (and their doctors) nervous. Another negative factor to consider: Many women in this age group are already battling a tendency to gain weight and will find the two- to four-pound weight gain per year associated with this form of contraceptive method unacceptable.

For more specifics on the pros and cons of each contraceptive method, see page 70.

WHEN CAN I STOP USING BIRTH CONTROL?

By the time we hit our forties, we are (or should be) the world's authorities on contraception. But the gap between knowledge and practice has become an abyss: 51% of pregnancies among women in their forties are unintended. In this respect, we are not getting wiser with age. We have succeeded in being second only to teenagers in contraceptive indiscretion. If you've already read the section on perimenopause, you may have the impression that your aging ovaries are behaving erratically and that if you're suffering from this much PMS, you couldn't possibly suffer an unintended pregnancy as well. But as the biological clock ticks on, you continue to experience the occasional release of eggs, which can, of course, be a target for wandering sperm. Yes, your fertility at age 40 may be much less than it was in your twenties, but don't kid yourself: It's not zero.

The traditional teachings of our contraceptive sages dictate that you continue to use contraception for six months to one year after the onset of menopause. The average age of this event is 51.7. But menopause may occur in 11% of women ages 45 to 49, while 30% of those of us who have not had a hysterectomy won't go through menopause until sometime between ages 51 and 54. How does this theoretical wisdom translate into contraceptive decision-making in the real world? If you have opted to stay on birth control pills in the perimenopause, you won't even know when you're officially in menopause. At the age of 50 or 51 you can go off your pill for two weeks and get your FSH checked. If it's elevated to menopausal levels (over 30 milli-international units per milliliter), congratulations, you're in menopause and can now consider switching to hormone replacement therapy and stopping contraception. (I offer the following caveat in deference to all the lawyers out there: On rare occasion, one FSH level can be spuriously high and in subsequent months there may be some fluctuation. So if you want to play it super-safe, you have to realize that hormone replacement therapy is not a contraceptive, and additional barrier methods for another six months might be needed for 110% protection and true peace of mind.) Those women who have not altered their perimenopausal transition with the Pill should obviously wait until they have had no period for six months to stop contraception.

Some women begin hormone replacement therapy during perimenopause. HRT is not a contraceptive and will not prevent your ovary from releasing an egg. So, at least initially, it would be wise to add on some form of barrier contraception. Eventually, when your FSH levels remain above 30 miu/ml on day two or three of your cycle, the chance of ovulation is low enough to consider throwing away that diaphragm and gels for good. I'm often asked by my patients who are menopausal and on cyclical HRT if because they get a "period" they can also get pregnant. This bleeding does not signify release of an egg. It is there only because of the arbitrary withdrawal of progestin that is part of this type of HRT. No, if you are menopausal you will not get pregnant.

Menopause, however, unless it connotes an additional pause from all sexual contact, does *not* mean that you can throw away those condoms. Many women who are experiencing this transition are also going through separation, divorce or widowhood and entering a whole new world of sexually transmitted microbes. The older you are and the less estrogen you have, the more vulnerable you are to HIV and other STDs. This is because sexual activity is more likely to cause minute tears if your vaginal tissue is thin and open a pathway for infection. At least 15% of women diagnosed with AIDS are over the age of 40.

I DIDN'T HAVE A CHANCE TO HAVE MY BABY. CAN YOU HELP?

I can try, but know that the odds aren't exactly in your favor. Thanks to the incessant tick-tocking of our biological clock, there is a 50% reduction in the rate of spontaneous pregnancies that result in live births among women by the age of 35, and a 95% reduction by the age of 45. In the United States, less than 1% of all live births (excluding those resulting from assisted reproduction) are to women over age 40. This number declines to 0.01% by age 47.

These figures are so woefully low because of a fertility triple whammy: Fortysomething eggs are difficult to fertilize in the first place. Our reproductive menopause (which can begin 10 years before actual menopause) dictates that the number and quality of our eggs has measurably diminished, and the pituitary hormones that direct the development and release of these eggs are not working in sync. Additionally, there have been all those years of wear and tear on your pelvis. Infections, endometriosis, surgeries and fibroids may have caused tubal or endometrial damage that can make it difficult for sperm to get to the egg or for a fertilized egg to implant in the uterus. Finally, chromosomal abnormalities in the fertilized egg are so prevalent that half the pregnancies that develop in a woman's mid-forties end in miscarriage. I know I've painted a bleak picture, but all hope is not lost. Let's consider what options you have so that you can take them as quickly as possible.

Your first move should be to have your FSH level tested on the third day after you've started your period. If the level is over 20 milli-international units per milliliter, and certainly if it's over 25 mu/ml, for several cycles in a row, you must face the fact that your own eggs won't get you pregnant. If you wish to keep trying, it should be with eggs from a younger donor. A normal FSH level is no guarantee that you can become pregnant, but it will allow you to attempt fertility therapy with your own eggs with some hope of success.

If you've never tried to get pregnant before, it's reasonable to start by timing intercourse to the most fertile part of your cycle. But if nothing happens after three to four periods, stop futzing around on your own and get thee to a doctor, ideally a reproductive endocrinologist. You should have all the tests I've listed on page 80, but at an accelerated rate. Aggressiveness may be key to success, which means that your therapy will probably entail expensive, high-tech procedures such as superovulation with intrauterine insemination, in vitro fertilization (IVF) or gamete intrafallopian tube transfer (GIFT). If in vitro procedures are used, your doctor may add on ICSI. (For more information on all of these therapies, see page 81.) In the best of clinics, pregnancy rates per IVF cycle for women in their early forties can be as high as 29%. But take-home baby rates fall to 16.5%. If a donor egg is used, live birth rates should be similar to those of the age group of the egg donor and can be as high as 40%.

Note that if you succeed in your goal and become pregnant, you should certainly have all the genetic testing recommended for women over age 35 (see page 88). Because of your age, you're considered high risk, especially if you have the added hazard of a multiple pregnancy resulting from all that fertility manipulation. You should be followed by an obstetrician who routinely sees high-risk patients.

I TOOK FERTILITY DRUGS. DOES THIS MEAN I'M AT INCREASED RISK FOR OVARIAN CANCER?

In order to answer your question, I have to ascertain whether the drugs allowed you to have a successful term pregnancy. If they did, you probably have absolutely nothing to worry about. If, on the other hand, you've had a history of infertility and you took medication unsuccessfully, you may face an increased risk of ovarian cancer. Chances are this is not due to the hyperstimulation of your ovaries with the drugs, but rather the result of the incessant ovulation that occurred when you didn't have a baby. Research shows that women who have not carried a pregnancy to term have a 1.5- to 2-fold increased risk of ovarian cancer when compared with women who have had at least one baby. That doesn't mean they were infertile—many didn't try to become pregnant.

There appears to be a mutation of a gene known as p53 in about half of ovarian tumors. This mutation has been shown to increase in proportion to a woman's lifetime number of ovulatory cycles. This may be why suppression of ovulation by pregnancy, breastfeeding or oral contraceptives protects against ovarian cancer later in life. The issue is whether being infertile or adding fertility drugs to this problem of incessant ovulation increases risk even more. The latest and probably best data come from a Danish study that found that among women who were infertile but never took fertility drugs, the risk of ovarian cancer was 2.7 times greater than that faced by women who had at least one baby. Fertility drug use by infertile women did *not* add to this risk.

In addition, according to this study, if you've had a baby but have had trouble conceiving another one, this secondary infertility does not increase your risk of ovarian cancer, even if you resort to taking fertility drugs. In other words, no matter what you've done or gone through, once you've had a term pregnancy, the possible damage of infertility is canceled out.

There has been tremendous warranted criticism of the earlier studies that caused such consternation over a suspected link between fertility drugs and ovarian cancer. But even this latest study is far from perfect. And in order to give total reassurance that these drugs have no effect whatsoever, I and all the other doctors involved in reproductive biology require surveys that follow large numbers of women for decades after they've taken fertility medications. While we're all waiting for these results, I would advise you to take advantage of birth control pills' ovary-protecting effect in your forties—whether or not you need the Pill for contraception—if you have a history of unsuccessfully treated infertility or if you've never had a baby.

I'VE BEEN DIAGNOSED WITH AN OVARIAN CYST. WHAT CAUSED IT, AND CAN IT TURN CANCEROUS?

First, a note of reassurance. Ovarian cancer is rare among women in your age group. Your lifetime risk of developing this disease is one in 70 (that's assuming you live well into your eighties). But your risk while in your forties is about one in 400. Furthermore, the term "cyst" usually connotes a simple and benign accumulation of fluid, including blood. There are myriad reasons as to why cysts develop. Doctors classify them as "functional" (having to do with ovulation and spontaneously resolving after a couple of cycles) and "nonfunctional" (caused by benign conditions or tumors). Even having one of the latter should not increase your future risk of developing ovarian cancer.

This is what you should know if your doctor does a pelvic exam and/or pelvic ultrasound and proclaims that your ovary is enlarged or has a cyst.

Functional ovarian cysts: These can develop when excess fluid accumulates during the development of the follicle in the first two weeks of the cycle (*follicular cyst*) or after ovulation, in the corpus luteum (a *corpus luteum* cyst, which may contain blood) or during pregnancy (a *theca luteum* cyst). From the time you start ovulating, you're at risk for these types of cysts. However, there seems to be a slight increase in their development during your later reproductive years. Follicular cysts are the most common type of functional cyst and rarely become larger than 8 centimeters. They can be present without causing any symptoms and be discovered during a routine exam. However, on occasion they make their presence known by rupturing, usually at midcycle, and causing significant pain that may mimic appendicitis. If unruptured, this type of cyst will usually go away by itself in four to eight weeks and should not require surgery.

Corpus luteum cysts are less common and are usually smaller. Because they contain blood, if they do tear there can be significant bleeding into the pelvic cavity and surgery is sometimes required. Rupture of these cysts usually occurs between day 20 and 26 of the cycle, often after intercourse, and—here's an interesting fact—this is more likely to happen on the right ovary. (Or perhaps the stats are stacked on the right, since this condition must be differentiated from appendicitis.)

Theca luteum cysts are the least common of the functional ovarian cysts and can occur on both ovaries during pregnancy. They are more likely to be stimulated to grow if levels of pregnancy hormone are very high, as they tend to be in multiple pregnancies and among women with diabetes and those who have used fertility drugs. These cysts, which can grow to 30 centimeters in diameter, are actually groups of smaller cysts clumped together. The good news is that they regress spontaneously.

In general, combined estrogen-progestin birth control pills seem to markedly reduce the chance of developing nonpregnancy functional cysts. There is a possibility, however, that triphasic pills may slightly increase your chance of developing this type of cyst. So if you have a tendency to form cysts, you may want to take the Pill, but make sure it's a monophasic one. Smokers have a twofold increased risk of developing functional ovarian cysts. So now you have another incentive to quit.

Nonfunctional ovarian cysts: These include several types, and although I'll dutifully list the possibilities, I don't think you need to be put through a complete pathology course. *Endometriomas,* also known as "chocolate" cysts because they are filled with old, brownish-colored blood, can enlarge to 8 centimeters in size and will not resolve on their own. *Dermoid* cysts are composed of a fascinating mix of fat, hair, glands and even teeth. They represent primitive cells that normally should have become the eggs in our ovaries but instead tried to form a new being without being fertilized. They account for two-thirds of benign ovarian tumors in women under age 50. Most are discovered between the ages of 30 and 43. Dermoid cysts will not go away on their own, and indeed have a 15% chance of twisting on their stalk or causing the ovary to twist. This causes severe pain and necessitates surgery. Although it is rare, 2% of dermoid cysts can become malignant, and this is more likely in your forties, so once a diagnosis is made, they need to be removed. *Serous cystadenomas* consist of a cyst divided into multiple compartments and account for 20% of benign ovarian tumors in women under 50. These cysts will not disappear on their own. Because 10% to 25% of these cysts become malignant, they must be removed and checked carefully to ensure that they are not cancerous.

The benign ovarian cysts that can grow to the largest size, sometimes filling the entire abdomen, are the *mucinous cystadenomas.* These are composed of multicystic structures that, as the name would imply, are filled with a thick, mucinous substance. These too must be removed and carefully checked because 5% to 10% can become malignant.

Adnexal cysts: Adnexa is a broad term that encompasses the fallopian tube and ovary. When your doctor examines you and feels a mass or cyst, it's sometimes difficult to determine whether it's coming from the ovary, the tube or both, so the word *adnexal* is used to describe it. An accumulation of fluid in the tube called a *hydrosalpinx* can occur as a result of scarring from pelvic inflammatory disease (PID). Sometimes this fluid becomes infected and an abscess develops in the tube and ovary. Just like any other abscess, this infection may need to be drained with surgery. Although it is not generally grouped together with pelvic cysts, you (and of course your doctor) should heed the fact that an ectopic pregnancy can form a blood-filled, cystlike structure in the tube or on the ovary, and therefore if you develop "something" in this area and your period is late, a blood pregnancy test is mandatory.

Okay, so you got more of a pathology lesson than you'd ever want or need. What should you and your doctor be doing once a tentative diagnosis of a cyst in your pelvis is made? Here are the steps according to chronology and invasiveness.

1. **Pelvic ultrasound**. This will determine the size of the cyst, whether it's completely fluid-filled or partially solid and whether blood is present in the fluid. If there is any concern about a cyst's cancerous potential, Doppler ultrasound can be used to measure the blood flow to the cyst. Malignancies tend to be fed by increased blood flow in multiplying blood vessels.

2. **Blood tests.** A complete blood count will help establish if the cyst is bleeding (your hematocrit and hemoglobin will be low) and if it is part of an inflammatory process such as PID (your white count will be high). The second important blood test that most of us have heard of by now is one to measure cancer antigen 125 (CA-125). This protein is elevated in 80% of women with ovarian cancer. But, unfortunately, it is elevated in many other conditions as well, including endometriosis, fibroids, PID, hepatitis, cirrhosis and certain other malignancies. This makes CA-125 testing alone a poor screening test for ovarian cancer. Having said that, if you have a mass and your CA-125 is in the 100s, this is cause for concern. If it is above 35 but below 100, it is more likely to indicate endometriosis. Another blood test you might need if you are not using reliable contraception or your period is late is, of course, a pregnancy test.

3. **Watchful waiting and possibly taking birth control pills.** If you don't have significant pelvic pain and your cyst appears to be a functional one, it's perfectly fine to wait for two cycles to see if it shrinks or disappears, especially if it is less than 7 centimeters in size. There is still some controversy as to whether the Pill will help it shrink more quickly. Many doctors, myself included, feel that it will and prescribe oral contraceptives during this waiting period.

4. **Laparoscopy.** If you're in severe pain and certainly if your falling hemoglobin and hematocrit indicate internal bleeding (this is beginning to sound like an episode of *E.R.* . . .), you have a surgical emergency and need immediate laparoscopy. The same is often true if your doctor has determined that you have an abscess. Laparoscopy will diagnose the problem and allow the surgeon to remove the cyst or drain it and control any bleeding. You may also need an elective laparoscopy if your cyst has not diminished in size after several

months with or without birth control pills, or if it appears to be a dermoid cyst, a sizable endometrioma, a mucinous cyst or a cystadenoma. Often the cyst can be removed without sacrificing the ovary; however, the ovary should be removed if the diagnosis of a mucinous cyst or cystadenoma is made, and in fact many doctors will remove both ovaries in this case, particularly if a woman is close to or in menopause. This is because these tumors can develop in both ovaries and can become malignant. Once the cyst is removed, it should be examined by a pathologist.

5. **Laparotomy**. This is a last resort and is usually preceded by a failed laparoscopy, in which the surgeon was either unable to safely complete the surgery through the scope or encountered severe bleeding or scar tissue, or the mass is highly suspicious. If a malignancy is confirmed, the surgery should be a total hysterectomy together with removal of the ovaries, tubes, lymph nodes and omentum (the layer of fat covering the intestines).

MY DOCTOR RECOMMENDS A HYSTERECTOMY. IS THERE ANY OTHER SOLUTION?

Traditionally, women were not offered alternative solutions. There was a nationwide "better take it out" hysterectomy hysteria that peaked in the 1970s, resulting in 725,000 women undergoing this procedure each year. The current incidence of hysterectomy has declined, but it is still hovering in the unacceptable 600,000 range, and your decade contributes the most to this number. The average age at which this procedure is performed is 42.7 years. There is a major need to diminish the number of these major surgeries, a goal that is certainly medically feasible. Both patients and doctors must redefine the reasons for hysterectomy and explore new avenues of uterus-preserving therapy. The uterus you save may be your own!

A hysterectomy is an invasive and pelvis-altering procedure no matter which surgical method is used. Although the mortality rate is low, it is not zero and ranges from 0.06% to 0.11%, depending on how it is performed and the health of the patient. Major complications, including hemorrhage requiring blood transfusion, the need for follow-up surgery as a result of damage to surrounding organs or life-threatening pulmonary clots or a heart attack, can occur in up to 4% of women. Minor complications, including fever, bladder infection, wound infections and pneumonia, accompany this surgery 20% to 40% of the time. There are also possible long-term adverse effects. The most obvious is that without a uterus, you can't reproduce. Then there is the possibility of developing "post-hysterectomy depression." Its true prevalence is unknown because many of the women experiencing this are really in the throes of hormonal shock due to the additional loss of their ovaries. However, women with a history of psychiatric problems, those who have never had children and those under age 35 appear to be particularly at risk. Having made these negative comments, I, the surgeon, have to add that when hysterectomy is truly necessary and alleviates pain, suffering or cancer, most women will come through this surgery with their psyches intact and feeling much better.

So when is a hysterectomy the right choice? Most gynecologic cancers are certainly an irrefutable indication for removal of the uterus, usually together with the fallopian tubes and, if necessary, the ovaries (see page 151). These include invasive cervical cancer, endometrial cancer, leiomyosarcoma (cancer of the uterine wall), cancer of the ovaries or fallopian tubes and, in some cases, invasive cancer of neighboring organs such as the bladder, colon or rectum. But these conditions account for only about 10% of all hysterectomies.

Fear of these conditions is often used to justify removal of the uterus prophylactically—"just in case." This is often accompanied by the accessory statement "You've finished having your children. What do you need your uterus for anyway?" I regretfully must report that statistics show that you're more likely to hear this statement (and get a hysterectomy) from male rather than female physicians and in the South as opposed to in the rest of the United States. This "useless uterus" excuse is often proffered when a woman is diagnosed with precancer of the cervix or carcinoma in situ (noninvasive early malignant changes in cervical cells). Be aware that less extreme uterus-conserving procedures such as cryotherapy (freezing), laser tissue destruction, LEEP (loop electrosurgical excision procedure) or cervical conization are often adequate and safe treatments for these conditions.

But by and large the bulk of hysterectomies (30%) are done for uterine fibroids. These benign tumors are present in at least a third of women in their forties, and for most of them the growths are silent and cause little if any adverse symptoms. The first sign may be your doctor's disapproving utterance at the time of your routine pelvic exam, "Oh dear, I think I've found a fibroid." These tumors require therapy only if they are very large (usually greater in size than a four-month pregnancy) and/or cause abnormal or heavy bleeding, pain or pressure. Being told that your fibroid has grown rapidly since the previous exam probably does not constitute a reason to run into the O.R. and have it removed. Fibroids tend to grow in spurts and stop. Moreover, the concept that this rapid growth indicates—heaven forbid—a malignancy is outdated and rarely accurate. I'll say it here and repeat it frequently when answering questions about pelvic growths: It is *highly* unlikely that a fibroid will become cancerous. And if a cancer such as leiomyosarcoma should occur, it probably did not arise from a fibroid.

The other mistaken excuse for immediate hysterectomy is that the tumor will get larger and surgery will become riskier. Wrong. There is *little* or *no* difference in surgical complication rates whether the uterus is removed abdominally when it's the size of a 12-week pregnancy or when it's as large as a 20-week pregnancy. (And it may never reach that size.) Certainly hysterectomy should never be considered as your only option if you want to use your uterus in the future for pregnancy. This may sound mildly absurd if you're in your forties. However, with new reproductive technologies allowing women to use donor eggs, you can consider a pregnancy as late as your fifties, provided you have an intact housing unit.

Okay. So you have a fibroid that is causing symptoms. What can you do to keep from sacrificing your uterus? If your chief complaint is abnormal or heavy bleeding and ultrasound has shown that the fibroid projects into the endometrium (a subserosal fibroid), it can be excised with hysteroscopic resection (see page 128). Should your doctor feel that its size would make this procedure difficult, GnRH analogs (Lupron or Synarel) can be used to shrink the tumor to an operable size. GnRH analogs can also be used if the fibroid is in the wall of the uterus (intramural). Six months of therapy will shrink some tumors by as much as 50% and will stop your periods (allowing your blood count to build up if you've become anemic) as well as control pain and pressure. The problem is that once you stop using a GnRH analog, the fibroid will rapidly return to its original size and your symptoms may recommence. There is the possibility of continuing the medication until menopause; however, due to our concern about menopausal symptoms and bone loss, long-term GnRH therapy should be accompanied by some form of hormone replacement therapy. Another drawback is cost. A monthly shot of Lupron averages $400. In general, I use GnRH analogs only in women for whom I plan to perform future surgery, either to build up their blood count and allow them to donate their own blood or bypass a transfusion altogether, or if I want to shrink a submucosal fibroid to facilitate its removal. Some of my patients who truly need to undergo hysterectomy choose to use Lupron in an attempt to shrink the fibroids sufficiently so that I am able to perform a vaginal rather than abdominal procedure.

Many women have been told that the Pill is a no-no if they have uterine fibroids of any size. In fact, it has often been blamed for the growth of these tumors. Yet if we consider that most fibroids grow rapidly in either the first trimester of pregnancy or in your forties during cycles of unopposed estrogen, it would logically follow that the Pill, with its even, continued dosage of low estrogen and progestin, would rectify any underlying hormonal imbalance and control fibroid growth. So use of the Pill in your forties is perfectly justifiable (provided you don't smoke) if your chief symptom is abnormal bleeding, or if you need contraception. It may even prevent further growth and keep your fibroids at their current manageable size.

A surgical alternative to hysterectomy for symptomatic uterine fibroids is myomectomy, or the removal of the growths. This is certainly the surgical therapy of choice for any woman who wants to get pregnant. How it's done depends on the size and position of the fibroid and the training of the surgeon. Generally, tumors that are less than 5 centimeters in diameter or those that are not deep in the wall of the uterus or entering the uterine cavity may be safely removed through a laparoscope, especially if they grow out of the uterine surface on a narrow stalk (pedunculated fibroids). However, larger or deeper masses may require extensive reconstruction to repair the uterus after their removal. This is probably best achieved with the hands-on technique requiring the opening of the abdomen (a laparotomy). A laser can be used with both techniques and may decrease bleeding and subsequent scarring. If the endometrial cavity is entered during fibroid removal, you will need a C-section for any future deliveries. Myomectomy has an 80% success rate in reducing heavy bleeding, pelvic pain and pressure. It may also be useful in treating infertile women or those who have recurrent miscarriages if the only abnormality that is found is a uterine fibroid. But your inherent tendency to grow benign uterine tumors remains, and there is a 20% chance that you will regrow fibroids that will require future surgery. The procedure can also result in scar tissue that can diminish your future fertility.

There is also a new technique called myolysis, or fibroid coagulation, in which a fibroid is drilled in multiple areas with special needles or a laser beam. This destroys the tumor's blood supply and causes it to shrink to about 50% of its original size. It can be done through the laparoscope and should be reserved for women whose fibroids are not too large. Doctors don't yet know how a "drilled" uterus will perform in future pregnancies.

Even less surgically invasive than myolysis is uterine artery emboliza-tion, a recently developed procedure performed not by your gynecologist but by an interventional radiologist. A catheter is run through an artery in your leg and is used to inject tiny synthetic particles into the vessels that supply blood to the tumors. Deprived of blood, the fibroids shrink by an average of 60%. This is not recommended for extremely large fibroids and, because it is considered highly experimental, is not yet covered by most insurers. Some women experience significant pain as the fibroids shrink, and in 2% of cases to date, ovarian failure and subsequent menopause have occurred. As with myolysis, the effect on future pregnan-cies is not yet clear.

The next leading cause of hysterectomy, accounting for 8% to 10% of these procedures, falls under the nebulous heading "chronic pelvic pain." Surgery of any nature should be considered only if the discomfort is severe enough to interfere with normal activities, or causes you to take to your bed for a significant amount of time each month. For more about the causes of pelvic pain, see page 95.

Hysterectomy is a last resort for pelvic pain. It should be considered only after you've undergone a complete workup, which should include laparoscopy, and after disorders of the bowel, bladder, spine and neuro-logic system have been ruled out. If the pain is found to be due to severe scarring, with or without endometriosis, your uterus should be removed only after previous attempts to remove the scar tissue and/or endometri-otic implants, or to control your condition with drug therapy, have failed. I, as well as most gynecologists, have treated patients with unexplained pelvic pain that did not respond to all attempts at therapy, and have finally resorted to hysterectomy. A study by the Centers for Disease Control and Prevention of 300 women who underwent this major surgery for pelvic pain of unknown origin found that after it was done, 60% were pain free. But that means 40% continued to have problems.

Another possible reason for a hysterectomy, pelvic prolapse, is not as common in your age group as it is after the age of 55. But because it is responsible for 10% to 15% of all hysterectomies, I want to mention it here. If the pelvic ligaments supporting the uterus, bladder and rectum are severely stretched or injured because of multiple vaginal deliveries or even a single prolonged and difficult delivery, these organs can descend to the point where they protrude into and even out of the vagina. This can result in a sense of constant pelvic discomfort, often described as a "pulling" sensation. It's also associated with frequent urinary tract infections and incontinence, and may even result in an inability to have normal bowel movements. Prolapse may also make intercourse difficult or painful. All of us who've had vaginal deliveries probably have some degree of prolapse, and just because our physician remarks on it during a Pap smear does not mean we require surgery. But if you are acutely aware of the prolapse because of its symptoms, vaginal hysterectomy, together with a procedure to resupport the bladder and rectum, is certainly an option. Unfortunately, surgically lifting a completely fallen uterus usually fails (it falls back down), so if this is the problem and you're not willing to use a pessary (see page 279), a hysterectomy is probably in order.

I NEED TO HAVE A HYSTERECTOMY.
WHAT KIND SHOULD I HAVE?

There are a lot of misconceptions about the terminology regarding hysterectomy. So let me play medical dictionary for a minute. A *total hysterectomy* means the removal of the uterus together with the cervix, and has nothing whatsoever to do with the ovaries. (If the ovaries are removed at the same time, a new term is used: *bilateral oopherectomy*. And since the tubes are usually removed as well, the correct terminology is *bilateral salpingo-oopherectomy*.) A *subtotal hysterectomy* is the removal of the uterus *without* the cervix, which is left in its normal place at the top of the vagina, where it aids in the vagina's support and possibly in your sexual response. As we complete this short course in pelvic surgical lingo, we also need to consider whether the procedure is done through an abdominal incision (*abdominal hysterectomy*), a vaginal one (*vaginal hysterectomy*), or a combination of the two, where a laparoscope is inserted through the belly button in order to view the procedure and help place instruments, but the uterus is removed through the vagina (*laparoscopic-assisted vaginal hysterectomy*).

Let's consider the vaginal-versus-abdominal issue. Seventy-five percent of all hysterectomies are currently performed through an abdominal incision, but which method you and your surgeon should choose will depend on whether you meet the following criteria, as well as your surgeon's expertise.

Abdominal hysterectomy should be performed in these circumstances:

- Invasive cervical cancer (this will require a radical hysterectomy, which includes removal of surrounding tissue, lymph nodes and a portion of the top of the vagina)
- Endometrial cancer that has invaded the uterine wall or the cervix, or has spread to other areas in the pelvis
- Tubal or ovarian cancer
- Large uterine fibroids that cannot be removed vaginally
- Severe pelvic scarring with or without endometriosis, which prevents safe separation of the uterus from adjacent organs with vaginal or laparoscopic procedures

Abdominal hysterectomy is not absolutely necessary but is reasonable if:

- Your surgeon is uncomfortable attempting to remove moderately large fibroid tumors vaginally or laparoscopically
- You have moderate scar tissue or endometriosis that might make other surgical methods more complicated
- You wish to conserve your cervix (Note: If a hysterectomy is done vaginally, the cervix is removed)

Vaginal hysterectomy is often preferable to abdominal surgery (when it can be safely performed) for several reasons. The first is "Look, Ma, no scar." But perhaps more significantly, the postoperative hospitalization, pain and recovery time are at least half that of abdominal hysterectomy. You can eat, walk, bend and even laugh almost immediately after surgery. There are fewer postoperative problems, and the risk of fever and chance that you will need a transfusion are halved. Most of my patients who have this procedure are nearly pain-free after a week and return to work after three weeks. It's sometimes hard to make them heed important instructions to avoid vigorous exercise, heavy lifting and intercourse until they are totally healed at six weeks. You're a likely candidate for this procedure if:

- You have simple pelvic and uterine prolapse
- You have noninvasive cervical cancer
- You have noninvasive early endometrial cancer (Note: In this case, it might be preferable to perform a laparoscopic-assisted vaginal hysterectomy, which will allow for removal and biopsy of certain pelvic lymph nodes to ensure they are negative)
- Fibroids are present, but your uterus is smaller than a 12-week pregnancy.

Laparoscopic-assisted vaginal hysterectomy (LAVH) allows your surgeon to directly view your abdomen and assess and remove scar tissue, tumors, nodes and other hidden or unsuspected dangers that might lurk in your pelvis. These could be missed or misjudged during a vaginal procedure, in which your doctor's view is limited, to say the least. It also makes it easier for the surgeon to find and remove your ovaries, although most of the time an experienced surgeon can reach and remove the ovaries with a simple vaginal hysterectomy. On the downside, many of the instruments that are used to perform LAVH are disposable and extremely expensive, and there does not seem to be compelling evidence that, overall, this procedure decreases complications or hospitalizations. You are a candidate for LAVH if:

• Your fibroids have made your uterus larger than a 12-week pregnancy, but your surgeon feels comfortable removing the tumors vaginally after extensive morcellation (in other words, the fibroids are cut into smaller pieces with a laparoscopically inserted instrument before they are removed)
• You and your surgeon have decided that your ovaries should be removed, but there is concern that this might prove difficult without the aid of the laparoscope because you've had previous pelvic surgeries or are suspected to have pelvic adhesions
• You've had previous surgeries for or documentation of endometriosis
• You have known or suspected pelvic adhesions
• Lymph nodes or other pelvic organs have to be evaluated or removed at the time of surgery (This would include some women with early endometrial cancer.)

If you've decided on abdominal hysterectomy, the next decision you'll be faced with is whether your cervix should be removed or saved. (Who said this would be easy? There's a veritable Chinese menu of options!) From my vantage point as a surgeon, the procedure is faster and less fraught with chance of bleeding, trauma to the ureters and postoperative pain if the cervix is left in place. The Europeans routinely do this; my American colleagues have been trained to automatically remove the cervix whenever performing a hysterectomy in order to eliminate any future possibility of cervical cancer. The latter approach would seem to negate the value of Pap smears. If you haven't developed precancerous changes by this decade in your life and you're not at high risk for cervical dysplasia or cancer (you don't have multiple partners, don't smoke and don't have a history of HPV infection or other STDs), it's perfectly legitimate to save your cervix and be screened like other women in your age group.

The specter of loss of sexual response and pleasure after hysterectomy haunts many women. Some equate the loss of the womb with the end of their femininity and sexuality, and this issue has been complicated by the fact that up to 60% of women over age 45 have their ovaries removed when they undergo a hysterectomy. For these women, the real trauma to their sexuality is most likely the sudden loss of ovarian hormones. Once this is factored out, it would appear that for most women, if sex was good before the hysterectomy, it will continue to be so after. And if a woman experienced pain during sex because of tumors, endometriosis or scar tissue, the discomfort will be gone and intercourse will improve.

Having said that sex will be fine (hopefully better than fine), I should report to you that the European "save the cervix" consensus is that this opening to the uterus plays a role in orgasmic response. There is a group of nerves in the area of the cervix through which pelvic sensation travels. This nerve bundle has even earned the right to its own name: the Plexus of Frankenhausen. And there is no question that the integrity of this plexus is interrupted when total hysterectomy is performed. Also, when the cervix is removed, the vagina may be shortened, which may result in discomfort during intercourse. Finally, there may also be a somewhat increased risk of subsequent prolapse of the vagina because the ligaments that fastened the cervix and the top of the vagina to the pelvis have been cut (although in all fairness, a good surgeon will reattach the cuff to important ligaments to help prevent this problem). So consider all these facts and decide what you fear the most: the extremely slight possibility that you will develop cervical cancer, or that loss of your cervix will change your sexual response and vaginal support.

SHOULD MY OVARIES COME OUT TOO?

The decision to remove your ovaries when you have a hysterectomy should be based on your risk for future ovarian disease and subsequent surgery versus the problems you will encounter after surgically induced hormone deprivation. Put simply, you have to weigh your fears. If at the time of hysterectomy your ovaries appear to be normal, simply having the surgery *without having your ovaries removed* decreases your risk of developing ovarian cancer tenfold. The average woman runs a 1.4% chance of having ovarian cancer in her lifetime, while a woman with normal ovaries at the time of a hysterectomy has only a 0.14% lifetime risk of the disease. No one knows why. Obviously, those women who are allowed to keep their ovaries comprise a select group: They show no pathology in that organ. But by viewing the ovaries of a woman in her forties, can a surgeon predict whether they will be cancerous 20 years later? Probably not. It's possible that removal of the uterus prevents contaminants or toxins from reaching the ovaries; it may also diminish blood flow and thus duration of ovarian activity—and the less you ovulate, the lower the risk of cancer.

But ovarian cancer is not the only fear. You don't want to go through this major procedure and then have to have another surgery because you later develop benign ovarian disease. Statistics show that this occurs in 1% to 5% of women, and half the surgeries are needed in the first five years after hysterectomy. The most common causes are endometriosis, ovarian cysts or a condition called residual ovarian syndrome. The latter occurs if the ovary is buried behind the peritoneum or gets covered by scar tissue that forms after the hysterectomy. During ovulation it can swell, resulting in chronic pain.

Finally, if your ovaries are active, which they should be in your forties, their removal is likely to result in hormonal shock. You not only have lost the estrogen and progesterone they produce, but you've also lost a substantial amount of testosterone. All this can lead to severe hot flashes, sleep disturbances, mood swings, short-term memory loss, vaginal dryness and loss of libido and sense of well-being, not to mention an acceleration of future risk of heart disease, osteoporosis and possibly Alzheimer's. Unless there is a contraindication, you should begin estrogen replacement immediately. (I place an estrogen patch on my patients in the O.R. at the time of surgery.) But that may not be enough, and testosterone therapy is also appropriate for most women. Unfortunately, our attempts to mimic what your ovaries once did have to proceed on a trial-and-error basis. There is no set formula, and many women never feel that they reach the exact hormonal balance that they had before their ovaries were removed. Add to this the concerns some women (and physicians) have regarding long-term hormone replacement therapy (You're taking estrogen? Aren't you worried you'll get cancer?) and we find that fewer than 40% of women who start treatment after hysterectomy and bilateral oopherectomy continue to take estrogen for five years. The stats on testosterone use are even worse.

So to make a long story about small organs short, you should probably consider having your ovaries removed, especially if you are over the age of

45, if you have a significant family history of ovarian cancer. Their removal is also probably indicated if you have a hysterectomy because of severe endometriosis. It's easier to make the decision if your peri-menopausal symptoms indicate that you are very close to becoming menopausal and your FSH level is elevated. Otherwise, it is perfectly legitimate to leave these unoffending organs in place.

I USED TO ENJOY SEX, BUT LATELY I'M JUST NOT INTERESTED. WHAT'S WRONG WITH ME?

The question is whether your lack of sexual enjoyment means you don't want to have sex or that once you have it, you don't find it pleasurable. Let's look at what's happening in your body as you go through the stages of sexual response. Hopefully, before there is sex, there is *desire*. Your libido is partially governed by your hormones, and surprisingly not by those deemed female (estrogen and progesterone), but by so-called male ones (androgens, including testosterone, dehydroepiandrosterone and androstenedione). Their production and your libido all started with puberty. But in your forties, the level of these male hormones can decrease by as much as 50%. For some women this means a noticeable loss of desire.

The second stage in your sexual response is *arousal*. This occurs thanks to increased blood flow and swelling of blood vessels in the labia, clitoris and vagina. Clear fluid from the engorged vessels is pushed into the vagina, resulting in lubrication. The chief hormonal requirement for this process is estrogen. As you traverse your forties and proceed to peri-menopause, your levels of estrogen fluctuate or diminish, and as a result, engorgement and lubrication can be hampered.

After arousal, there is *orgasm*, a phenomenal event associated with rhythmic contractions of muscles in and around the vagina as well as an increase in breathing and heart rate. And finally, there is *resolution*, when your body returns to its resting, nonaroused (but hopefully content) state.

In order to determine the source of your problem, you and I have to figure out which of these stages has gone awry. Many of my patients in their forties tell me that they are simply "not in the mood," although they enjoy sex once they start and are capable of reaching orgasm. The next step is to determine whether the source of this libido loss is psychological (stress, fatigue and depression are chief culprits), related to relationship problems, due to med-ical issues (such as medication use, disease, surgery, chemotherapy, radiation or pain) or hormonal. Is this lack of libido constant, occurring even when you're well rested or on vacation? Is it global (no one or no fantasy turns you on)? If so, then the source of your problem could be hormonal and you should have your testosterone checked, both total blood levels as well as the portion that is free (not bound to a protein that prevents it from doing its job). Low levels of free testosterone can be carefully treated with very small amounts of testosterone, administered in the form of a cream, gel, ointment or lozenge placed under the tongue. If perimenopause is also causing your estrogen levels to vacillate, and especially if you are going to take testosterone in any form, it might be worthwhile to even out your estrogen level with low-dose birth control pills. (For this purpose, triphasic ones might be best.) Another option is very low doses of estrogen replacement therapy. I frequently prescribe low-dose estrogen patches together with a testosterone lozenge. I could go on, since I've written a whole book on this subject. But perhaps you could just read it—it's called *I'm Not in the Mood: What Every Woman Should Know About Improving Her Libido*.

If your lack of libido is only situational and you're feeling much lustier when you're relaxed and away from normal stresses, hormone supplements won't help—supplemental rest will, and a vacation is just what the doctor ordered, although I doubt your insurance will cover it.

If erotic movies, books or fantasies fuel your desire but your partner doesn't, it might be worthwhile to explore your relationship together, perhaps with a professional therapist.

Should none of the above explain your situation, it's time to look for a medical cause. Thyroid abnormalities, anemia, autoimmune diseases and many other chronic medical conditions can deplete your libidinous urges and should be diagnosed and treated. The stages of our sexual response are intricately linked, so that if one is out of order, it can produce a negative domino effect. If your arousal response is not there, especially if vaginal dryness results in pain, you're not going to want to initiate something that is not pleasurable, and your libido can suffer. So although estrogen by itself is not considered a pro-libido hormone, it is a pro-*arousal* hormone. It may suffice to use a vaginal estrogen cream in your forties to facilitate genital blood flow and relieve dryness. And of course, once you're menopausal, consider more comprehensive estrogen replacement therapy.

The last possible scenario is that you've lost interest because you're no longer achieving orgasm. Although low free testosterone levels might be implicated in this response and it's worth testing them, boredom with your sexual routine or inadequate stimulation may be to blame. It might be worthwhile to talk about this problem with your partner and perhaps jointly explore books, videos or sex paraphernalia, or even consult a qualified sex therapist.

I FOUND A LUMP IN MY BREAST. WHAT'S THE NEXT STEP?

Don't panic. Most breast lumps are not cancerous. Indeed, benign fibroadenomas account for 10% of lumps, cysts for 25% and fibrocystic masses for at least 40%.

The first thing to do is determine whether you have felt this in the past and it's changed, or whether it is something you've been vaguely aware of, and that comes and goes with your periods. In the latter instance, you can certainly wait for your next period and recheck your breasts when they're least lumpy—once your menstrual bleeding has stopped. If the lump has disappeared, it is most likely a sign of fibrocystic changes (see page 66). If, however, this appears to be a brand-new lump or it does not change over the course of your cycle, it will warrant further assessment. Before your doctor's more experienced fingers check the lump, you may be able to ease your anxieties. Benign tumors tend to be soft, smooth and moveable with fairly distinct borders. Those that occur with fibrocystic changes may be multiple, rubbery and tender with less distinct borders. Cancerous lumps are typically hard, rough-edged and immobile.

Having said all this, neither you nor your doctor have Superwoman's X-ray fingers, so you'll need to have additional diagnostic testing. First, if you haven't had a mammogram in the last nine months to a year, you need one on both breasts. But make sure you inform the radiologist of the lump and where it's located in case special views are needed. (The mammogram should always be done before your doctor attempts to make a rapid diagnosis by aspirating fluid or cells from the area with a needle. This trauma can make a mammogram appear very suspicious.) Additionally, an ultrasound of the breast should be ordered to ascertain if the mass is fluid-filled (cystic) or solid. If the mammogram is negative and the ultrasound shows that the mass is a simple cyst, you can wait and repeat the ultrasound in three to six months, provided the cyst is small (roughly less than 2 centimeters). Benign cysts can either decrease in size or remain unchanged.

If, however, there is any questionable finding on the mammogram, or if the cyst is large or has any suspicious characteristics, it should be aspirated and the cells in its fluid examined by a pathologist, particularly if the fluid is discolored or bloody. Once it's deemed benign, the cyst can be rechecked in four to six weeks. Should it recur, grow larger or cause pain, it should be surgically excised. This can often be done under local anesthetic.

If the ultrasound shows that the mass is solid, that still does not mean it is malignant. The most common benign solid tumor of the breast is a fibroadenoma. Although these painless, mobile lumps are found in all age groups, they are most likely to appear during your twenties or early thirties. But because these lumps are solid and you are in your forties, if one is found it should be biopsied. Some surgeons are comfortable doing a fine-needle aspiration or a core biopsy, but if the results are at all inconclusive or suspicious, the entire mass should be surgically removed. Other doctors, including myself, recommend that the entire mass be removed from the outset because of your age.

Having described all the reassuring outcomes, I can't ignore the worst-case scenario. If the mammogram is suspicious or the mass appears irregular on ultrasound, biopsy or excision is absolutely necessary. This can either be done the old-fashioned way—the surgeon will make an incision and remove the mass—or it can be performed using one of several newer, less invasive methods such as Mammotome, which uses a gunlike device to sample breast tissue. If suspicious cells are found with this smaller technique, a larger open excision of the area is necessary. If a malignancy is identified, in most cases an even larger excision or lumpectomy is in order. This may surgically suffice for 70% of cancers (the rest will require mastectomy). You will also need to have some nearby lymph nodes removed to see if the cancer has spread. I'll go into this in greater detail on page 232.

HOW OFTEN DO I NEED A MAMMOGRAM?

In my opinion, you need one annually starting at age 40. Let me tell you what my opinion is based on. First, there are the Swedish women, whose westernized lifestyle, and thus their risk of breast cancer, is very similar to our own. (Having spent some time in Sweden, I concluded that their summer lifestyle is less stressful than ours, but their long, dark winters make up for it.) Their medicine and meticulous follow-up are above reproach. Hence research coming from this country must be taken very seriously. Four Swedish studies showed a 35% to 44% decrease in deaths from breast cancer among women who had yearly mammograms in their forties. A broader analysis of all published studies showed a 16% to 24% decrease in mortality among women ages 40 to 49 who had screening mammograms. Statisticians consider the 16% not to be significant; however, if some of the Canadian studies, which involved old mammographic equipment, are excluded from this analysis, the 24% figure predominates and frequent screening for younger women wins. And as the quality and sensitivity of mammographic equipment improve (and particularly if digital mammographic equipment becomes available), the detection and survival rates will probably be even more convincing.

Although I promised to spare you from a multitude of studies, I'll make an exception for mammograms and load up additional ammunition: A recent study at the University of Chicago showed that 90% of women under age 50 whose cancer was found by a mammogram were alive and recurrence-free five years after diagnosis. This number fell to only 77% if the cancer was detected after the woman or her doctor found a lump. It appeared that a mammogram was even more important in these younger women than in those over age 50: 87% of the older group survived without a recurrence for five years after a lump was detected during a manual exam. A mammogram will detect these cancers when they are half the size of what can be felt during a manual exam.

I have to reiterate at this point that the incidence of breast cancer significantly increases with age, and during this decade your odds of being diagnosed with the disease go from 1 in 217 at age 40 to 1 in 93 at age 45. By age 50, your risk is 1 in 50. Breast cancer is particularly likely to be invasive and deadly in a woman's younger years. And although "only" 2% of those women who develop the disease get it in this decade, this accounts for fully 20% of the total breast cancer mortality number each year.

Breast cancer in younger women develops a greater blood supply and grows and spreads faster than a malignancy in an older woman. This in itself is a reason to consider yearly rather than every-other-year screening. In your age group, there's more to be missed if you wait two years between X-rays. My recommendation for yearly mammogram is in line with that of the American Cancer Society, the American Medical Association, the American College of Obstetricians and Gynecologists and the American College of Radiology. The only major group that has not wholeheartedly endorsed universal screening in your age group is the National Cancer Institute, which is still waffling and advises having the test every one to two years.

Now that I've (hopefully) convinced you to have a mammogram every year, I have to add a negative caveat. Your relatively dense, firm breasts in your forties (I know you don't think they're as firm as they used to be, but I'm speaking from a mammographic point of view) create a veritable diagnostic jungle. It's sometimes very difficult to pick up early cancers in women with dense breasts, and as a result 25% of cancers in women in their forties will be missed, versus 10% in an older age group. Some researchers feel that adding ultrasound to mammography may improve the odds, but this practice is still controversial for women who have no palpable mass or abnormality on X-ray.

That's not the only drawback. You are also at risk for what's called a "false positive" finding—in other words, an abnormality found on your mammogram is in actuality nonmalignant. Unfortunately, the only way for you and your doctor to be sure that it's not cancer is to have additional tests, which may entail more X-rays, as well as ultrasounds and even biopsies—not to mention the emotional anguish associated with this process. For mammographic lesions that cannot be felt or seen on ultrasound, stereotactic biopsy, in which the needle is guided by X-ray images, may be the only way to make that final diagnosis.

Your chance of enduring a false positive workup is one in 12 each time you have a mammogram during this decade. When it comes to biopsies, the number of cancers detected per biopsy performed is one in four. For many of us this is an acceptable price to pay for early detection and therapy, not to mention peace of mind when results are negative.

WHAT CAN I DO TO PREVENT BREAST CANCER?

If there was a clear picture of cause and effect for this malignancy, I would simply list the causes and tell you to eliminate them whenever possible. But the only factors for which we have a consensus regarding importance are ones that you currently have absolutely no control over. These include a family history of women who had multiple and/or early breast or ovarian cancer, which indicates a possible presence of a hereditary gene for breast cancer (Ashkenazi Jewish women may be especially "chosen" for this risk). Other important factors: your age at the onset of your first period (menstruation before age 11 increases risk), when or if you had children (having your first child after age 25 or never giving birth equal elevated risk), when you'll go through natural menopause and whether you received radiation or chemotherapy at a younger age.

But I don't want to leave you feeling that you're entirely at the mercy of your medical history. Here's what we know you can do that might (and I stress the word "might") help diminish the chance of developing this disease. These recommendations assume you're of average risk—women whose family history or gene-testing results place them at high risk will get special advice in the chapter titled "Your Genetic History."

Curtail your alcohol intake: For the past 15 years, epidemiologists have warned us that there is an increase in risk of breast cancer among women who regularly consume alcohol. This substance has been found to cause a rise in blood estrogen levels, possibly by diminishing estrogen's metabolism or increasing its production. It's possible that the spurts of estrogen that may occur after you imbibe a drink are more harmful to the breast than constant exposure to lower levels, whether they be natural or pharmacologic. This suspected link has received far less attention than the warnings regarding estrogen replacement therapy's purported tie to breast cancer. Could it be that the liquor industry has more money to spend on promoting alcohol than drug companies have to spend on the promotion of ERT? Or is alcohol considered "natural," whereas estrogen is not? Maybe we're just in denial because we enjoy our wine (and its effects) and are delighted at the prospect that it may decrease our risk of heart disease. Whatever the excuse, the bottom line may not be "bottoms up." According to the oft-quoted Harvard nurses' study, three alcoholic drinks per week increases breast cancer risk by 30% to 60%. The risk seems to be even higher—250%—among women under age 55 who have no other risk factors for breast cancer and who imbibe just one or more drinks a day. There are other studies that seem to be more reassuring when it comes to light drinking (no more than one drink a day). But even they show that when the level of drinking increases, so does the risk of breast cancer (24% greater for women who have two drinks a day and 38% greater for those who have three drinks a day, when compared to women who do not drink).

The most recent attempt to reach a conclusion by combining the results of six studies found that women who consumed approximately three to seven glasses of wine, two to five bottles of beer or two to four shots of liquor per day had a 41% higher risk of invasive breast cancer than teetotalers. Each daily drink increased breast cancer risk by 9%.

So my advice is to limit your alcohol consumption to no more than one drink a day. And even then, you have to play favorites with your organs and choose between your breasts and your heart. A drink a day may help keep heart attacks away, but there are a lot of other steps you can take to lower your chances of cardiovascular disease. (And you can get the same cardiac benefits of wine with unfermented grape juice!)

Take your vitamins: Getting your folic acid from a multivitamin supplement may be especially relevant if you've ignored my previous recommendation to reduce your alcohol intake. The Harvard nurses' study showed that consuming at least 450 micrograms of folate per day appeared to mitigate alcohol's adverse effects on breast cancer risk. Indeed, among women who had roughly one drink a day, multivitamin users experienced a decrease in breast cancer risk of 26% when compared to drinking women who didn't down their multivitamins. It may be that alcohol causes a mild folate deficiency, and this in turn may influence genetic changes that lead to cancer.

Don't gain weight: Adult weight gain is obviously something you would prefer to live without. The question is whether living with it will increase your risk of breast cancer. The answer is "probably." Weight gain after the age of 18, and certainly in your forties and beyond, has not been shown to elevate your risk of premenopausal breast cancer. But it has been correlated with both a greater than average risk of postmenopausal breast cancer and death from this disease. (When obese postmenopausal women develop a tumor, it may go undetected longer and may grow and metastasize more quickly.)

The reason we aren't seeing more premenopausal breast cancer in obese women is that they are more likely to skip ovulation and to have irregular cycles. So their bodies—and most important, their breasts—are bombarded with less estrogen and progesterone from their ovaries. But once these women go through menopause, this ovarian factor is canceled, and their fat cells become the principal purveyors of estrogen. This continuous high level of estrogen exposure may be the culprit behind their increased incidence of cancer. Overweight women also produce more insulin, and more insulinlike growth factor, which is similar to the growth factors that have been found to promote breast cancer.

Postmenopausal women who gained more than 40 pounds in adulthood and who do not use hormone replacement therapy (which will override their fat cells' estrogen production) may have approximately double the risk of breast cancer of women who did not gain weight. In the nurses' study, weight gain alone was felt to be responsible for roughly 16% of postmenopausal breast cancers, while hormone replacement therapy alone accounted for just 5%. When the two factors were combined, they were associated with fully one-third of postmenopausal breast cancers! This certainly means you should avoid weight gain. Whether it means you should avoid estrogen if you're heavy is still debatable (among other things, estrogen may help reduce the risk of heart disease).

Limit your fat intake . . . maybe: High levels of dietary saturated fat—from meat and dairy products—have been shown to cause molecular damage to breast cells and certainly increase the risk of breast cancer in animals. And another form of fat, trans-fatty acids—found in processed or packaged foods containing hydrogenated oils—has also been implicated in causation of breast cancer. On the other hand, monounsaturated fat such as olive oil has been declared protective. And the traditional Japanese diet containing half the fat we consume is likewise associated with a risk of breast cancer that is one-fourth that of American women. But when women move from Japan to the United States (or remain in Japan and eat like Americans), the difference in risk disappears. While it could be argued that part of Japan's advantage is that its diet is very high in soy products, fat seems to be a factor as well.

The question is also whether it's the total amount of fat, the type of fat or what the fat does to our weight that truly affects our risk. Nobody knows for sure. Recent reports from the Harvard nurses' study gave those of us riding the low-fat, right-fat bandwagon food for thought. The researchers found *no* increased risk of breast cancer with increased intake of *any* fat, whether it be animal, vegetable, polyunsaturated, saturated or trans fat. Moreover, they found no protective effect from olive oil and actually reported a slightly increased risk of breast cancer with consumption of omega-3 fat from fish. The study's conclusions have been criticized by everyone from cancer advocates to olive oil manufacturers and fishermen. The researchers only considered the previous 14 years of dietary intake, and it is possible that a study of younger women who were followed for a longer period of time would have rendered different results. Since we know without a doubt that the wrong fats in the wrong amount can boost your risk of heart disease, obesity and cancers in other parts of your body, my advice would be to limit your overall fat intake to 30% of calories (ideally less) and make sure that most of this fat is monounsaturated.

Eat more soy protein We've all heard that if we are going to be nutrition-ally correct, we need to discover the joy of soy. This wonderful legume contains natural plant estrogens, or *phytoestrogens*, that have been touted as a cure-all for menopausal symptoms, heart disease, osteoporosis and (the clincher) as a dietary agent that can prevent breast cancer. There are actually three classes of phytoestrogens: *bioflavins, lignans,* and *coumes-tans.* The first class includes soy products, lentils, kidney and lima beans. Lignans are found in the fiber of such foods as whole grains, berries, fruits, and vegetables. Particularly famous for its lignan-bearing properties is flaxseed. *Coumestans* are present in alfalfa and seed sprouts and fodder crop such as clover (so cow's milk, which may pass on the phytoestrogens of clover, could also be an indirect source of phytoestrogen).

Soy's attributes are due to three major substances called *isoflavones*, and these are *genistein, diadzein,* and *equol*. All of these, from a molecular point of view, look remarkably like the estrogen our ovaries make, estra-diol. The thought is (as usual, I can't make pure declarative statements since the researchers are still arguing) that these phytoestrogens bind to estrogen receptors and compete with your body's own estrogen, prevent-ing the latter from taking its rightful place and stimulating cells that, on occasion, might be cancer cells. Moreover, some studies have shown that phytoestrogens may increase levels of sex hormone–binding globulin (SHBG) so that a portion of the estrogen that is in the body would be bound up and rendered inactive and unable to bind to those cells. Finally, lignans may also inhibit an enzyme that converts prehormones made by our adrenal glands and fat cells to estrogen, and thus reduces the total amount of circulating estrogen in our bodies. Whatever the mechanism, it appears that women in Japan who have a traditional diet rich in soy prod-ucts (tofu, miso and soybeans) have one-fourth the incidence of breast cancer of women or Japanese women living in western countries who "succumb" to our phytoestrogen-less diet. The breast protection features of lignans are even less clear. So far, they have only really been demon-strated in rats. When female rats were injected with carcinogens and fed flaxseed, they had an almost 50% decrease in their tumor development. Whether it will do the same for women has yet to be shown in any signifi-cant study.

Based on these facts, can we now isolate the right phytoestrogen, put it in a powder or pill, and deliver the same phytoestrogen bang we would get from the natural product? No one knows. It could be that the actual veg-etable or its fiber contains other factors or vitamins that work in a necessary synergy to bestow breast health. Certainly not all soy protein concentrates are created equal. Some are processed by alcohol extraction, and this can remove the phytoestrogen. So make sure that if you're using a soy protein product, it contains genestein and diadzein. The amount of phytoestrogen we should aim to consume (again based on Japanese diets) has been estimated to be between 20 and 60 milligrams a day. Many soy beverages contain 20 milligrams of isoflavones, as does four ounces of tofu. If you add one or the other, or both, to your minimum five portions of fruits and vegetables a day and add one to two tablespoons of flaxseed in baked goods or cereals, you may be doing that "dietary something" that's within your control to decrease your risk of breast cancer. At the very least, it won't hurt.

Exercise: The majority of studies on the connection between recreational exercise and breast cancer have shown anywhere from a 12% to a 60% reduction in risk among both pre- and postmenopausal women. The thought is that physical activity may change hormone production (in fact, intense exercise will shut down hormone production altogether), prevent weight gain and improve immunity so that your body destroys abnormal cells more efficiently. But there is such a mishmash of what the researchers considered "physical activity" that it's difficult to tell you how much time, frequency, duration or intensity of activity you need to minimize your risk. One of the most comprehensive (and comprehensible) studies came out of Norway, where 25,000 women were followed. Those who exercised four hours a week had at least a 37% reduction in their rate of breast cancer, and this protection grew to 72% in women who were lean. Frankly, this study has been a major impetus for the many hours I have committed to walking like a caged gerbil on my treadmill.

Stop smoking: The median age of breast cancer patients who smoke is eight years younger than that of nonsmokers with breast cancer, according to a Danish study. Several other studies have indicated that smokers are at increased risk of breast cancer, and the more cigarettes smoked, the greater the risk. Some women—a majority of Caucasian women and those of Middle Eastern descent, as well as 35% of African-Americans and 20% of Asians—have a gene that impairs their ability to detoxify certain carcinogenic substances found in cigarette smoke. Breast cancer rates may be higher in these women. Since gene testing is not a criteria for cigarette sales and lung cancer is even more predominant than breast cancer, once again, I'll beg you not to smoke.

Consider taking tamoxifen if you're at high risk: This is such a big subject that I've devoted an entire section to it below.

Having made my anti-breast-cancer recommendations, I want to give you a short list of things that have been touted or rumored to cause breast cancer but that, in reality, do not. The first is abortion. Certain special-interest groups have suggested that abortion, especially at a young age, increases future risk of breast cancer. But thoughtful analysis of old and new statistics has refuted this. Birth control pills have also gotten a bad rap. There is no correlation between Pill use in our forties and ultimate risk of breast cancer. However, some data have shown that birth control pill use at a very young age, especially in African-American women, may lead to an increase in premenopausal breast cancers.

One of the strangest ironies of our heightened breast cancer awareness is a fear of the very instrument that has allowed us to diagnose this disease earlier and improve survival rates: the mammogram. First to the physical: The squishing and mushing of the breast in that machine may be uncomfortable but, provided you don't have a breast implant (and even with an implant if proper pressure is applied), it is not harmful. Then there's the concern about radiation. Yearly mammograms give an average dose of 0.2 rads per breast. This is less than the exposure you get from flying round-trip from New York to Los Angeles or living for a year at a high elevation location such as Denver, Colorado.

Finally, there's caffeine. It may cause lumpiness and breast pain, but there are no data whatsoever linking it with an increased risk of breast cancer.

SHOULD I TAKE TAMOXIFEN?

Zeneca, the pharmaceutical company that markets the breast cancer prevention drug tamoxifen under the brand name Nolvadex, has helpfully created a computer program called the Gail model. This program (also available in noncomputerized slide-rule form) incorporates many of the factors that can increase your risk for breast cancer so that you can calculate your risk of developing breast cancer over the next five years as well as over your lifetime. It also allows you to compare your risk to that of the average woman of your age and race. The program takes into account the following risk factors: your age (the older a woman is, the greater her risk); age of menarche; your age at the first live birth of a child; whether any first-degree relatives (mother, sister or daughter) have had breast cancer; whether you have had a previous breast biopsy; and finally, whether you have had documented atypical hyperplasia (abnormal cells) on a breast biopsy. Each of these factors is evenly weighed. This may surprise you, since, like most women, you may view a family history of breast cancer as the most important risk factor. You have to remember, though, that as many as 80% of breast cancers occur in women with no family history of the disease.

Since I cannot include a computer program in this book, you'll need to examine your own risk factors with your physician, who can compute your risk, or you can log on to www.nolvadex.com or call 1-800-34-LIFE-4 and compute your risk yourself. If your five-year risk is 1.67% or higher, you are considered at high risk of developing breast cancer and perhaps should consider using tamoxifen as a preventive therapy. Unfortunately, the Gail model does not include some important risk factors that I've already discussed, including a personal history of breast cancer, ductal carcinoma in situ or lobular carcinoma in situ, as well as obesity and alcohol use. Moreover, it doesn't consider whether you have any second-degree relatives with breast cancer or the age at which any relative was diagnosed with breast cancer (a diagnosis before age 50 can be particularly significant). Finally, the model doesn't incorporate age of menopause or whether a woman has used HRT. So there may be some women who, according to the Gail model, fall into the no-risk category when in fact they are at risk.

The recent Breast Cancer Prevention Trial demonstrated that five years of tamoxifen use decreased risk of developing breast cancer in women age 49 or younger by 44% (among women ages 50 to 59, the decrease in risk was 51%; for those 60 or older, 55%). Risk was also reduced by 56% in women with a history of lobular carcinoma in situ, and by 86% among those with atypical hyperplasia. Overall, tamoxifen reduced the risk of noninvasive breast cancer by half. It reduced the occurrence of estrogen-receptor-positive tumors (those whose growth is stimulated by estrogen) by 69%, but no difference in the occurrence of estrogen-receptor-negative tumors, the most aggressive type, was seen.

So if this drug is so wonderful, why don't we all just go on it at some point in our forties or fifties? First, we're not sure how long the drug renders protection. The Breast Cancer Prevention Trial followed women for just 69 months. We also don't know whether the type of breast cancer you might develop would be estrogen-receptor positive or negative. Finally, this drug has side effects: It can increase the risk of stroke, pulmonary embolism and deep-vein thrombosis, although in the trials these events occurred more frequently in women age 50 and over. It also more than doubles a woman's risk of endometrial cancer, although the cancer is so rare that a doubling of risk isn't cause for major alarm. Additionally, the cancers caused were localized and easily treatable. You should not try to conceive while on this drug because its effects on a fetus are unknown, and you should be using a nonhormonal means of contraception. Before and certainly after menopause, tamoxifen has been shown to significantly increase hot flashes and bothersome vaginal dryness. But other quality of life issues such as depression, fluid retention, nausea, skin changes, diarrhea, weight gain and weight loss have not been shown to be significantly increased. There may be, however, a marginal increase in development of cataracts among women who take tamoxifen. The good news is that the drug also helps prevent bone loss, and a reduction in hip, wrist and spine fracture has been documented among users, especially those over age 50. At present, doctors are not recommending that tamoxifen be combined with HRT when you become menopausal. Simultaneous use of both therapies has not been sufficiently studied, and their long-term effect is unknown.

An antihormonal cousin of tamoxifen, raloxifene, which is also a selective estrogen-receptor modulator, or SERM, has been shown to decrease breast cancer risk in menopausal women who have osteoporosis. But at this point it has not been proven to reduce the incidence of breast cancer among women at high risk of the disease. An ongoing study is comparing raloxifene to tamoxifen and may give us an alternative breast cancer–preventive therapy, but the results will not be available for a number of years.

Many of my patients at high risk for breast cancer, especially those who have had genetic testing that revealed the presence of a breast cancer gene, have asked me if they might be best off by having both of their healthy breasts removed, a procedure called bilateral prophylactic mastectomy. A recent study found that this radical approach did indeed reduce the incidence of breast cancer by an estimated 90%. (The reason this number isn't 100% is that the surgery cannot guarantee removal of every single breast cell. Some tumors still developed in the chest wall, but they were not associated with metastases.) After 14 years, the risk of death from breast cancer was reduced by up to 94% in very high risk groups, 100% in moderate-risk groups. This is a very major surgery, and although there are excellent methods for reconstructing the breast, the breasts will always lack erogenous sensitivity and "normal" feeling. You have to weigh the effect of this irreversible surgery on your body and body image against how threatened you feel by this disease.

DO MY BREAST IMPLANTS POSE A THREAT TO MY GENERAL HEALTH?

I'm going to have to give you an extended medical "probably not," depending on a fairly complicated compilation of breast augmentation factors: What kind of implants were used? How long have you had them? Are you asking whether they threaten your health now or in the future? And why did you get implants in the first place?

If your implants were inserted in your twenties or thirties, there's a good chance that they are silicone-filled (90% of implants inserted before the early 1990s consisted of a silicone envelope filled with silicone gel; only 10% were filled with saline). However, 1992 was a very bad year for silicone implant manufacturers. That's when the FDA announced that there was a lack of evidence supporting the safety of these implants and ordered the devices taken off the market. The only exception was for use in clinical studies or for women seeking reconstruction after breast cancer surgery. The agency had already received numerous complaints of health risks believed to be associated with the implants, so it asked doctors and manufacturers to report adverse reactions. Between 1985 and 1996 there were more than 100,000 reports of problems possibly linked to silicone implants and more than 23,000 involving saline-filled implants. The FDA, surgeons, epidemiologists, advocacy groups, implant manufacturers and of course lawyers are still debating these reports, leaving you in an unfortunate state of gel- or even saline-filled murkiness. Here's what we do know:

Surgical Risks
Even though you've already dealt with these risks when you initially had this surgery, you should know about them in case you're considering having old implants replaced with new ones. They include:

• Infection
• Hematoma (a large blood clot that may require surgical drainage)
• Hemorrhage
• Skin necrosis (tissue death due to insufficient blood flow)

Implant Risks

- *Capsular contracture* (hardening of the breast due to scar tissue). This occurs more frequently if the implant has a smooth-walled outer shell rather than a textured one, and if it is filled with saline instead of silicone. There's little good published data, but on average, about half of women with implants will have this problem.
- *Leak or rupture.* This can range from pin-size holes to large tears. But even when the outer envelope remains intact, silicone can seep or "bleed" into surrounding tissue. The silicone shell becomes weaker over time, and studies have shown that an average of 89% of women can expect to have both implants intact after 8 years, 51% after 12 years but only 5% after 20 years. The rates of implant disruption appear to be similar in women with and without symptoms such as discomfort, hardening or an unevenness in the contour of the implant.
- *Loss of sensation in the nipple or breast.* Exactly how often this problem happens after implants are inserted under breast tissue is unknown.
- *Shifting of the implant from its original position.* Here again, the number of women who experience this problem is not known.
- *Interference with mammography reading that may hamper cancer detection.* Depending on the way the mammogram is performed, there is a 25% to 35% decrease in the visible areas of breast tissue. The view may be further limited by scarring around the implant and hardening of the implant, which curtails compression in the first place. (Because mammograms have been associated with implant rupture, there is a tendency to limit compression and perhaps compromise the quality of the picture.)

General Health Risks

This may be one of the most controversial issues I have to deal with in your decade, if not in the entire book. There is a huge discrepancy between what our legal system has deemed a liability risk and the risks that are validated by scientific data. The chief concern is that rupture, leakage or even the presence of intact silicone implants in the body puts women at increased risk of autoimmunelike disorders. Symptoms that have been suggested to be associated with an autoimmune reaction include joint pain and swelling, skin tightness, redness or swelling, swelling of hands and feet, headaches, rash, swollen glands, muscle weakness, fatigue, general achiness, increased vulnerability to colds and flu, hair loss, memory problems, irritable bowel syndrome and nausea and vomiting. Many of the well-publicized reports linking silicone implants with health problems were anecdotal and involved small numbers of women. This evidence, however, was enough to support a major lawsuit against one implant company, Dow Corning, which eventually settled for a sum of $4.4 billion. But even as this suit was under way, five major studies and at least as many minor ones found no association or only an insignificant link between silicone implants and these autoimmunelike responses. Some researchers have suggested that there may be a small group of women with genetic factors that make them susceptible to a syndrome resulting from exposure to silicone. The problem is that this constellation of symptoms occurs in just 1% of the general population, so even if the risk is doubled, it's still a fairly rare condition—one that would only show up in studies of tens of thousands of women.

So at this point, if you have no symptoms of an autoimmune disorder, you don't have to live with the sense of impending immune disaster. Nor do you have to have your implants removed for this reason alone. (A note of reassurance: Your risk of breast cancer is no higher than that of implant-free women.)

A Plan for Implant Monitoring and Maintenance

Your implant monitoring and your breast monitoring have to go—you should excuse the expression—hand in hand. When you get your mammogram, make sure it's done by a technician who has experience with implants and knows how to position your breasts properly. But by all means do not let fear of compression and rupture dissuade you from having your annual X-ray. Rupture is rare, and you don't want to allow one foreign body to impair early detection of another truly foreign body: cancer.

Although mammography is the state of the art for breast cancer monitoring, it isn't the definitive method for detecting ruptures or leaks. If globules of silicone have spread into breast tissue, or the implant is weakened and bulging, a mammogram should pick it up. But the test will not show small tears or seepage, nor will it allow your doctor to assess the integrity of the implant's outer shell. Ultrasound can detect rupture 50% to 74% of the time. But the state of the art in terms of implant evaluation is magnetic resonance imaging, which will depict a leak inside or outside the capsule wall in more than 90% of cases.

Should you be screened for rupture? And what should you do if it's found? Certainly if you have local complications such as breast deformity, pain or silicone "lumps" outside of the implant, you should be checked. If rupture is confirmed, the implant should be removed. Some plastic surgeons recommend prophylactic removal of implants within eight years of placement to avoid the increasing risk of rupture as the device ages. This would negate the need for monitoring with ultrasound or MRI. On the other hand, it means having surgery every eight years. Women who have systemwide autoimmune-type symptoms may want to be screened for rupture, or may simply elect to have the implants removed in hopes that their symptoms will dissipate.

And what if you fall within the majority of women who have no symptoms or signs of rupture? It now appears that an awful lot of these women may actually have a silent rupture. Whether screening is either advisable or feasible remains, well, questionable. Based on information available in 1992, an FDA panel recommended that if an implant is known to have ruptured, it should be removed. So you and your doctor will have to weigh the risks and benefits of this expensive testing, realizing that if a rupture is discovered, you may feel compelled to have surgery.

Note: If your implants have become capsulated and your breasts feel very hard, you should not undergo any form of manual compression of the breast in an attempt to break up the scar tissue. This "closed capsulotomy" can cause rupture and tears. Your choice is either to live with this scarring or have the implants removed.

Finally, with any implant removal comes the question: Should they be replaced with a new pair? If implants are not reinserted, your breasts will sag, and while you can have them surgically reduced or lifted, extensive visible scarring will probably result. Many surgeons today replace silicone-filled implants with saline ones, but these too can rupture or undergo encapsulation.

WHAT TESTS SHOULD I HAVE?

Here are the examinations, tests and procedures I advise for my patients in their forties:

Examination/test/procedure	How often
Blood pressure	At least every two years
Cholesterol test	Nonfasting total and HDL test every five years

Examination/test/procedure	How often
Fasting plasma glucose	Every three years
Thyroid hormone test	Every five years
Pelvic exam & Pap smear	Annually; Pap at doctor's discretion after three negative tests
Rectal exam	Annually
STD testing	At your/your doctor's discretion
Clinical (physician) breast exam	Annually
Breast self-exam	Monthly
Mammogram	Annually
Electrocardiogram	Every five years
Bone mineral density	At your/your doctor's discretion
Immunizations	Tetanus booster every 10 years
Eye exam	Baseline exam at age 40, then every three years
Skin exam by dermatologist	Every two years
Skin self-exam	Annually

WHAT CAN GO WRONG AT MY AGE?

Weight Gain

Many of us in this decade begin to feel that the "F" in forty (and, eventually, fifty), stands for *fat*. The pounds just seem to appear, and their insidious addition that begins in our twenties now becomes very apparent as we collectively cry, "Where have all our flat stomachs gone?" Understanding and treating obesity remains one of medicine's greatest challenges. We (patients and doctors) approach this condition burdened by the weight of self-guilt and societal blame. After all, isn't this really just a personal failure to control one's appetite, eat the right foods, get off that ever-widening tush and exercise? No! Weight gain is caused by a huge number of factors that range from physiologic, neurologic, biochemical, environmental and psychosocial to cultural and, of course, genetic.

If your family pattern is to be obese or to gain weight with age, the genes you inherited may be responsible. The amount of food you need to achieve satiety or the way your body metabolizes calories is overwhelmingly genetic. Anger at your weighty relatives won't help. They, and you, are the result of evolutionary changes in metabolism that allowed for important conservation of calories through drought, famine and war. The thin were simply less likely to survive. Pursuit of food—you know, the hunting, gathering, farming and other physical stuff that your ancestors spent most of their time doing—has also programmed your vital needs and metabolic deeds. Cars, supermarkets, restaurants and fast food have just not been factored into your genetic metabolism. Whatever we as modern women do about our individual energy requirements, the laws of physics still prevail; the calories we put into our bodies need to be used up, or we end up storing them. For every 3,500 calories we neglect to burn off, we accumulate one pound. Here's how we use up those calories and what happens as we get older:

1. **Metabolic rate.** This is the energy needed to maintain basic body functions while we rest. It constitutes 60% to 70% of our daily caloric expenditure. Unfortunately, this decreases 4% to 5% with each decade, or by about 100 calories in our forties and another 100 calories in our fifties.
2. **Eating.** Our entire digestive process takes only about 10% of our calories. Maybe we should chew more (our ancestors did).
3. **Physical activity.** This can range from 10% of our total calories if we're sedentary to 50% if we're training for a marathon.

Many of us become less physical in our forties. Menopausal women also tend to decrease their leisure-time physical activity when compared to women of the same age who are not yet menopausal (if we're having wild hormonal fluctuations in perimenopause, which affects our emotions and sleep, we're also less likely to be in the mood to exercise). And, to add hormonal insult to poundage, as our estrogen levels fluctuate and then decline, we begin to lose lean body mass. Fat replaces muscle, and since fat doesn't metabolize calories as well as muscle, the unused calories get deposited as—you guessed it—more fat, and we've entered a vicious cycle. If our intake of calories exceeds our energy expenditure by just 2% a day, after one year we'll gain five pounds.

One more female weight factor is pregnancy. We average a three-pound gain with the birth of each child. When you put this all together, it renders the following stats: The typical American woman puts on 20 pounds between ages 25 and 50. At least half the adults in this country are overweight or obese, and women are more prone than men to plump with age.

Medical science is a mean (I'll refrain from adding the term *lean*) machine when it comes to counseling us on what constitutes being overweight. In the past we used height-weight tables based on a 1983 weigh-in of women with indoor clothing and one-inch heels who were autocratically assigned to averages that were deemed medically okay. But doctors and life insurance companies eventually determined that these averages were overages, and the lowest mortality rate was found in women who weighed 10% to 20% *less* than average and who, most important, did not gain weight after the age of 18. The Harvard Nurses' study found that women who gained *only* 11 to 17 pounds doubled their risk of diabetes and increased their risk of coronary artery disease by 50%. If they gained 17 to 25 pounds, diabetes increased by 250%, and if they exceeded a 45-pound weight gain in their fifties, they increased their risk of hypertension and heart disease by a factor of 3 (300%), diabetes by a factor of 10, and gallstones by a factor of 4, compared to women who gained only 10 pounds. Moreover, one-third of cancer deaths in these obese nurses, especially breast, ovarian, uterine and colon cancer, and half of cardiovascular deaths (heart attack and stroke) were attributed to obesity.

We are no longer supposed to just get on a scale and compare ourselves to the women in the old height-weight tables. Two other methods of weight computation that you can use to calculate your body's fat correctness are the Body Mass Index (BMI) and Waist-to-Hip Ratio. The former accounts for height and correlates well with your body fat and health risks; the latter is a reflection of the amount of weight or fat you have accumulated in your critical abdominal region. To compute your BMI, divide your weight in pounds by your height in inches squared, then multiply the total by 704.5.

If your BMI is 25 or greater, you are in the overweight category. If your BMI is 30 or more, you are considered obese, and if it's 35 or more, extremely obese. (Use a calculator or just look at the following table to get an approximation of where you fit.)

BODY MASS INDEX

Height	Normal weight (at or less than)	Overweight (at or above)	Obese (at or above)
4'10"	115	119	143
4'11"	119	124	148
5'	123	128	153
5'1"	127	132	158
5'2"	131	136	164
5'3"	135	141	169
5'4"	140	145	174
5'5"	144	150	180
5'6"	148	155	186
5'7"	153	159	191
5'8"	158	164	197
5'9"	162	169	203
5'10"	167	174	209
5'11"	172	179	215
6'	177	184	221
6'1"	182	189	227
6'2"	186	194	233
6'3"	192	200	240
6'4"	197	205	246

The weight picture gets even more complicated, since total fat content may not be as important as where the fat has accumulated. The worst type of weight gain is measured by your belt. If your waist-to-hip ratio (your waist measurement divided by your hip measurement) is above 0.8, your apple shape is more than cosmetically rotten. It means that you have an increased risk of heart disease. Ratios of 0.80 to 0.84 increase your risk by 26%, 0.84 to 0.9 by 50%, and if you are above 0.9, your risk rises by a whopping 330%! In the future, you might be able to just use a tape measure around your waist to calculate your risk. A new study suggests that if your waist measures 30 inches or more, your risk of coronary artery disease doubles, while a waist measurement of 38 triples risk.

It's not just a matter of whether you carry fat around your waist—it's a matter of how deeply it's deposited. Internal abdominal fat appears to be associated with insulin resistance and subsequent development of diabetes and heart disease, whereas the fat under your skin (which you can pinch or cinch with your belt) seems to be less dangerous. So those fat-fold measurements that were so popular at our gyms may be less than prophetic.

By now, between getting on the scale, standing as tall as possible for your height calculations, and sucking in your gut to measure your waist, you may have found that no matter how you arrive at the final figure, your figure is overly ample. The question is whether you have indelibly set your future health risks with the pounds you've gained since age 18, or will losing weight at this point in your life make a difference?

The answer to the latter is a resounding "Yes," and to spur you on in your weight- and health-altering quest, here are some encouraging statistics: Every 2.2 pounds of weight loss can prolong your life by three to four months. Weight loss will decrease development or severity of diabetes, hypertension, coronary heart disease, high cholesterol, joint disease in the hip and knees and gallbladder disease. And you don't have to come down to what we used to call "ideal" body weight (unfortunately, some of the waist data I gave you makes it appear that only a Barbie doll has the ideal body). We really have to rephrase our goal and call it a "healthier" weight, or the weight at which the complications of obesity are reduced or avoided. A 10% weight loss can produce a significant drop in blood pressure after just six months. And a 5% to 8% weight decrease can reduce triglyceride levels and raise good HDL levels. Bringing your weight down may also have a positive effect on your heart, reducing the thickness and mass of the chambers that are valiantly trying to pump blood to your overweight body. Another incentive comes from those joints that bear the brunt of your weight: A reduction of 2 BMI units (or about 11.2 pounds) will decrease your risk of knee osteoarthritis by more than half. Weight loss can also reverse snoring and the associated decreased breathing, or apnea, during sleep.

So here's what you can do about weight gain: If your current weight is healthy and you don't want it to rise with age or menopause, you should decrease your caloric intake by 100 to 200 calories a day from what you consumed in the previous decade. In your total caloric count, maintain a healthy balance. That means less than 30% fat; less than 10% calories from saturated fat; fewer than 300 milligrams of cholesterol; at least five servings of vegetables and fruits; and six servings of cereals, pasta and legumes. Make sure your complex carbs come from whole grains rather than processed ones. My advice is to stay away from the white stuff: white bread, rice and potatoes. Depending on how they're processed and cooked, these can have a high glycemic index, which means they raise blood sugar and call for a greater outpouring of insulin and fat. Carbs that have a low glycemic index and are better for your fats and fat deposition include whole wheat pasta, whole grain breads, beans, peas, barley and certain fruits such as apples. Make sure you get 25 to 35 grams of dietary fiber (which you will achieve if you eat whole grains, legumes, fruits and vegetables) and either don't drink alcohol or limit your consumption to less than one ounce a day.

You also need to continue or start exercising. Combine both aerobic exercise, which will burn calories, with resistance training to maintain or acquire muscle mass. The former can be accomplished with just 30 minutes of exercise a day: walking briskly, cycling, swimming, doing general calisthenics or playing tennis; you can even "cheat" and aerobicize in three 10-minute intervals. For the latter, invest in barbells and some ankle weights; use them for arm and leg reps for 15 minutes three times a week. And, your back permitting, add sit-ups to this exercise routine.

Finally, consider controlling your fluctuating hormones with low-dose birth control pills in perimenopause, and estrogen replacement therapy if you are menopausal. Women who take estrogen after menopause develop less abdominal obesity than women who do not.

If you are overweight and want to do something about it, consider a long-term plan. Crash diets are doomed. You can't sustain tremendous diet restrictions for long, and when you stop, the weight will come back. Your body is consistent, even if your diet isn't, and when you seriously reduce calories it will fight hard to maintain the weight and fat content it's used to. It learns to burn fewer calories while you are dieting, and when you go back to more normal eating and rest from overly rigorous exercise, the pounds will not only return, they may increase. Your weight yo-yo doesn't come just up to its previous level; it often goes higher.

Diet plans that promise instant svelteness and eternal happiness or ads that show you skinny models consuming foods that are low-fat and imply that you will never get fat as long as you consume these products are too good to be true. My response to all of them is: "It's the calories, stupid." If you want to get to a healthy weight, you need to develop a low-calorie but nutritionally adequate eating plan, combined with a sustainable level of physical activity. This should then be followed by a balanced way of eating for years to come.

During your weight-losing phase, your goal should be to drop no more than one to two pounds a week. Since one pound of body fat contains

3,500 calories, that means it's necessary to reduce the amount you consume by 500 calories a day to get a one-pound-a-week weight loss (or
1,000 calories to lose two pounds). The following equation will help you
determine how many calories you need in order to either maintain your
weight or lose it. You should never consume fewer than 900 calories a day
without medical supervision.

*Calculating Daily Calorie Requirements for Weight Maintenance and
Weight Loss*

YOUR DAILY CALORIE REQUIREMENT FOR WEIGHT MAINTENANCE EQUALS:

[(7 × your body weight in kilograms) + 800] × 1.2 (if you're not very
active), 1.4 (if you're moderately active) or 1.6 (if you're very active)

(To find your weight in kg, divide your weight in lbs by 2.2)

If you want to lose one pound a week, subtract 500 calories from this number; to lose two pounds a week, subtract 1,000 calories.

Here's a sample calculation for a sedentary woman with a height of 5'2"
inches and weight of 165 pounds (75 kilograms):

(7 × 75) + 800 × 1.2 = 1,590 (maintenance); 1,090 (to lose 1 lb per
week)

Obviously, if you want to raise the number that is listed under your energy
requirement so that you don't have to subtract all of those great-tasting
calories, you simply have to raise your activity level. Moderate activity
would be considered 30 minutes of the following.

• Walking briskly
• Cycling for pleasure
• Swimming, moderate effort
• General calisthenics or conditioning exercises
• Rapid sports or table tennis
• Golf (but walk, don't ride, the course)
• Fishing with standing and casting (and, hopefully, pulling in some fish)
• Canoeing, leisurely pace
• Housecleaning (our surroundings should get something out of this)

- Mowing the lawn while pushing (not riding) a power mower
- Home repair
- Painting

High activity includes 30 minutes of:

- Walking uphill or with a load
- Cycling fast or racing (more than 10 mph)
- Swimming, fast
- Conditioning exercise such as stair-climbing at a fast pace or using a ski machine
- Singles tennis or racquetball
- Fishing in a stream
- Canoeing, rapidly (3 to 4 mph)
- Moving furniture
- Mowing a lawn with a hand mower

So now that you know how much to eat, the next and, for most of our tastebuds, most crucial question is what to eat. Here is where many authors deliver an ode to protein or even fat, while putting up hex signs to ward off carbs. I don't totally disagree with the protein part. As a matter of fact, we need more protein when we lower our caloric levels, because some of the amino acids that make up protein are needed to maintain our blood glucose levels and provide energy. Although many of these diets, if rigorously followed, will initially induce a fairly rapid weight loss, they may also cause dehydration, breakdown of protein and loss of muscle mass. The "eat fat and eliminate carbs" approach can lead to an unhealthy metabolic state and raise lipids, which ultimately can cause heart damage. So, eater beware. At some point you should reintroduce the food groups that are known to be healthy: fruits, whole grains and red, yellow and leafy green vegetables. Sugar, processed starch and saturated fat can stay out. You do need a minimum of fat, 3.6 grams a day. The USDA Food Guide Pyramid is still the best way to get the right proportion of food groups, but go to the minimal number for each.

As you lose weight, your kidneys will excrete more fluid, so it is important that you hydrate with more than one liter of water a day.

The key to getting all of your nutritional needs met without oversupplying weight-gaining calories is portion control. Most of use have the wrong idea of what constitutes a portion. More is better, or at least we are getting more for our money. Hence the jumbo size of our burgers, fries and "gulps" of huge, sugar-filled sodas. This American largesse has enlarged our waists and endangered our health. We wonder how the French or Italian women manage to look so good. Well, take a look at the amount of food on their plates! Their portions are what we would consider appetizer size. So think of what you eat as a combination of appetizers. Spread them out; eat them six times a day rather than the full-size American meal consumed three times a day. A serving of protein is not one-quarter of a chicken; it's only three ounces, or half of a chicken breast, or one chicken leg with thigh. Nor is it a whole steak, but the equivalent of a piece of cooked meat that is 3 × 3 inches and ¼ inch thick. Fish should have the same dimensions, or if it's flaked, it should fill a cup. Milk products are also excellent sources of protein and carbs; remember that a portion is 8 ounces of milk, one cup of nonfat yogurt, one-half cup of nonfat cottage cheese, or one ounce of cut cheese. When you eat eggs, if you want to maintain the protein and cut the cholesterol, use two egg whites instead of one large whole egg. In the fruit and vegetable department, a serving of fruit is one medium fruit, three-fourths cup of fruit juice or one-half cup of chopped or cooked vegetables or canned fruit (but that usually contains a lot of sugar). So if you have a

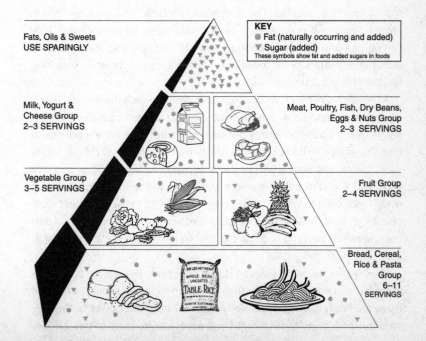

KEY
● Fat (naturally occurring and added)
▼ Sugar (added)
These symbols show fat and added sugars in foods

Fats, Oils & Sweets
USE SPARINGLY

Milk, Yogurt &
Cheese Group
2–3 SERVINGS

Meat, Poultry, Fish, Dry Beans,
Eggs & Nuts Group
2–3 SERVINGS

Vegetable Group
3–5 SERVINGS

Fruit Group
2–4 SERVINGS

Bread, Cereal,
Rice & Pasta
Group
6–11
SERVINGS

small glass of fruit juice, one apple, a small salad and the equivalent of one cup of vegetables (steamed broccoli will do it), you've had your five healthy servings. As far as those six or more servings of grainy stuff, a portion equals just one slice of bread, one-half cup of nugget or bud-type cereal, one-half cup of cereal such as oatmeal, and only one cup (not a bowl) of cereal flakes. You can also get your grains through one cup of cooked (hopefully whole grain) rice or pasta. Starchy vegetables also count as grains, but a portion is just one-half cup (potatoes, corn, yams or sweet potatoes). So think small or cute, or whatever brings you to three ounces or half-cups full when you prepare your meals. Remember, you don't have to be a member of the "Clean Plate Club." If need be, eat half of what you're served by chefs or overgenerous hosts.

Also try to keep yourself out of temptation crises. Eliminate junk, fatty foods or sweets in your house, or at least make sure they are out of sight. Stock up on and keep healthy foods visible and limit your eating to one or two rooms in the house (don't eat in the bedroom, family room or while watching television).

Don't start out with unrealistic expectations. Go for a decrease of 5% of your body weight, and once you've lost that much, you can set a new goal of an additional 5%. Reward yourself with a new dress or something other than a chocolate sundae. The true health rewards from your new lower weight come with maintenance. So if you've been on a less-than-1,200-calorie diet and lost those pounds, you can increase your caloric intake, but only by 100 to 150 calories a day. Make sure you maintain your new level of physical activity.

Although I don't want to discount your desire to look thinner, ultimately your physical fitness may have a greater impact on your mortality than losing weight. If you are obese with a BMI of greater than 30, a moderate to high fitness level will lower your mortality risk by as much as 70%. If you're "just" overweight with a BMI of 25 to 30, you can benefit by as much as 50%, and if you're not overweight at all, you will still lower your risk of dying (compared to women in your age and weight range who don't exercise) by at least 50% with moderate exercise. In simple terms, the difference between being fit and unfit at *any* weight means a difference of at least 50% in mortality rates.

Having told you what you can do on your own, I now have to address the issue of better dieting through chemistry (e.g., diet pills), or, to be more medically correct, antiobesity agents. I have the power of the prescription pad, so why shouldn't I just save you from all of this calorie-counting, food-grouping deprivation and physical exertion? Isn't there a pill that will control your appetite, speed up your metabolism and let you continue the pleasure of good-tasting fat intake without the associated weight gain? Many of my patients feel that svelte is svelte and it doesn't matter if it's natural, pharmaceutical or surgical. The drug companies would love to patent an ideal medicinal cure for obesity. And I would pre-scribe it if it were ideal. But antiobesity drugs are not one-course therapies like antibiotics. Whatever you take, you'll have to continue taking, and once you stop, the weight will usually return. Long-term studies need to be conducted to show whether these drugs work, or if they work but cause serious side effects. We've been disappointed and harmed in the past.

The medical miracles of fenfluramine (Pondimin, the "Fen" in "Fen-Phen") and dexfenfluramine (Redux) ended in a disastrous medical recall. The pharmacology of these agents was theoretically wonderful. Our feed-ing behavior is controlled through neurotransmitters that include serotonin, norepinephrine and dopamine. When they are released by the brain, they either decrease appetite or increase the sense of satiety. Pondimin and its newer cousin Redux caused serotonin levels to rise, and were effective in controlling appetite, but as time went on and women became thinner on these drugs, reports increased that those who took them were at risk for developing a thickening of the heart valves and serious heart disease. (One study found that one-third of patients on these drugs had cardiac abnormalities, but subsequent reports have found a much lower, even insignificant, risk of cardiac damage.) But the damage was done. The drugs were withdrawn from the market, and many of my patients, instead of worrying about the possibility that these medications could result in their becoming skinny corpses, bemoaned the loss of the drugs that were making them thin. I did worry, and I made a lot of referrals for cardiac testing.

A second drug, phentermine (Adipex-P or Fastin), which was prescribed together with fenfluramine, remains on the market. It raises dopamine and norepinephrine levels and can also reduce appetite and increase sati-ety, but when taken alone does not seem to curb carbohydrate intake. If you had major success with Fen-Phen in the past and can't keep your weight down without it, you might want to have your doctor prescribe just the phen part. Some diet specialists are now substituting Prozac or other SSRIs that can increase serotonin levels in combination with phentermine, but there are little data on this technique. Because it may foster a serotonin overload, which is what could have caused the coronary valve disease seen with Fen-Phen, this may be hazardous to your future heart health.

A more recently approved antiobesity agent that selectively decreases reuptake of serotonin as well as norepinephrine and dopamine, but doesn't cause their release, is sibutramine (Meridia). Meridia has been found to decrease food intake by enhancing feelings of satiety and, at least in animals, it also raises energy expenditure. Studies have shown that for patients on low- or very low calorie diets, weight loss with Meridia was significantly better than with a placebo (averaging about 5.5% to 7.5% after a year). Most of the weight loss occurred in the first six months and remained essentially unchanged thereafter. The problem is that when the drug was discontinued, the weight came back, so the "thereafter" if you're taking these medications may need to be "forever after."

Now, on to the possible side effects (you *knew* this was coming). Meridia can increase both systolic and diastolic blood pressure by 1 to 2 mm/Hg and pulse rate by approximately four beats per minute. This is not very much and can probably be ignored, but in some patients, blood pressure and pulse rate can go much higher, and this obviously has to be monitored carefully. If you already have a history of poorly controlled hypertension, abnormal heart rhythm, coronary artery disease or stroke, you should not use this medication or should do so only under strict medical supervision. There is also a warning that you should not take it if you are already on a MAO inhibitor antidepressant or use any recreational drugs.

Unlike the medications that work on our brain neurotransmitters, the latest antiobesity drug doesn't act centrally at all. In fact, it barely enters the body. This is orlistat (Xenical), which, when ingested, remains in the gut, where it blocks absorption of about one-third of fat intake. Because the fat remains in the stool, it causes some unpleasant side effects such as flatulence, increased defecation, abdominal pain, greasy stools and, probably the most embarrassing of all, fecal incontinence (this occurs in about 2% of those using this drug). The more fat you consume, the worse these adverse symptoms, so simply being on the drug may be an incentive to cut the fat and help you lose weight. But even though about 30% of fat is not absorbed, weight loss is improved only by about 5%. The good news, however, is that weight loss that occurs with orlistat is also accompanied by beneficial lipid changes above and beyond what we would expect to see with weight reduction alone. And even after two years, orlistat continues to help keep the weight off (although, once more, pounds rebound if the drug is discontinued). Because vitamins A, D and E are absorbed with fat, you need to supplement these while on this therapy.

This is what is currently available to help you lose weight. But there will be more. Research continues furiously as pharmaceutical companies try to develop the right drug for your pounds and their profit. You don't necessarily have to resort to these products to lose the 5% to 10% body weight that can dramatically impact your health and longevity. Don't let the media (or even this long section in my book) cause you to despair. You can repair the damage that weight gain has caused your present and future health.

High Blood Pressure

High blood pressure rapidly becomes a "woman's thing" as we begin the next half of our lives. Over 50 million Americans have hypertension, and 60% are women. Although "just" 11% of Caucasian women are hypertensive in their forties, the number rises to 33% in our fifties and becomes a whopping 50% in our sixties. The stats are much worse for African-American women, one-third of whom are already hypertensive in their forties and whose ranks swell to nearly 75% in their sixties. These troubling statistics become even more alarming when we consider the fact that one-third of women with hypertension are unaware of their condition, and only one-fifth have received adequate therapy. Our estrogen probably protects us from hypertension during our reproductive years, so that we're far less likely than men to develop this disease. But once we're menopausal, we establish parity, and by our fifites, we overtake the opposite sex in the incidence of this disorder. Not only are we more likely to have the problem, we're also more prone to complications such as stroke (59% of women versus 39% of men). We are twice as likely to develop heart attack and heart failure (this is especially true in women whose blood pressure does not decrease at night, a phenomenon called "non-dipping"). The Harvard Nurses' Health Study showed that women with hypertension were six times more likely to have a fatal heart attack than women whose blood pressure was normal.

Based on this awesome data, it certainly behooves us to make sure that this silent disorder is diagnosed. So here is a blood pressure primer: When your blood pressure is checked, two numbers are given. The first (or to be mathematically precise, the nominator) is your systolic pressure. It represents the pressure in your vessels when your heart contracts. The second number (or denominator) is the diastolic pressure and shows the resting pressure in your arteries when your heart is not contracting. If your arteries are narrowed or partially blocked by plaque (atherosclerosis), or if they are less pliant and thickened (arteriosclerosis), the pressure in your vessels increases, and your heart has to pump harder to force blood through. This can damage and weaken the arteries (and may result in rupture, which, if it occurs in the brain, will lead to stroke), or it can promote the bruising of blood cells so that they clump together and form clots that can then block the blood supply to the heart, brain or kidneys. Heart failure may occur when the muscle of the chamber of the heart that pumps the blood to your body thickens or undergoes hypertrophy, as it pushes harder and harder against those nonpliant vessels (this is termed *left ventricle hypertrophy,* or LVH). If you are obese, your heart has to increase its effort even more, and at some point it can no longer meet your body's demands. Half the women who develop LVH subsequently suffer a heart attack or stroke. To further complicate this tense picture, and your life, if you have other risk factors for cardiovascular disease such as diabetes, high cholesterol, kidney disease or you smoke, you compound your risk for heart failure and heart attack.

You can do something about diagnosing this silent menace: Have your blood pressure checked at least every two years, more frequently if it's elevated or you are under therapy. Make sure it's taken when you are seated and your arms are at heart level. Rest at least five minutes before your blood pressure is taken, and don't smoke or ingest caffeine in the half-hour before your exam. Don't consider one blood pressure reading a complete pass/fail: It's more like a grade in school that, when poor, requires study, in the form of follow-up testing and therapy.

Grade	Systolic Pressure	Diastolic Pressure	Follow-up If No Other Risk Factors	Treatment
Optimal	<120	<80	Recheck in 2 years	None
Normal	<130	<85	Recheck in 2 years	None
High Normal	130–139	85–89	Recheck in 1 year	Lifestyle modification

Hypertension

Stage I	140–159	90–99	Recheck within 2 months	Lifestyle modification (up to 12 months)
Stage II	160–179	100–109	Get evaluation and care within one month	Drug therapy
Stage III	>180	>110	Get evaluation and care immediately	Drug therapy

In the past, women were told to worry only if their diastolic pressure was up. It's now clear that the systolic pressure may be an even more important cardiovascular risk factor and should definitely be aggressively treated even if it's the only value that's high. Don't feel that you are in a state of impending stroke if you are told, after just one reading, that your blood pressure is high. About one-fourth of women diagnosed as having hypertension in a doctor's office have normal readings when at home, a phenomenon known as white coat hypertension. (I suspect that as office care becomes more clinical and less personal, we'll see a burgeoning of such suspicious readings.) So it may be worthwhile for you to invest in a home blood pressure monitor. There are many automated digital devices; the ones that check the pressure in your arm rather than your finger are preferable. You should also occasionally bring the device to your doctor's office to make sure it's properly calibrated.

If your blood pressure falls into the Stage 1 hypertension category, or even it it's high normal, it's time you took the following steps (and as far as exercise goes, *stepping* is literal) to bring these numbers down:

· Increase your aerobic activity to 30 to 45 minutes at least five times a week (rapid walking will do it, as will using a stair-climbing machine, taking step classes or climbing stairs)
· Stop smoking
· Lose weight if you're overweight (just a 10% loss will provide major benefits)

- Reduce your sodium intake to less than 2.6 grams of sodium, or less than 6 grams of sodium chloride (salt) per day (Note: You are more likely to be salt-sensitive if you have a family history of hypertension. Salt restriction alone will lower blood pressure in one-third of women with hypertension, especially African-American women. Don't add salt to your food; look for sodium-free products and avoid salty prepared foods as well as ketchup, soy sauce and monosodium glutamate.)
- Maintain adequate calcium and magnesium intake (1,200 to 1,500 mg of calcium a day and 500 mg of magnesium); use supplements if necessary
- Maintain an adequate potassium intake of 90 millimoles per day
- Limit your alcohol intake to no more than one drink per day
- Reduce your consumption of dietary saturated fat and transfat, as well as cholesterol (A new approach to dietary therapy called the DASH [Dietary Approaches to Stop Hypertension] diet has been found to substantially lower blood pressure. It's rich in fruits, vegetables and fiber, and saturated fat is replaced by low-fat dairy foods.)

If these measures don't reduce your minimally elevated blood pressure in six months to a year, if you have other significant cardiovascular risk factors or if your initial pressure after several readings is greater than 160/100, it's time to consider drug therapy. Proper medication can reduce the incidence of heart attack and stroke as well as death from them by as much as 36%.

The first medication that is usually prescribed is a diuretic and, indeed, this alone may be effective, especially in women over 60 and African-American women. Good news: It may also decrease development of osteoporosis. But when this single therapy is not sufficient, a beta-blocker is usually added. Because one agent can improve the effect of the other, using two drugs may allow you to reduce the doses and the side effects.

There are two other types of medication. The first, angiotensin converting enzyme (ACE) inhibitors, appear to be more potent in white women with hypertension as well as in those with diabetes. The second group of medications are calcium antagonists, which have been shown to work well in African-American women as well as in women with angina (chest pain caused by spasm of arteries in the heart). A final encore to this symphony of available medications: Once you've gone through menopause, estrogen appears to sensitize your system to many of these drugs, so if you add hormone replacement therapy (HRT), you may be able to lower your doses of antihypertensive medication. Hypertension is certainly not a contraindication to use of HRT. And since this disorder is a major risk factor for heart disease, I certainly recommend that you consider HRT in addition to traditional blood pressure therapy for future cardiac protection.

Headaches

Finally—a unisex problem. But is it? The answer is no. Women are two to three times as likely as men to suffer from migraine headaches and are also more prone (to a lesser extent) to develop tension headaches. Hence the separate inclusion of headaches in this book. And since headaches of all kinds peak in our late thirties and forties, it's a fitting end to this chapter (the reading of which, I hope, has not given you a headache). As is the case with most of our bodily discomforts, there are a small multitude of causes for headaches. The most prevalent are *tension headaches,* which almost half of all women experience in this decade. Three percent of us have them chronically, which means the pain occurs more than 15 times a month for at least six months, according to the International Headache Society. (Yes, there is a medical society looking out for our head welfare.) This type of headache is caused by the tightening of muscles in the back of the neck and scalp. The pain is a steady ache without throbbing and occurs on one or frequently both sides of the head. The pain often begins in the afternoon or evening, when the day's tension has accumulated in your muscles. It can last just 30 minutes or up to 7 days! Tension headaches may be made worse by movement, but if you feel nausea or sensitivity to light or sound, you're probably having a migraine. Studies suggest that people with recurrent tension headaches experience more stressful events, are more sensitive to stress and have a lower pain threshold than those lucky individuals who are headache-free.

So aside from avoiding stress and becoming less sensitive to it, what are your options? If your headaches occur occasionally, go for the nonprescription painkiller such as aspirin, acetaminophen, ibuprofen or naproxen sodium. Products that combine painkillers with caffeine seem to be more effective. But beware of success: If you use even low doses of these analgesics almost daily, you may develop a chronic "rebound" headache—and you won't break out of this headache bind until you totally withdraw from all painkillers and caffeine for a few weeks.

If your headaches are chronic, recurring almost daily (and aren't the result of a nonprescription drug), you may need to consider a prescription drug to prevent them. The most effective is amitriptyline, a tricyclic antidepressant. Chronic headaches are certainly depressing, and underlying depression may contribute to them, but this drug increases the pain threshold, and that's why it works so successfully.

Your head pain may also respond to muscle relaxants or antianxiety medications). These can help stop a vicious cycle in which prolonged muscle spasm causes headache and provokes anxiety, which in turn increases pain and muscle tension. Several medications put these benefits together by mixing a painkiller with an antianxiety or muscle relaxant drug. These include Fiorinal and Fiorocette (that also contain caffeine) as well as Axocet and Midrin.

Migraine headaches are the next most common type of headache, occurring in up to one-fourth of women, with the highest prevalence after puberty and again between the ages of 35 and 45. Women are two to three times more likely than men to be *migraineurs*. Their agony generally lasts from 4 to 72 hours. If a family member suffers migraines, your chance of having the headaches is four times greater than normal.

Migraines are pulsating, occur on one side of the head and are aggravated by movement. They really make you feel sick, with nausea and even vomiting. Light and sound may intensify the pain. There are two types of migraines—the more frequent (brilliantly known as "common") migraine and the less frequent one, migraine with aura, which occurs in one-third of sufferers. An aura consists of vision changes (you might see bright or dark spots) and numbness on one side of the body. These symptoms usually develop over several minutes and can last up to an hour before the headache strikes.

Doctors used to give a very simplistic explanation for this type of headache, attributing the aura to a constriction of blood vessels around the brain, and the headache to the vessels' subsequent swelling. But neurophysiologists feel we aren't giving migraine its due unless we talk about something called "cortical spreading depression" (CSD). This is not a source of unhappiness, but a wave of depolarization or "depression" of electric brain cell activity that the researchers feel causes the aura. The ensuing headache is believed to be due to activation of fibers that run through the trigeminal nerve, a major cranial nerve that supplies sensation to the front half of the head. It sends signals to the large central brain vessels as well as the smaller ones in the outer lining of the brain (the dura).

Brain proteins then released from the nerve fibers cause the vessels to swell and fluid from these vessels to flow out into the surrounding tissue. (I know this description is painful.) But the therapies I've described above are based on their ability to prevent release of the neuroproteins by the trigeminal nerve and block the inflammation and swelling of the blood vessels. This cascade of events can be instigated by fluctuating estrogen levels. Stabilizing these levels with estrogen, either in the form of birth control pills (see page 60) or hormone replacements (see page 215) may prevent the headaches' onset.

I would be committing a neurological injustice if I didn't briefly include some other types of headaches in this section. So here they are, with a desription of the cause and treatment of each:

Headache Type	Symptoms	Prevention/Treatment
Cluster headache	Extreme pain near eye; tearing of eye, nose; flushing of face. Pain often develops during sleep and may last for several hours.	Prevent with prescription steroids, ergot medications, calcium-channel blockers and lithium; treat attacks with oxygen, ergot medications, sumatriptan (Imitrex) or intranasal anesthetic.
Temporal arteritis	Boring, burning or jabbing pain caused by inflammation of the temporal arteries. Pain, often near ear, during chewing. Rare before age 50.	Steroids after diagnosis confirmed by biopsy.

Headache Type	Symptoms	Prevention/Treatment
Sinus headache	Pain across nose-bridge that often grows worse over the course of the day. May be accompanied by fever, congestion.	Treat infection with antibiotics; relieve pain with decongestants.
Caffeine withdrawal headache	Throbbing pain occurring for several days after consumption of large amounts of caffeine.	Prevent by avoiding excess caffeine.
Exertion headache	Brief, pain episodes following physical activity, such as exercise or intercourse, or after sneezing or coughing.	Identify the cause of headaches, then prevent with alternative forms of exercise. Avoid jarring exercise. Treat pain with aspirin or propranolol.
Eye strain headache	Pain on both sides of forehead caused by eye strain.	Prevent by correcting vision.
Hypertension headache	Morning headache that diminishes over the course of the day; pain may occur in a "headband" pattern.	Prevent and treat by controlling blood pressure.
Arthritis headache	Pain in back of head or neck that worsens with movement.	Anti-inflammatory drugs and muscle relaxants.

Headache Type	Symptoms	Prevention/Treatment
Aneurysm	Sudden migraine-like headache that may become unbearable with double vision, stiff neck or even unconsciousness.	Prevent by controlling blood pressure; discovered early, aneurysm can be treated with surgery.
Tumor	Progressively worsening pain, disturbances in vision, speech, personality, balance or coordination. Extremely rare.	If possible, treat with surgery or radiotherapy.

Most of these headaches can be diagnosed and treated without major tests such as MRIs or CT scans. But there are some symptoms that require a workup, and you may need to get to your doctor (or a hospital) quickly. These include aura symptoms that always occur on the same side of your body, especially if they continue for more than an hour. A sudden change in the duration or frequency of your migraines also requires a doctor's attention. Get immediate help if you experience a sudden, unbearable headache that causes double vision or stiff neck to make sure that the cause is not an aneurysm, prestroke or hemorrhage. The same goes for headaches associated with blurred vision (not seeing spots), speech problems, seizures or difficulty with balance, which should be thoroughly investigated to rule out the rare possibility of a brain tumor.

These are words of caution and are not meant to cause you to react the way my own daughter does: Every time she gets a severe headache she calls to inform me that she probably has an aneurysm!

MY TOP 10 LIST FOR STAYING HEALTHY IN YOUR FORTIES

1. Stop smoking.
2. Decrease your daily caloric intake by 100 to 200 calories.
3. Exercise regularly (30 minutes of moderate activity almost every day).
4. Substitute complex carbohydrates (whole grains, fruits and vegetables) for simple ones such as white bread, potatoes and white rice.
5. Take a multivitamin and consume 1,200 mg of calcium from foods or supplements daily.
6. Moderate your alcohol and caffeine consumption as well as your sun exposure.
7. Establish destressing routines such as hot baths, meditation, reading and other pleasurable activities.
8. Seek help if stress or depression becomes unmanageable.
9. Build and maintain strong emotional bonds with your family and mate.
10. Cultivate and express your sexuality.

YOUR FIFTIES

BY THE TIME we get over the shock of becoming forty, we've reached the big five-oh. My totally nonmedical advice is to take this birthday for all it's worth—begin with major moaning (so you get great presents) and end it with a great party. And then, lo and behold, once the festivities are over, you wake up the next day realizing you're no different and you can now progress from dreading to dealing with and enjoying the rest of your life.

There's no question that this decade is dominated by menopause. Estrogen depletion has been blamed for every bodily change, symptom and illness that women experience in their fifties. The expression "It's your hormones, my dear" is often used as a diagnosis in lieu of blood tests for anemia, diabetes, autoimmune disease, thyroid dysfunction and electrolyte imbalance as well as electrocardiograms, gastrointestinal testing, bone density exams, MRIs and CT scans.

Having protested so much, I don't want to negate my subspecialty. Hormones are amazingly important and can impact our sense of well-being and health. The average age of menopause is 51. It signals the end of our ovarian supply of follicles and a loss of 80% to 90% of our estrogen production. At the same time, there can be a loss of testosterone, although it is not as complete. Menopausal symptoms are natural and occur in up to 90% of us. They can make you feel miserable, or you may be one of the lucky ones who can shrug them off. But what this lack of estrogen is silently doing to your body's systems should not be dismissed or ignored.

Superficially, and most noticeably, your skin becomes thinner, slowly loses its collagen and elasticity and becomes drier and prunier. Dryness also occurs in the vagina, perhaps the most obvious of the many changes that are going on in the urogenital tract. The labia lose fat, the lining of the vagina becomes thinner, smoother and less elastic and there is a decrease in blood flow to the area. As a result, lubrication is diminished. The same estrogen-sensitive cells that form the lining of the vagina are present in the lower portion of the urinary tract, and as these cells change, you may become more vulnerable to bladder infections and continence problems.

Throughout the body, muscle is replaced with fat, which tends to lodge around your disappearing waistline. You experience a weight-gain triple whammy: Fat does not burn calories as efficiently as muscle does, so even if you remain at the same weight, you'll burn calories as your fat mass increases. Meanwhile, your basal metabolic rate also decreases due to age (this occurs at a rate of about 5% per decade) and estrogen loss (which can curtail your energy use by about 100 calories per day). This means that you need to cut at least 200 calories from your daily intake just to maintain your current weight. Another alternative: exercise. This will maintain your muscle mass and help you burn off those 200 extra calories.

Exercise (which seems to be the magic word for this decade) will also help diminish the effect of estrogen loss on your bones. Our bones are not the static structures you might imagine upon viewing a Halloween skeleton. They are living tissue that is constantly being broken down by special bone-eating cells (osteoclasts) and being rebuilt by other, more constructive cells called osteoblasts. This equilibrium is upset by age. After 30, we don't build bone mass anymore; at best we can hope to maintain what we have. After the age of 50, there is a 0.5% loss of bone mass each year in both women and men. But once we're menopausal, loss of estrogen empowers the bone destroyers and significantly weakens the bone builders, so that in the first seven years after menopause there can be a 3% to 6% loss of bone each year and a 1% loss every year thereafter. Women who failed to reach their peak bone density by age 30 will start this decade at a grave bone disadvantage, and indeed, 20% of women will have clinical osteoporosis in their fifties.

We lose our cardiac estrogen superiority over men in our fifties. It was our estrogen that kept us from having heart attacks in our forties. This hormone helped prevent a rise of total cholesterol and the bad plaque-causing cholesterol LDL, while also maintaining beneficial levels of good HDL cholesterol, which coated our vessels like Teflon and prevented plaque formation. This hormone also had a direct effect on our heart muscle, encouraging it to utilize oxygen more efficiently and pump more effectively. It protected the lining of our small arteries and allowed them to remain more pliable. It helped prevent clot formation too. When we lose our estrogen, we lose these benefits and begin to gain cardiac equality with men—not exactly the kind of equality we, the women of the sixties, envisioned when we burned our bras. At this age, we're still not being felled by heart attacks at the same rate as men, but we'll catch up with and even surpass them in the decades to come.

Then there's the brain. Its neurochemical production, neuronal synaptic continuity and general well-being have survived perimenopause, but this has definitely been a dress rehearsal for the advent of menopause. Once estrogen production is on hiatus, there is an effect on the production, utilization and breakdown of the neurotransmitters in selected areas of our brain—chiefly those that govern short-term memory and word recall. Estrogen loss may also be a factor in the development of Alzheimer's disease later in life.

Lack of estrogen in the hypothalamus of our brain also causes our inner thermostat to malfunction. The "mal" translates into hot flashes and subsequent sleep disturbances. Estrogen also can ultimately affect serotonin levels, which help govern our sense of well-being. This may cause a menopausal malaise, although I should make it clear from the get-go that menopause is not a psychiatric disorder, nor has it been shown to increase our chance of developing depression.

Enough already with our ovaries and hormone production. There are other glands that are changing. We're more likely to develop thyroid problems, especially low thyroid, or hypothyroidism. Nodules and thyroid tumors are more prevalent after 50 and should be checked to make sure they are not cancerous. Our pancreas may now be exhausted from its half-century of churning out insulin, especially if our need for this hormone has increased due to obesity. As a result, the incidence of Type 2 diabetes increases in this decade; this in turn is a major risk factor for heart disease, particularly for women. Our adrenal glands are feeling the effect of age as well and produce less DHEA, a weak male hormone that is converted to testosterone and estrogen by the body.

Our immune system does not emerge from this decade unscathed. The ongoing need to fight and destroy foreign invaders may, with time, confuse or overstimulate immune reactions to the point that the immune system turns on itself and begins to attack healthy cells in our joints, skin and other connective tissue. Rheumatoid arthritis, scleroderma and Sjögren's syndrome peak during this decade. Some researchers blame falling estrogen or even testosterone levels.

Your gastrointestinal system may begin to show its age, and you are more likely to develop weakening or hernia in the walls of the esophagus near the entrance of the stomach (hiatal hernia) or in the colon (diverticulosis). You're also entering the prime time for colon polyps, which can be precancerous.

Having given this list of our failing body parts, let me reassure you that the picture, certainly from a psychological point of view, isn't all bleak. We're wiser, we know who we are, the kids are out of the house and many of us have reached goals we set for ourselves decades before and are in the midst of a renaissance, setting new goals.

If your forties was a time to discover how your body's systems work, your fifties is a time when you have to start caring for—and even repairing—them. What's so wonderful is that we now have tests and therapies available that can delay or prevent many of the less-than-desirable changes that can occur in our fifties. I know they've worked for me. With the proper nutrition, regular exercise and the right lifestyle, all of us can help ensure that although we're over fifty, we're not over the hill.

HOW DO I KNOW WHEN I'M IN MENOPAUSE?

It's like labor. You'll *know*. The key, of course, is that you'll stop having your period. But the diagnosis is a retrospective one: You have to experience at least six months of no periods to qualify as being menopausal. (The founding fathers of medicine said there had to be a menses moratorium of at least a year, but I prefer not to wait that long to bestow the title.) If you've had a hysterectomy, changes in your nonexistent menstrual cycle won't help you determine whether you're in menopause. Other symptoms will, and are shared by 90% of women whether they have a uterus or not. These include hot flashes, sleep disturbances, vaginal dryness and short-term memory loss. The same hypothalamic temperature-control mix-up that causes hot flashes may also be responsible for sleep disturbances. Changes in internal body temperature may disturb REM (dream) sleep, and although you may never consciously awaken or be aware that you're having nighttime hot flashes, they interrupt your normal sleep pattern and wonderful dreams. As a result, you may walk around like a sleep-deprived zombie, feeling fatigued, depressed, confused and forgetful. The majority of women will find that these symptoms abate within two to five years, but for 15% of us, the symptoms continue for life.

If you don't have a uterus or you're in your early fifties and you're experiencing these symptoms, you don't need hundreds of dollars' worth of blood tests to confirm this diagnosis. However, if you still occasionally get a period or you're under age 50 and your symptoms of menopause have been dismissed, it might be helpful to prove the condition with a blood test that measures follicle stimulating hormone (FSH). Levels over 30 milli-international units per milliliter, especially if they persist over the course of several tests, will signal that your ovaries are not producing estrogen and that you're in menopause. This is a more reliable indicator than estrogen blood levels because some menopausal women persist in making small amounts of estrogen, and if you're not menopausal, there are times in your cycle when estrogen levels will be low.

Many women, especially those who have read my previous arguments in favor of Pill use during perimenopause, will miss the usual clues of menopause because they are taking birth control pills. The estrogen and progestin in the Pill will supersede any hormonal changes taking place in the ovaries. The end result of being on the Pill through your forties is that you don't get hot flashes, you won't miss periods (although they may be lighter) and you'll have no other signs of impending menopause. So you can continue in ignorant bliss until you begin this decade. At this point, you can stop the Pill for two weeks (instead of the one week when you stop the active Pill so you'll get your period) and then have a blood test to measure FSH. If your FSH is at a menopausal level, you then have to decide whether you want to go from birth control to hormone control with replacement therapy. Many of my patients are so happy on the Pill that they dread having to convert to HRT. There are very little data as to whether postponing this conversion is good or bad for you. However, most researchers agree that continuing the Pill in the first year of menopause is not harmful as long as you have no underlying contraindications to Pill use. Some of my patients continue to have low FSH levels until their mid-fifties, and I've allowed them to stay on the Pill (I check their FSH yearly).

I would hope that during perimenopause you gave some thought and even had some conversations with your doctor about the issue of hormone replacement therapy in menopause. But if this transition appeared out of nowhere and you've procrastinated about preparing yourself, it's time to face the hormonal facts and make an informed decision.

SHOULD I TAKE HORMONES?

To take or not to take? That is the question. But unfortunately, many women are not even discussing this with their doctors. Fewer than half of all menopausal women seek treatment for menopause. It isn't just a question of not asking, either—it's also a question of not being told. Only 44% of women say they've received adequate information about HRT from their doctor. This may be why even if a woman is given a prescription, there's a 33% chance she won't fill it. Moreover, one-fifth of users discontinue HRT within nine months of starting it, and 10% must feel that it works in miraculous spurts, because they only take it intermittently.

Now let me return from these disturbing statistics to your question. Whether or not you should take estrogen is dependent on your symptoms and risk of certain diseases. This risk is in turn based on your lifestyle, your family history and your personal medical history. Finally, you have to weigh your fears. Let's look at each of these issues.

Menopausal Symptoms

Pros: Estrogen is magic when it comes to alleviating hot flashes. Indeed, two-thirds of women begin this therapy for hot flash distress. Once the flashes are gone, sleep improves and that zombie state virtually disappears. Estrogen also greatly reduces vaginal dryness and keeps the vaginal lining thick and well supplied with blood. I can tell the difference between a menopausal woman who takes estrogen and one who does not simply by inserting a speculum. This rejuvenating effect on genital health extends to the urethra and bladder, and women who take estrogen may have better bladder control as they age. From a vaginal point of view, estrogen is a microbe-normalizing substance, and normal flora translates into fewer vaginal and bladder infections.

Estrogen is also a memory-normalizing substance. It helps hot-wire neurons, effects levels of neurotransmitters, increases blood flow and improves activity in the memory centers of our brain. Pictures confirming this have been captured with MRIs after fewer than 21 days of estrogen therapy. But most women don't need an MRI to appreciate that they're no longer fumbling for words or forgetting what they did yesterday. Estrogen's effect on mood may be more subtle, however. Estrogen increases the rate of destruction of a brain enzyme called monoamine oxidase (MAO). MAO breaks down serotonin, the brain's feel-good chemical. So less MAO means more serotonin. This may be why women who take estrogen experience mood improvement. That doesn't mean, though, that clinical depression will significantly respond to estrogen. But I should add that studies show that depressed women can lower their dosage of antidepressants if they also take estrogen.

Cons: When it comes to menopausal symptoms, there are no adverse effects from estrogen. But in all fairness, only 15% of women have disabling symptoms. I advise these women to go ahead and start estrogen replacement for immediate relief, then decide in the years to come whether they want to continue estrogen long-term for its other health benefits. I remind them that the prescription isn't written on a stone tablet and that they can change their minds at any time.

The other 85% of women range from "I guess I can cope" to "this is a breeze." Certainly, if you fall into the latter category, you may not have a pressing impetus to start this drug. Your decision should then be based on whether you need or would benefit from estrogen in the long term.

Risk of Disease

Pros: Here's the big picture: It's been estimated that hormone replacement therapy can increase life expectancy for almost all postmenopausal women, some by more than three years. This is due to its protective effect against the following diseases.

CARDIOVASCULAR DISEASE

Estrogen safeguards our heart. Most studies have shown that it decreases the risk of fatal heart attack, our number one killer, by 50%. (Although in all fairness I have to add that the researchers generally looked at women who took estrogen and compared them to women who didn't, and the "takers" may have been healthier to begin with and may also have maintained a healthier lifestyle.) But numerous tests, including angiograms and coronary CT scans, have also shown that estrogen replacement therapy significantly diminishes plaque formation (atherosclerosis). And there is no contesting this hormone's positive effect on cholesterol levels. This is probably less than half of the story, however. The other half of estrogen's cardiac benefit is thanks in part to its ability to keep blood vessels supplying the heart open and prevent their spasm. Estrogen also prevents platelets from sticking to one another and forming clots on top of plaque. In short, our hearts and the blood vessels supplying them are probably as estrogen-receptive as our reproductive organs.

OSTEOPOROSIS

Women who take estrogen for a minimum of 10 years after menopause have at least half the risk of hip fracture of women who don't take the hormone. Estrogen prevents bone resorption by inhibiting the activity of bone-eroding osteoclasts. It's never too late to start estrogen—the hormone helps even if osteoporosis is already present. Less life-threatening but certainly vital to quality of life is the effect estrogen has on tooth loss. Women who take estrogen are 38% less likely to lose their teeth than women who don't take it, probably because teeth are anchored in the jawbone, which can be vulnerable to osteoporosis. Brushing and flossing may not be enough.

ALZHEIMER'S DISEASE

The purists still debate whether this disease should be put in the "risk is absolutely and positively decreased by estrogen" category. Based on the prevailing evidence, I think it belongs there. Estrogen replacement has been shown to be associated with a diminished chance of developing Alzheimer's and even general dementia by anywhere from 29% to 54%, depending on duration of use and dosage. There are several postulated explanations for estrogen's effects. The first is that it restores choline acetyl transferase activity. This enzyme synthesizes acetylcholine, the major neurotransmitter that is deficient in Alzheimer's disease. Estrogen also helps maintain levels of important chemicals in the hippocampus, the part of the brain that undergoes degeneration in those with Alzheimer's disease. Estrogen also improves cerebral blood flow. Finally, it possesses both antioxidant and anti-inflammatory properties, both of which help protect against protein plaque formation in the brain, a hallmark of this disease.

COLORECTAL CANCER

Decreased risk of developing this cancer has not quite made it onto the definitive list of estrogen's attributes. However, if results of the studies on the subject are pooled, it appears that ever having used estrogen therapy decreases the risk of colon or rectal cancer by about 20%, and that current use reduces risk further, by about 36%. Estrogen may work by helping to minimize secretion of bowel-irritating bile acids.

Cons If your risk of developing a disease as a result of estrogen cancels out your chance of living longer and better with estrogen, you may not want to start or continue hormone replacement therapy. Here are the conditions that create concern among many women and their physicians.

BREAST CANCER

Of all the diseases that are affected either positively or negatively by estrogen, breast cancer is the most controversial. More than 50 studies have attempted to confront this issue. About half show no increase in breast cancer risk in women who take estrogen, and the other half do. The Harvard Nurses' Health Study found a slow increase in risk with each year of hormone use, up to a roughly 30% elevation among women who took estrogen for more than five years. Other analyses pooled data from many studies and found that an increase in risk took longer to appear and ranged from 10% to 50%. The newest look at this issue comes from the Iowa Women's Health Study of more than 37,000 women. Researchers found that only 5% of breast cancers were linked with estrogen, and these cancers were the type that are considered low-risk and highly curable. In other words, 95% of tumors were *not* estrogen-linked.

Also on the reassuring side is the huge study undertaken by the American Cancer Society, which followed more than 420,000 women for 10 years and found that those who ever took estrogen had an overall 16% decrease in breast cancer mortality when compared to women who never took it. The earlier a woman started taking estrogen, the less likely she was to die of breast cancer. Women who started estrogen before age 40 had a 34% decrease in their risk of death from breast cancer. The problem with comparing this study to the ones I cited earlier is that the ACS researchers only looked at mortality—not incidence. Women who develop breast cancer while on estrogen have been found to have a more manageable and less invasive disease than women of the same age who get breast cancer while not on estrogen. The knowledge that one's chances of survival are better with estrogen won't negate the devastation that accompanies this diagnosis and therapy.

ENDOMETRIAL CANCER

Unopposed estrogen (estrogen taken alone, without progestin or progesterone) causes stimulation of the uterine lining and a five- to eightfold increase in the risk of uterine cancer. Even small amounts of a progestational agent will cancel out this risk, so if you have your uterus and take estrogen, the unequivocal recommendation is to add this second hormone. Instead of estrogen replacement therapy (ERT), you need hormone replacement therapy (HRT).

GALLSTONES

ERT is associated with a twofold increase in gallbladder disease due to gallstones. This is because estrogen concentrates and diverts cholesterol from our liver into bile for excretion. The higher the cholesterol content of the bile, the greater the chance of forming irritating cholesterol stones.

BLOOD CLOTS

Clots that form in veins deep in the legs are called *deep vein thromboses* (DVT). These can travel to the lungs, heart or brain, a process called *thromboembolism.* In rare cases, this can be fatal. HRT (estrogen plus progestin) has been reported to double or triple the risk of this condition. This may seem confusing because I've already told you that estrogen prevents clot formation. But that prevention applies to the arteries of the heart, not to the deep veins of the leg.

What does all this mean when you're weighing pros and cons? The bottom line is that hormone replacement therapy should increase the average life expectancy of most menopausal women. The only women who may not reap these benefits are those who are at greatest risk for breast cancer and at lowest risk for heart disease and osteoporosis. Even among those at high risk for breast cancer, the presence of just one risk factor for heart disease (see below) tips the scale in favor of hormone replacement therapy.

Lifestyle Factors

This is where you have to own up to previous abuses of your body.

Abuses that may signal a special need for estrogen:

SMOKING

If you've smoked regularly in the past or are a smoker now, you have committed a grave osseous (bone) sin and are at risk for osteoporosis. The dire consequences of smoking continue: It has placed you at risk of high blood pressure, coronary artery disease and stroke. Smoking's effect on bone is permanent, but if you've been a nonsmoker for at least four years, your heart disease risk should return to normal for your age group.

OBESITY

On the plus (-size) side, having more fat may increase your production of estrogen after menopause and is probably somewhat protective against

Alzheimer's disease and osteoporosis. But the downside is huge: Your cholesterol, insulin levels and blood pressure are probably all unhealthily high, increasing your risk of heart disease. Add to this your significant risk for diabetes and the cardiac insult becomes even greater.

Abdominal (male-pattern) obesity is a more significant threat to your heart than fat in your tush and your thighs. There is evidence that estrogen can minimize the tendency of fat to collect around the beltline, so if you're having to let out the waistband of all your clothes, it may save you tailoring expenses, not to mention your heart.

LACK OF EXERCISE

You may have spent the last four decades exercising your brain, but if you didn't use your muscles too, you have created a bodily situation that, quite frankly, is unfit for health and longevity. The data are overwhelming: At any given age, someone who is out of shape is twice as likely to die as someone who is fit. This difference is largely due to aerobic exercise's protective effect against heart disease. But weight-bearing exercise, with or without an aerobic component, is also essential for preventing bone loss and osteoporosis. So if your past routine has not included at least 30 minutes a day of moderate exercise (see page 176) and weight bearing exercise, your fitness quotient is low. This means you're at elevated risk of heart disease and osteoporosis, and, once more, estrogen can help (although it won't excuse you from exercise).

NUTRITIONAL FAULTS

Too much fat, or the wrong kind of fat (the saturated or "trans" kind) may elevate your cholesterol level—especially the "bad" LDL cholesterol and triglycerides—and ultimately put you at risk for heart disease (see page 293). So assess your past and current fat intake and factor it into the estrogen equation. (I'm not suggesting, however, that you take estrogen so that you can eat cheeseburgers with abandon.)

There's another dietary factor to consider: Like many American women, your diet may have been woefully deficient in calcium. Or you may have other past risk factors that demineralized your bones, such as a history of missed periods or an eating disorder. If a bone density scan shows that you're starting off this decade with low bone mass, you may want to take the most potent antiosteoporosis drug we currently have, estrogen.

Family History

A family history of any of the following can be factored in on the pro side for estrogen action.

Heart disease: If your grandfather, father or brother died of a heart attack before age 55, or if your grandmother, mother or sister died of one before age 65, you have an increased risk for heart disease. However, you don't have to wait for your relatives to drop dead to know they have cardiovascular disease. If they have been successfully treated with cardiac medications, angioplasties or open heart surgeries, you are also at risk.

Osteoporosis: Was your grandmother or mother stooped with a dowager's hump, or did she suffer a fractured hip? If your mother broke her hip, your risk of hip fracture doubles; if she broke her hip before age 80, your risk is even greater.

Alzheimer's disease: Having one or more relatives who developed Alzheimer's before age 65 places you at increased risk of being diagnosed as well.

Colon cancer: If you have a family history of colorectal cancer, and particularly if you have a first-degree relative (parent or sibling) with the disease, you are at increased risk of getting it yourself.

We also have to consider family history when we look at reasons not to take estrogen.

Breast cancer: If you have a first-degree relative (mother, sister or daughter) with breast cancer who developed the disease before menopause, you're at increased risk. The question is whether estrogen will exacerbate any tendency you may have inherited to develop breast cancer. According to a study conducted by the American Cancer Society, estrogen has the same protective effect against death from breast cancer among women with a family history of breast cancer as it does for women with no family history. (Women who take estrogen before age 50 have a 16% lower risk of death from breast cancer; those who take the hormone after age 50 have an 11% lower risk.)

When it comes to women who have inherited one of the breast cancer gene mutations, BRCA1 or BRCA2, the effects of estrogen on cancer risk are still unknown—researchers are just beginning to identify and follow these women.

The bottom line is that each of us has to weigh all of our risks and fears when making the estrogen decision. There are enough data out there to raise concerns about estrogen's cancer-promoting (as opposed to cancer-*inducing* effect). To be less technical: Estrogen may coax slow-growing cancer cells that are already present in a nascent form in the breast to go forth and multiply. But it doesn't convert benign cells to malignant ones. Moreover, it appears that estrogen may ultimately prevent cancer cells from spreading aggressively. This would explain why women who develop breast cancer while on hormone replacement therapy are 32% less likely to die than women who develop the cancer and who do not take estrogen.

Personal History

You can't blame everything that happens to you on your ancestors. Your past and present health also have to be factored into your estrogen decision. Once more, we'll look at this disease by disease.

Heart disease: High cholesterol levels, high blood pressure, diabetes and obesity are all conditions that tremendously increase your risk for cardio-vascular disease and heart attack. I advocate estrogen if you have one (or more) of these conditions. But my position isn't necessarily shared by the entire medical community. The American Heart Association recently recommended that cholesterol-lowering drugs be considered instead of hormone replacement as the first line of drug therapy for reducing high cholesterol levels in postmenopausal women. They did not, however, dismiss it as a valuable therapy for heart disease prevention.

In the past I advised women who have had a previous heart attack to take estrogen. After all, we had evidence that the hormone decreases death in women with previous coronary vascular disease. There are also some very convincing studies demonstrating that estrogen placed under the tongue has the same blood-vessel-relaxing effect as nitroglycerine during an attack of chest pain brought on by heart vessel constriction.

However, the HERS (Heart and Estrogen-progestin Replacement Study) found that one type of hormone replacement regimen, Premarin plus Provera, initially increased death rates in women who began taking the medication shortly after a heart attack. Most of these deaths were due to increased clot formation. This risk came down after four years but was not enough to convince one and all that the therapy was warranted. Many physicians feel that the initial increase in recurrent heart attacks should not be used to blanketly dismiss *all* hormone replacement therapy; it's possible that forms of estrogen other than Premarin, and natural progesterones (as opposed to Provera, a synthetic), would have different effects. Even the authors of the study commented that women who are currently taking estrogen after a heart attack should not stop while we wait for further long-term studies. As a result of this study, if one of my patients who was not on estrogen suffers a heart attack, I talk to her and her cardiologist about transdermal estrogen (the patch). It may have a smaller effect on clotting factors and if she needs HRT, I prescribe a natural rather than synthetic progesterone.

Osteoporosis: No one disputes estrogen is a benefit to women with low bone density or osteoporosis. Even if we consider all the other bone-building drugs that are currently on the market, estrogen still comes out ahead.

Alzheimer's disease: There are a few small studies hinting that estrogen replacement may diminish the degree of dementia in women who have been diagnosed with Alzheimer's disease.

Colorectal cancer: There are no definitive studies showing that women already diagnosed and treated for colon cancer fare better on estrogen therapy. But laboratory tests have shown that activation of estrogen receptors in colon cancer cells suppresses tumor development. We also know that the production of bile acids that may promote malignant changes is decreased when we take estrogen. Since having had colon cancer is perhaps the greatest risk for having it again, I feel comfortable prescribing estrogen to women who have been treated for this disease.

Breast cancer: The traditional advice to a woman who has had breast cancer is not to take estrogen, the fear of course being that it would seek out and stimulate any cancer cells that may have been missed during treatment. But several recent studies suggest that estrogen use does not adversely affect long-term outcome in cancer survivors. It may be too early to categorically reverse the conventional recommendations. However, I do prescribe it to patients who had very small tumors, negative lymph nodes and/or whose tumor was found to be estrogen-receptor negative or who have been free of cancer for five or more years. This is especially the case if they are having severe menopausal symptoms or are at significant risk for cardiovascular disease. There is no sense in saving a woman's life from breast cancer only for her to die of heart disease.

Endometrial cancer: If the cancer was found early, before it spread beyond the uterine cavity, there is probably no reason to withhold estrogen replacement therapy if you want it or need it. Only 1% of patients with this early-stage cancer have a recurrence, and if it happens, it usually occurs within three years of diagnosis and treatment. If a woman's initial cancer is more advanced, however, I suggest use of a potent progestin, Megace, to inhibit the growth of any stray malignant cells. But if she remains cancer-free after three to five years, I and many other gynecologists have no qualms about prescribing estrogen.

Gallstones: If you already have gallstones, it's possible that estrogen may make your condition worse. But if you've had your gallbladder removed, the level of concern is greatly diminished. To be on the safe side, I would prescribe estrogen in patch rather than pill form. This allows the hormone to initially bypass the liver so that it has less effect on the cholesterol content of the bile and thus on stone formation.

Blood clots: The pharmaceutical companies have been very careful about advising against estrogen for women with a history of abnormal clot formation in the deep veins of the legs or pulmonary embolism (clots that travel to the lungs). But many physicians consider this blanket prohibition inappropriate. Instead, these doctors feel that we should look at whether a woman has an underlying clotting problem that may increase her general risk of these conditions (venous thromboembolism). If, in addition to her own history of clots, she has a family history of the problem, she should be tested to see if the following clotting factors are elevated: Leiden factor, protein C, protein S and fibrinogen. If any or all of them are, she should probably not take estrogen, although some doctors will prescribe it if the woman agrees to also take an anticlotting medication.

In the past, I've been fairly cavalier in prescribing estrogen to my patients who tested negative for abnormal clotting factors, although I gave them the patch in order to minimize the effects of estrogen on clotting factors produced in the liver. But recent studies, including the Nurses' study and the HERS study, have shown a two- to threefold increased incidence of venous thromboembolism among women on HRT. I'm still prescribing the patch, but I share my concerns over these risks with patients so that they can be fully informed when participating in the decision-making process.

Fibroids: There is a myth that estrogen replacement therapy will cause fibroids to grow larger. There's no question that fibroids tend to shrink once you're menopausal and have no estrogen on board. But the amount of estrogen used in replacement therapy has not been found to cause significant growth. You won't die of a fibroid, but you might die from a heart attack. That said, you should know that if your fibroid projects into the uterus, you may experience heavier or more irregular bleeding on hormone replacement therapy, especially if the progestin component is given in a cyclical fashion. You might be better off taking continuous-dose therapy—but more on that below.

Autoimmune diseases: Since some doctors blame falling estrogen levels for autoimmune disorders that peak in this decade, will supplementing estrogen help if our tissues are already under an auto-attack? No one knows for sure. Women with lupus are often treated with steroids that can place them at high risk for osteoporosis, so having osteoporosis might be reason enough to start HRT even if its effects on lupus are not clear. Studies to date show that HRT doesn't appear to make lupus better or worse, but women's overall health may benefit from taking estrogen. When it comes to rheumatoid arthritis, estrogen, given at adequate doses, may help alleviate morning stiffness and joint pain. As for Sjögren's syndrome, there are little data, but vaginal dryness is a significant symptom and there's every reason to expect that estrogen would help relieve it.

Liver disease: We're bombarded with warnings about hepatitis. There are several types: A, B, and C. Each of these can lead to chronic liver disease, although hepatitis A is least risky and hepatitis C is most risky. If you have a history of hepatitis and question the use of estrogen, relax. As long as your liver function and liver enzymes are now normal—something that can be checked with a simple blood test—there are no contraindications to the use of estrogen. Abnormal liver function is a warning sign that warrants additional tests, perhaps even a biopsy, to check to see if the disease is active, in which case you probably should not take estrogen. If I know a patient has a history of liver disease, even if she has normal enzymes, I'm more likely to prescribe an estrogen patch rather than a pill because hormones delivered by patch will initially bypass the liver.

Asthma: If you have asthma, you've probably had a chance to note whether your symptoms intensified at ovulation or in the two weeks before your period, when estrogen and progesterone levels rose. Women whose symptoms follow this pattern may be susceptible to a worsening of the disease if they take HRT. There have been reports that both estrogen and progestins may exacerbate the condition. But many women with asthma have taken steroid drugs to control their symptoms; as a result, they have low bone mass or osteoporosis. So for them, estrogen could be advisable. They may have to try various forms of HRT until they find one that is most tolerable. My experience is that they usually do well with estradiol products and natural progesterone in a vaginal gel. (For more about specific therapies, read the next question.)

WHAT TYPE OF HORMONE REPLACEMENT IS RIGHT FOR ME?

A major topic of conversation among women in their fifties is not only "to take or not to take hormones?" but which kind and whose doctor has prescribed the newest, most natural and lowest effective dose. I'm always asked, "What's the best?" My more audacious patients even ask me what I'm taking! There is no "best"—this is not "one prescription fits all" therapy. I have to tailor my prescription to each and every woman depending on her previous history of PMS, headaches, insomnia and weight gain, her menstrual bleeding patterns, her reaction to past birth control pill use, her risk factors for disease, her current health profile and her menopausal symptoms. Sit down, take a deep breath and relax. It takes time and patience to sleuth out what's right for you.

The Many Faces of Estrogen

I've always felt that there is one word that raises our collective health consciousness: *natural*. Let me first reassure you that as far as your body is concerned, all of the estrogens currently used in hormone replacement therapy are natural. When the endocrinologists and I say "natural," we're not referring to where the hormone came from but whether it is treated like natural estrogen once it's in our bodies. "Natural" means that this estrogen is metabolized just the way our own ovary-produced estrogen is and broken down to less potent estrogens called estrone and estriol. Some of these estrogens are further deactivated when they are attached to a sulfate molecule by the liver. It is these reworked estrogens that are released to our blood and enter cells in our body, where they do their thing.

The difference between the estrogen used in estrogen replacement therapy (ERT) and the kind found in birth control pills (ethinyl estradiol) is not how it is made—extracted from either animals or plants or cooked up in a lab—but how it is processed by the liver. The estrogens in ERT are extensively broken down, while those in oral contraceptives are not—they degrade very slowly; because of this, they are at least five times more potent. That is why the Pill is able to block ovarian hormone production and stop ovulation.

Continuing our natural history lesson . . . Originally, many of the estrogens used in ERT are derived from natural sources such as plants, namely soy and wild yams, and the urine of pregnant mares (although some purists do not consider urine a natural source). But once the hormone is extracted or made from scratch in the lab, it has to undergo chemical processing to produce the pill, patch or cream that is the final product. There is (you should pardon the expression) a natural tendency to condemn this chemical processing. But without this system that isolates, enhances, purifies and condenses estrogen, we'd have to ingest impossibly huge quantities of soy or drink mares' urine to get the dose of estrogen we need. And yams? Forget about it—our bodies don't even have the enzyme needed to extract the estrogen found there. (For more information on what benefits we can get from these foods—mares' urine excepted—see page 162.)

Here's a look at the different types of estrogen that are made by pharmaceutical companies and approved by the Food and Drug Administration.

Pills

Conjugated equine estrogen (Premarin): I'm starting with this product because estrogen therapy was introduced with it about 55 years ago, and it's been used in most of the American studies that look at long-term effects of estrogen. Premarin is a mixture of a number of different estrogens obtained from mares' urine. Equine estrogen is a very potent antioxidant, meaning it neutralizes harmful free radical molecules that promote development of plaque in our arteries. It may even be better than human estrogen at improving our cholesterol profile. However, it can elevate triglycerides, so in women for whom this is already a problem, I generally recommend the estrogen patch. Premarin also raises a woman's level of sex hormone binding globulin (SHBG), the protein that binds up estrogen and testosterone. Some researchers feel this may be good when considering breast cancer risk because less free estrogen circulating through the body means less available to affect receptors in breast cells.

Premarin is the preferred mode of therapy for many doctors simply because they're comfortable with it and it's paid for by most insurance companies. It's available in four different doses, ranging from 0.3 milligram to 1.25 milligrams. The most commonly used 0.625 milligram dose has also been brilliantly combined with progestin into an easy, once-a-day pill (Prempro) or in cycle packs of separate estrogen and progestin pills (Premphase).

Some of my patients object to taking Premarin because of claims that the pregnant mares are mistreated. I can't argue for or against this concept, but if they feel this is an issue I simply prescribe another form of the hormone.

Micronized estradiol (Estrace): This is the type of estrogen that is frequently used in Europe. "Micronized" means that the estradiol in this pill is chopped into thousands of tiny pieces to allow for better absorption. Some patients and doctors prefer this form of estrogen because it is the one our ovaries produce.

Esterified estrogens (Estratab, Menest): This is processed from plant sources, and the manufacturers proclaim this loudly on every package. Its chief component is estrone sulfate, one of the forms of estrogen that's produced in our body after we metabolize estradiol. Taking estrogen in this form allows the body to skip a step in the metabolic process. Whether this has any physiologic advantage is unknown, but my patients like the idea that this product comes from plants. I like the fact that Estratab is also available combined with testosterone (Estratest). Another new plant-derived estrogen, Cenestin, contains a slow-release conjugated estrogen and is similar in its action to Estratab.

Estropipate (Ogen, Ortho-Est): This estrogen is prepared from purified crystalline estrogen made in the lab. Once in our bodies, it acts like estrone. This formulation is a little weaker than the same dose of Premarin or Estrace.

Patches

17 (beta) estradiol (Alora, Climara, Estraderm, Vivelle): These contain estradiol synthesized in the lab. The patch, worn on the abdomen or buttocks, delivers a steady dose of hormone, which is absorbed through the skin. Estraderm was the original patch introduced in the United States. Since its very successful debut, the other patches with new and different adhesive and release systems have appeared. But the chief difference between them is their dosages and how often they need to be changed. Estraderm and Vivelle are changed twice a week. The manufacturer of Vivelle recently introduced the Vivelle Dot, which is worn on the abdomen and, amazingly, gives the same amount of estrogen as the regular Vivelle patch, even though it's about as big as a postage stamp—less than half the size of the other patches. Climara and Alora are changed once a week. Climara has the lowest-dose patch on the market. In the past, women who were very estrogen-sensitive or who wanted very low doses sometimes resorted to cutting a patch in half. That's no longer necessary.

These patches give only estrogen, and if you have a uterus, you need to take progestin to protect the lining. Women who loved the ease of patching up their hormone problems objected to having to remember to add on a progestin pill. Their objections have recently been overruled with CombiPatch, which supplies both estradiol and the synthetic progestin norethindrone acetate. The only drawback is that this patch is currently available with only one dosage level of estradiol. Women who need a lower or higher dose are out of luck. But there are two available dosage levels of progestin so that you can go to the higher dosage if you experience breakthrough bleeding on the low-dose patch.

Low-Dose Estrogen

Some women are extremely sensitive to the traditional doses of estrogen (0.625 mg of conjugated equine estrogen or esterified estrogens, 1 mg of estradiol or 0.05 mg estradiol patch). They develop breast tenderness, bloating and nausea as well as breakthrough bleeding at these hormone levels. Indeed, half of women on estrogen stop taking it, largely because of these symptoms. There is also some concern as to whether the amount of estrogen a woman takes might be linked to whether or not the hormone has the potential to encourage the growth of breast cancer cells or trigger abnormal clotting.

Lower-dose estrogen formulations (0.3 mg of conjugated equine estrogen or esterified estrogen, or 0.05 mg of estradiol or a 0.025 estradiol patch) are currently available. These low doses may relieve many menopausal symptoms, particularly if these aren't severe. Low-dose estrogen appears to preserve bone in most women, though it doesn't increase bone density to the same extent that higher doses do. (Even with the traditional 0.625 mg Premarin or its equivalent, 5% to 10% of women will lose bone density and may require double this dose in order to preserve it.) So if you're starting HRT and have significant osteoporosis, you may want to opt for the higher dose. If your bone mass is low to normal and you go on low-dose estrogen therapy, it's a good idea to have your bone density measured in two to three years.

With regard to heart disease, the lower the dose of estrogen, the less your lipids will improve. Despite this, or maybe because a little improvement plus estrogen's effect on coronary vessels goes a long way, the Harvard nurses' study showed that 0.3 mg of Premarin provided the same overall cardiovascular protection as 0.625 mg. We have no idea whether lower-dose estrogen will ultimately have a protective effect against risk of Alzheimer's disease. To make sense of all these milligrams, I think it makes sense to consider taking these demi-doses if you want just enough estrogen to get you through your symptoms, especially if you have trepidations about taking the hormone in the first place. This petite dose may also be right if you're petite in size.

Low-dose therapy is also an option for women who decide to go on HRT after breast cancer or who've had significant breakthrough bleeding on traditional doses. Although it is less likely to cause endometrial buildup and certainly results in less breakthrough bleeding, at this point most doctors, including myself, still recommend that women who have a uterus take a progestational agent even if they are on low-dose therapy.

Vaginal Estrogens

Conjugated equine estrogen (Premarin Vaginal Cream); micronized estradiol (Estrace Cream); estropipate (Ogen Cream); dienestrol (Ortho Dienestrol Cream); estradiol (Estring, a vaginal ring): The creams are generally inserted with applicators twice weekly. They act locally in the vagina to combat atrophy by building up its lining and improving moisture and lubrication. The absorption of the cream results in blood levels of estrogen that are much lower than those obtained with estrogen pills, so you can't expect the systemwide benefits of estrogen that you would get with either patches or pills. The ring, which can be left in place for up to three months, produces an almost negligible rise in blood estrogen levels. It may be the product of choice for women who want the least possible trace of estrogen in their bloodstream. You can put it in and take out by yourself, removing it during intercourse if you wish (though most couples don't know it's there). And it's not as messy as a cream.

Skin Creams and Gels

Estradiol: I promised to tell you here about FDA-approved products made by pharmaceutical companies. But I must make one exception if I'm to cover all our estrogen bases. Estradiol gel is very popular in Europe, where women rub it on their arms, shoulders or abdomen. However, it is not currently sold in the United States by any manufacturer, although companies are working on bringing it to market. In the meantime, it is being made by compounding pharmacies, which take the raw ingredients for estrogen

cream and concoct it in small personalized batches. They will not, however, do this without a prescription from your doctor. Dosage control with
a cream or gel may be more difficult than with pills or patches. I think that
once this product is proven to give adequate and controlled amounts of
estrogen and becomes readily available, many women will be happy to use
it and forgo the telltale badge of menopause (the estrogen patch). There
could also be a local skin advantage to using a cream or gel.

HOW SHOULD I DECIDE BETWEEN THE PILL AND THE PATCH?

Each has its own mode of hormone delivery and action. When you take
an estrogen pill, the hormone is absorbed and passes directly to the liver,
where it is metabolized. This is called first bypass. This is good if you want
your estrogen to immediately stimulate the liver to produce higher levels
of good HDL cholesterol and lower amounts of bad LDL cholesterol. The
estrogen from a patch or gel will find its way to the liver, but it takes three
to six months of sustained use before HDLs go up and LDLs go down, and
even then the change is not as impressive as it is with the pill.

There is one other way that these two forms of estrogen differ when it
comes to your cardiovascular risk. Oral estrogen increases triglycerides,
which have been found to be an important predictor of heart disease risk
in women, while the patch does not.

When it comes to estrogen's protection against cardiovascular disease,
we have to remember that lipids are not the only factor. More than half of
estrogen's heart benefits are through a direct effect on the heart muscle
and the arteries. These appear to be the same regardless of whether you
use the pill or the patch.

The fact that the estrogen from the patch is not initially introduced into
the liver means that it has less effect on clotting factors produced by this
organ. So if you have a history of clots or a disease that poses an increased
risk of clotting, this may be the safest way (albeit not a 100% safe one) for
you to get your estrogen.

Aside from these two major issues, there are other considerations in
choosing a pill or a patch. I'll summarize them here:

You Might Prefer the Patch If . . .

· You tried the pill and it caused nausea. (This is not common and can
often be diminished if you take the pills with meals.)

- You have daily variations in your hormone levels with pills that cause ups and downs in symptoms like hot flashes. (When you take the pill, estrogen levels peak after 2 hours and drop 14 to 18 hours later; the patch results in steadier blood levels.)
- You have a history of migraines or your headaches worsen with oral estrogen. (Again, this is maybe due to fluctuations in estrogen levels with the pill.)
- You have had or are at risk for gallbladder disease.
- You smoke. (Shame on you. Smoking lowers estrogen levels and interferes with the hormone's HDL benefits more in women taking oral estrogen than in those who use the patch. When oral estrogen is combined with nicotine, the risk of abnormal clotting may also increase.)
- You try the pill and your blood pressure unexpectedly increases. (This may be due to an elevation of a substance called renin, which does not occur with the patch.)
- You take oral estrogen and don't get relief of your menopausal symptoms. (Some women just don't absorb oral estrogen adequately.)

You Might Prefer the Pill If . . .

- Your HDL and LDL levels are off, but your triglycerides are normal.
- You prefer taking one pill a day and getting your estrogen replacement over with.
- You don't want any visible sign that you're using ERT.
- You develop a rash or itching with the patch. (This can occur in up to 9% of women. Sometimes switching to a different brand of patch may alleviate the problem.)
- You perspire a lot or take lots of hot baths and the patch won't stick.
- You want to take a form of estrogen that is extracted from a plant.

DO I NEED PROGESTERONE?

Yes, if you have a uterus. In all the excitement of the introduction of postmenopausal estrogen supplements more than 50 years ago, nobody thought to consider nature's wisdom. During our reproductive years, when we're cyclically correct, we produce varying amounts of estrogen and, after ovulation, an all-important two weeks' worth of progesterone. Not only is this a pro-gestational hormone, preparing the endometrium for possible implantation and pregnancy, but it also protects the uterine lining from an unopposed onslaught of estrogen. Estrogen, when left to its own devices, causes glands in the endometrium to grow, multiply and even become malignant. That means if you have a uterus, you need to add progesterone to your estrogen therapy.

Back in the old days of hormone replacement therapy, the only types of progestational agents available were synthetic. Chemists added molecules to progesterone in order to improve its absorption and stability. These new compounds were called progestins and are still the most widely used. They include medroxyprogesterone acetate (MPA), which is sold under the brand names Provera and Cycrin. It also composes the "Pro" of Prempro and the "Phase" of Premphase. Another progestin, norethindrone acetate, is sold as Aygestin, while its chemical cousin, norethindrone, is sold as Micronor. All of these progestins have been amply tested and, with the right doses, will provide endometrial protection. By the right doses, I mean the lowest effective dose, which is 2.5 milligrams of MPA daily (or 5 mg for 12 days a month); 2.5 milligrams of norethindrone acetate 12 days a month; or 0.35 milligram of norethindrone daily. (I'll go into more detail about the combinations and permutations of the different regimens below.)

The endometrium-protecting success of these progestins has not always been matched by their "feeling good on this medication" success. Progestin can cause side effects such as bloating, breast tenderness, headaches, irritability, sleeplessness and depression—you know, those PMS-like feelings you thought you'd said goodbye to once you were in menopause. Moreover, there was concern that adding progestins to estrogen might diminish the latter's beneficial effect on cardiovascular disease. An optimistically acronymed study, the PEPI study (which stands for Postmenopausal Estrogen-Progestin Intervention trial), demonstrated that indeed progestins slightly undermined estrogen's positive effects on the cholesterol profile. No one knows yet if this translates into a significant decrease in heart protection for women in the real world.

Most of my patients are far less concerned about the results of the PEPI study than they are about the fact that when they take any form of progesterone, they may still have periods or unexpected bleeding. There is a sense that we've earned the right to be pad- and tampon-free once we've gone through menopause. There are ways to minimize this side effect, but unfortunately it takes trial, error and some bloodshed to get it right. But more on that below.

If the word "synthetic" or the PMS symptoms I've described above have caused some progestational consternation, I can offer a natural option: micronized natural progesterone capsules. Once researchers figured out how to chop natural progesterone into thousands of tiny pieces and suspend it in oil, women could take it in capsule form and it would be absorbed properly. The initial offering of this preparation was through compounding pharmacies, but in the last couple of years it's been made available under the brand name Prometrium. Many women feel that this form of progesterone causes fewer PMS-type symptoms than the synthetic version. The PEPI study demonstrated that in the right doses (100 mg daily or 200 mg 12 days a month), this natural progesterone is as effective in protecting the lining of the uterus as MPA. A possibly important added bonus: Micronized natural progesterone does not impair estrogen's good effect on the lipid profile to the same extent that MPA does.

Natural progesterone, especially in high doses, causes drowsiness. I hesitate to call this a side effect because one of the symptoms of menopause is insomnia. Some women welcome anything that will help them doze off and remain asleep. But obviously we want to do our dozing at night—so the suggestion is to take it at bedtime.

Some of my patients are so progesterone-sensitive that no matter what preparation they take, they feel lousy. (Many had severe PMS or menstrual migraines before they entered menopause.) There is a new, localized way of protecting the endometrium with a natural progesterone vaginal gel (Crinone). Only small amounts of the progesterone in this gel get into the bloodstream, and because it is placed vaginally, it appears to be routed directly to the endometrium, where it has been shown to have a very strong progestational effect. As a matter of fact, the 8% progesterone gel has become the progesterone of choice in building the lining during infertility therapy. The lower-dose 4% version has been FDA approved for use with estrogen in younger women who don't menstruate because of low estrogen production. Approval for use in menopausal women is pending; in the interim many doctors (including myself) feel comfortable prescribing it as long as we monitor the uterine lining with an annual ultrasound exam. The gel comes in prefilled applicators. It should be inserted every other night for 12 days a month (a total of six applicators).

IF I DECIDE ON HRT, HOW DO I DETERMINE WHICH REGIMEN IS RIGHT FOR ME?

To bleed or not to bleed is a big question, but there are other issues that make this a custom-made decision. Let's look at the options.

The Cyclical Regimen

Once doctors figured out that in order to protect the uterine lining, hormones should be given in a way that re-creates our natural cycles, they invented a cyclical therapy, giving estrogen on days 1 through 25 each month and a progestational agent on days 14 through 25. Days 26 to 30 were deemed hormone-free, and most women would get a period. (Although if you're on this therapy long-term, it's possible the bleeding will cease.) The advantage to this therapy is that you know when to expect your period; the drawback is that you get it. Moreover, some women experience hot flashes, headaches and other symptoms of estrogen withdrawal on their five days off. The ups and downs in progestin levels may prompt PMS symptoms.

In an effort to reduce progestin-related suffering, some doctors prescribe a higher dose of progestin (10 mg of MPA) for 14 days in a row every three months. Theoretically this allows you to enjoy unopposed estrogen for two and a half months and still get the necessary uterine protection. The only problem is that when you do bleed, it tends to be heavier.

The Continuous Regimen

There's been an attempt to prevent bleeding and other drawbacks of cyclical therapy by improving upon nature and giving steady doses of both estrogen and a progestational agent throughout the month. You don't need to slough or "clean out" your uterine lining every month in order to protect it against endometrial cancer—opposing estrogen with progestin/progesterone on a daily basis is as effective as doing it cyclically. This consistent hormone balance prevents the uterine lining from buildup and indeed keeps it thin and happily nonactive. Lack of hormone fluctuation is also more likely to keep you in a happily PMS-less state and free of hot flashes and headaches throughout your cycle. Unfortunately, it may take your body a while to adjust to this hormonal equilibrium. Many women continue to have distressing breakthrough bleeding for the first six to nine months, and may become prematurely disenchanted with this form of HRT. In an attempt to decrease this bleeding, some doctors prescribe what I call the "Sabbath off" continuous therapy. In other words, you take estrogen and progestin/progesterone Monday through Friday and leave week-ends hormone-free. However, this decreases your total dose of estrogen—and possibly its protective effects, particularly those on your bones—by roughly 30%.

Because I have found that breakthrough bleeding is more likely to happen in the early years of menopause, I tend to start patients out with cyclical therapy and then switch to continuous dosing after at least a year of uterine "obedience." Even then, there can still be breakthrough bleeding.

IF I TAKE HORMONES, WILL I GAIN WEIGHT?

For most women, menopause is not associated with a weight-gain pause—there is an average three- to five-pound increase in weight in the first few years of estrogen deprivation, regardless of whether or not you take ERT. So don't blame these pounds on estrogen—blame it on menopause. Will ERT improve or worsen this gaining mode? Several studies have shown that it makes no difference. In fact, women taking estrogen are generally thinner than those who refrain from using ERT. This may simply be due to the fact that they take better care of themselves and exercise. It's also possible that doctors are less likely to prescribe estrogen to obese women in the first place. I recommend the patch, especially low-dose patches, to women who have a history of weight gain or who are concerned about it. A number of my patients who've switched from oral to transdermal estrogen have noted a minor change in weight or their ability to lose excess pounds, and there is some research data supporting their experience.

SHOULD I ALSO TAKE TESTOSTERONE?

By now—unless you've skipped the last 20 pages—you are an estrogen expert. But there's another hormone you should know about. It too is depleted, but gradually, starting in our forties. It's male hormone, also known as androgen. Our adrenal glands produce relatively weak androgens in the form of dehydroepiandrosterone (DHEA) and androstendione, and very small amounts of the more potent testosterone. Our ovaries are responsible for the rest of our male hormone production during our reproductive years. A little-known fact: Before menopause, most of our estrogen is derived from male hormone produced by the follicles in our ovaries. I like to proclaim that in women, estrogen is the end product of male hormone production. Men have not taken this evolutionary step.

By the age of 40, male hormone production from the adrenal glands has decreased by half. After menopause, there is additional loss—our remaining production is cut in half once we've used up our ovarian follicles. Most of us don't notice this loss, primarily because we have also lost our estrogen. I know this sounds weird, but estrogen increases production of sex hormone binding globulin, a protein that attaches to testosterone and renders it—I'll use a less-than-P.C. term here—impotent. So your free testosterone level, which is what counts, may be unchanged or even higher after menopause. (This may account for what has been euphemistically called "postmenopausal zest.")

This state of androgen well-being may not last. Roughly six years after menopause, the ovarian tissue that was responsible for your remaining male hormone production is often exhausted, and levels fall. (If your menopause was caused by surgical removal of both ovaries, you most certainly enter an androgen pause.) Free androgen levels can also be ruined by ERT, especially the oral kind, which boosts SHBG production.

So should you consider testosterone replacement as a part of hormone replacement? The answer depends on how you feel in general, and especially on how you feel about your sex life. From the get-go (puberty), male hormone has been a major proponent of your sexual desire and response. When you lose your free, active testosterone, there is a global deactivation of your libido—nothing or no one turns you on. Many of my patients have also expressed a sense of feeling dead from the waist down, with a lessening or complete lack of orgasmic response. If this sounds familiar, don't expect the problem to be fixed by estrogen alone. Adding testosterone should make a difference. You may also find that your menopausal symptoms, especially hot flashes, are not adequately controlled with ERT. The answer may not be more estrogen but additional testosterone. Finally, testosterone has good bone-building credentials and may provide additional benefits to women with osteoporosis. There are even some preliminary data showing that lean body mass is increased (in other words, fat is decreased) in women who take estrogen and testosterone together. The purists might suggest that prior to starting androgen therapy, you have your level of free testosterone checked with a blood test. I'm not strict—if a woman is menopausal and has no libido and generally feels crummy, even with ERT, I don't require her to spend $100 on this test before I'll let her try testosterone. I do, however, test her baseline cholesterol profile and liver function so I can cautiously monitor these once she's begun therapy.

You can accomplish testosterone replacement in several ways. There is a combined estrogen-testosterone pill (Estratest and Estratest H.S., which stands for half-strength). The smaller dose contains 0.625 mg esterified estrogen and 1.25 mg of methyltestosterone. (Methylating prevents testosterone from being broken down into estrogen by the liver.) This dose is sufficient for most women. Indeed, many women need half the amount of testosterone found in this pill to reach their libidinous goals without side effects, and so I have them take Estratest H.S. one day and an estrogen-only Estratab the next. (Note: Taking testosterone does not protect the uterine lining, so women who have not had a hysterectomy will still need to take a progestin.)

Currently, Estratest is the only prescription testosterone product approved by the FDA, and even then the approval is only to aid estrogen in combating resistant menopausal symptoms. But there are also testosterone products made by compounding pharmacies that are available by prescription and can be combined with any HRT regimen you might be on. These include methyltestosterone troques (lozenges) that can be placed under the tongue. The usual dosage I prescribe is 0.5 milligram to 1 milligram per day. There is also natural testosterone in pill, lozenge and liquid form. Although natural sounds great, this form of testosterone is quickly converted to estrogen and so does not always produce the desired response. Then there are testosterone ointments, creams and gels. These can either be applied to the labia, where they'll be absorbed locally and restore thickness and sensitivity, or rubbed on skin elsewhere on the body for systemwide absorption.

There is a conservative skepticism, even among menopausal experts, about adding testosterone to HRT. These authorities are so intent on promoting healthful estrogen replacement that they have deemed libido and sense of well-being less critical. They are also rightfully concerned about testosterone's effect on a woman's lipid profile because studies have shown that the hormone, especially in high doses, can decrease production of good HDL cholesterol in the liver, even as it also lowers total cholesterol and "bad" LDL levels and triglycerides. The good news is that at least in monkeys, testosterone does not completely undermine estrogen's benefits to the heart. But whether we can use short-term research on monkeys to predict long-term effects on women is debatable, and no lengthy studies on women exist. Using testosterone in the form of a lozenge or cream may diminish its effect on the liver, and thus on cholesterol levels.

Most of the "Why would you ever want to take a male hormone, anyway?" response springs from old data linking very high doses of testosterone to liver damage and enlargement of the clitoris. The doses now used to reestablish the testosterone levels you had in your twenties and thirties are generally too low to engender these worrisome effects. In some particularly testosterone-sensitive women, however, acne or male-pattern hair growth can occur with these doses. If this begins to happen, you can reverse these changes by switching to an even lower dose or stopping the medication.

ERT allows many of my patients to feel much better. TERT—testosterone/estrogen replacement therapy—has some of them proclaiming with glee, "I've got my old self back!"

I DON'T WANT TO TAKE ESTROGEN. WHAT OTHER MEDICATIONS CAN I CONSIDER?

The answer depends on your health goals.

Relieve hot flashes: There are a few prescription drugs that can do this. The standard nonhormonal medical therapy for hot flashes, night sweats, insomnia and restlessness is Bellergal, which constricts blood vessels, preventing the flush. It also contains phenobarbital, which sedates and may help regulate the brain's temperature control system, as well as belladonna, which has a relaxing effect. Unfortunately, phenobarbital is addictive, and belladonna causes dry mouth and dizziness. In my experience, after a couple months of use, this medication provides no more benefits than a placebo. I find that another drug, clonidine, is generally more effective. It comes in pill or patch form. Side effects include dry mouth and dizziness, as well as constipation. This drug was developed to treat high blood pressure, so if you have this problem, you'll be treating two conditions with one medication. But if you have normal blood pressure, you may find that you feel faint when you suddenly stand up.

Maintain heart health: If your cholesterol levels are already abnormal (greater than 240 mg/dl), you should definitely consider cholesterol-lowering statin medications such as Lopid, Lipitor or Mevacor. You're also a potential candidate for one of these drugs if your total cholesterol level is borderline high (200 to 239 mg/dl) and your triglycerides are over 150 mg/dl and your HDL level less than 45 mg/dl. In the past, doctors may have told you that these levels were not great, but you could live with them.

Now the current wisdom suggests that you could actually die from them, so earlier and more stringent therapy is advised. And if you already have heart disease, the statins (lipid-lowering drugs) may reduce your chance of dying of a heart attack, even when your cholesterol levels are considered normal.

The two so-called "designer" estrogens or SERMs (selective estrogen receptor modulators) will also have a positive effect on the cholesterol profile, albeit a far less potent one than estrogen. Tamoxifen is the drug of choice to prevent recurrence or decrease significant risk of breast cancer. Raloxifene is used to treat osteoporosis in postmenopausal women.

Another heart disease risk factor that you should control early and aggressively is hypertension. Diuretics and/or beta-blockers are in order for the former. For details, see page 183.

Maintain or improve bone mass: There are currently several drugs that are called "antiresorptive" because they prevent a process called resorption, where bone-eating cells create small cavities in the bone. While the bone-eating cells are held at bay, bone-building cells can continue filling up existing cavities, ultimately increasing bone mass. The very best antiresorptive drug is estrogen, but if you can't or won't use it, there are other contenders: the biphosphonates, SERMs and calcitonin. The most-prescribed biphosphonate is alendronate (Fosamax), which can increase bone density by 1% to 3% a year and nearly halve the rate of future fractures. If a bone density test shows you already have osteoporosis, you should start at the therapeutic dose of 10 milligrams a day; if your bone mass is low and you don't want it to go lower as a result of menopause, you might consider a preventive dose of 5 milligrams per day. This medication must be taken first thing in the morning, at least half an hour before you eat or drink anything but water. Because it can irritate the upper gastrointestinal tract, you have to remain upright (you can't lie down) after ingesting the drug. An older medication, etidronate (Didronel), is an option for women who can't take alendronate because of gastrointestinal upset. This medication should be taken at periodic intervals (14 days every 3 months). Too much or continuous dosing can cause bad bone production. It may not be quite as effective as alendronate, but it remains a viable therapy with few or no side effects. The SERM raloxifene (Evista) may be easier than Fosamax for some women to take. It can be taken at any time of day, with or without food, and doesn't cause GI upset. It promotes increases in bone density and a decrease in the risk of vertebral fractures. A possible added benefit is that it has been shown to decrease breast cancer risk in postmenopausal women who have osteoporosis.

An alternative for women who are at least five years postmenopausal and who, for whatever reason, don't want to take one of these oral medications is calcitonin, a nasal spray. It produces a slightly lower boost in bone density than the biphosphonates and Evista, but appears to protect against fractures just as well. There are also two experimental therapies that actually stimulate bone-building cells, parathyroid hormone and slow-release fluoride. These may eventually prove to be excellent options. With all of these medications, it is essential that you continue to get ample amounts of calcium—1,500 milligrams a day—as well as 400 to 800 international units of vitamin D.

I WANT TO GO THROUGH MENOPAUSE "NATURALLY." WHAT ARE MY ALTERNATIVES?

This is one of the questions that I'm most frequently asked, not only in my office but at many social events. (Frankly, I'd rather discuss politics or literature, but I'm not given the option.) This quest for an alternative is not surprising considering that at most, only 30% of menopausal women in the United States take HRT. I've found that many women are angry with the medical establishment because they feel doctors have dismissed this question. Others still love (or at least accept) their traditional M.D.s but want to use so-called alternative herbal or natural medicines because these therapies match their own values and philosophical orientations when it comes to their health. As a result, women are fleeing their doctors' offices in droves and taking their bodies to alternative practitioners. Two-thirds of women end up using some form of complementary medicine for menopausal complaints. (Even more amazing is the fact that almost three-fourths of women using estrogen *also* were seeking extra help from an alternative source!) My feeling is that a woman shouldn't have to leave my office unsatisfied. If you're properly informed about estrogen and decide not to take it, it's my responsibility to help you get relief from your symptoms and feel better.

My orthodox, traditional training has taught me to seek proof that a therapy works, in the form of a double-blind, crossover, placebo-controlled study. This simply means that the therapy in question was administered to a group of patients who didn't know whether they were getting the therapy or placebo (nor did their doctors). Meanwhile, a placebo was given to a similar group of patients. After an appropriate period of time, the groups were switched. Their responses were recorded throughout the trial. Alternately, I look at long-term studies on large populations to see whether a given substance or therapy influenced the development of a disease. Finally, when I prescribe a medication, I know that there is the Great One out there—the FDA—watching the drug's safety and purity and making sure the manufacturer's claims of efficacy are accurate.

Unfortunately, when it comes to most alternative remedies, we don't have this kind of proof. Natural medicines can't be patented, and there is no financial incentive to carry out the kinds of tests I'm looking for. Nor does the FDA require these tests. Having said this, I realize that women in other cultures have for hundreds, even thousands, of years used alternative therapies for symptoms of menopause. But when we attempt to do the same on our own, and especially when we mix them together with prescription drugs, we may end up with significant side effects. Here is what's available and what I tell my patients.

Herbs

Black cohosh: This is the only herbal remedy for menopausal symptoms that is recognized by the German Commission E, the most established body overseeing herbal medicine. (It's sort of an FDA for herbs.) There are a handful of studies that compare an extract of black cohosh, a forest plant, to estrogen or a placebo. Unfortunately the trials weren't "blind"— women knew what they were taking. Some of the studies were of very short duration, and some of the estrogen "controls" had unusually little improvement in their symptoms. But reports were made and they stated that this herb decreased hot flashes, sweating, headache, heart palpitations, nervousness, sleep disturbances and even bad moods.

A standardized form of black cohosh is sold under the brand name Remifemin. Standardization means that the manufacturer has taken steps to ensure that the product contains the actual dose of extract stated on the label. The suggested dose is one to two tablets twice daily. Although the manufacturer states that studies show no estrogenlike effects on the endometrium, I don't know that we have a complete endometrial bill of health with long-term use of this product. Mild gastrointestinal complaints, headache, dizziness and weight gain have been reported in a few of the studies. There are also reports that black cohosh may elevate liver enzymes, suggesting it might adversely affect the liver. If you decide to try this therapy, see your doctor for a pelvic exam at least once a year and report any unusual bleeding immediately. A liver function test may also be in order. The Commission has recommended that it not be taken for more than six months. The American PDR (*Physician's Desk Reference*) for herbal medicines states that "estrogen-like effect cannot be upheld any longer due to more recent results of research."

Dong quai: This is made from the root of a Chinese plant and is used in Chinese medicine for menstrual irregularities and menopausal symptoms. It is believed to relieve nervousness, dizziness, insomnia and forgetfulness. It's possible that the belief that it works is the crux of its success: In a recent study, dong quai was no more effective than a placebo at relieving hot flashes, nor did it have any estrogenic effect on the uterine lining or vagina. Practitioners of traditional Chinese medicine criticize this study, saying dong quai is almost never prescribed by itself but rather in conjunction with four or more other herbs. A note of warning: It can cause excessive bleeding if used with anticoagulants (including aspirin), and it sensitizes the skin to sun exposure and even skin cancer.

Ginseng: Another herb used by the Chinese to treat everything from menstrual disorders to depression, insomnia, sexual dysfunction and general old age. My experience with patients who have tried ginseng has been borne out by recent studies: Ginseng doesn't appear to be any better than a placebo at relieving hot flashes, but it may have a slightly uplifting effect on your general sense of well-being. (This is obviously a very subjective report and may be a placebo effect.) There are no good studies to tell us how much to take, but there is evidence that ginseng can, especially when taken with hormone therapy, cause uterine bleeding.

Chasteberry (vitex): This produces anti-male-hormone effects (hence the appellation "chaste") in men, but paradoxically, it's been purported to enhance libido in women. If it binds up receptors for male hormone, this doesn't seem possible. Because of this antihormone activity, it's also supposed to help treat breast pain. Herbal medicine practitioners recommend it for vaginal dryness and depression during menopause, but there are no reliable data that chasteberry is truly effective.

Soy: I've already given you a lengthy lesson on soy, its health properties and its possible effect on breast cancer risk (see page 162). But can the isoflavones (weak plant estrogens) in soy relieve hot flashes? Studies show that it is only slightly better than a placebo. But since it's healthy and will also improve your cholesterol profile, I would certainly urge you to try it. Aim for 20 to 60 grams of soy protein a day (you can get 30 grams from two cups of soy milk or six ounces of tofu). You can also take your soy protein in powder or pill form; however, it's not clear whether extracting the protein and putting it in a powder or pill undermines any health-promoting effect it may have.

Red clover: This plant is another rich source of isoflavones, and its plant estrogens are being used to produce the dietary supplement Promensil. The average American consumes only 2 to 5 grams of isoflavones daily, chiefly from beans and peas; people in Asian countries, however, average 40 to 80 milligrams per day. Promensil provides 40 milligrams of isoflavones in a daily tablet. Its manufacturers claim that it may be superior to soy supplements because it contains four isoflavones while soy has only two. The first placebo-controlled U.S. trial of Promensil was recently completed. It found that the frequency and intensity of hot flashes were reduced by roughly half.

Gingko: This has been shown to improve short-term memory and concentration in people with early Alzheimer's disease. There is also evidence that it helps treat circulatory disorders and mood swings. It may accomplish this by acting as an antioxidant and preventing cell damage. Since short-term memory loss may occur with estrogen loss, gingko may help as a menopausal therapy. I take it (as does my husband, whose occasional lapses in memory have nothing to do—we think—with his hormones.) The recommended dose is 120 to 240 milligrams of standardized gingko leaf extract a day. Possible side effects include gastrointestinal disturbances, headache and skin reactions. If you take more than the recommended dose, you may become restless and not sleep well. It can promote bleeding, so if you're using anticoagulants (or even aspirin), be careful not to exceed the recommended dose, and to stop if any bleeding occurs. It's probably a good idea to stop gingko, as you would stop aspirin, the week before any planned surgical procedures.

St. John's wort: A little esoterica: This plant is said to have real spots, symbolic of the blood of St. John, which appeared on its leaves on the anniversary of the saint's beheading—hence its name. *Wort* is simply an old English term for plant and has nothing to do with viral skin lesions (or frogs). The extract inhibits the reuptake of the neurotransmitter serotonin in a way similar to drugs such as Prozac, Paxil and Zoloft. I've included it as an alternative menopause remedy because (a) 20% of us experience depression at some point in our lives and (b) estrogen depletion has been associated with mood changes and a sense of the "blahs." St. John's wort has been shown to be effective in improving mild to moderate depression in up to 75% of patients after four to six weeks of use, and may also be helpful for seasonal affective disorder (SAD). Because the side effects are much less than with traditional SSRIs, German doctors now prescribe this extract 20 times more frequently than Prozac. The recommended dose is 300 milligrams three times daily. It can cause sun-induced skin reactions and should not be used together with SSRIs, although some doctors have found that if depression does not respond to St. John's wort alone, adding gingko (80 mg 3 times daily) helps. Obviously, when neither of these suffice, it's time to see a psychologist, psychiatriast or psychopharmacologist for more extensive therapy and prescription antidepressants.

SAM-e: Supplements of S-adenosyl-methionine, a substance that occurs in the body as a by-product of amino acid metabolism, are being touted as an antidepressant and antiaging elixir. This newcomer to the world of natural antidepressants has been studied extensively in Europe, but no good trials have yet been done in the United States. Like St. John's wort, it may offer relief for mild depression, but it's no substitute for professional help.

Evening primrose: The seeds from this plant are rich in gamma linoleic acid (GLA), which is a fatty acid produced by the placenta and found in breast milk. It has been recommended for breast pain, PMS and menopausal symptoms, but in recent studies has been found to be no better than a placebo.

Valerian root: This has been used for ages as a tranquilizer. It contains a gamma aminobutyric acid (GABA) derivative (a similar compound has also been found in chamomile). This herb has been approved by the German Commission E as a "sedative and sleep inducing preparation." Once more I include it as a menopausal alternative because sleep disorders are common in menopause. The herb is generally thought to be safe but has been linked to four cases of severe liver damage as well as headaches, excitability, uneasiness and heart function disorders. The usual dosage is one to two commercial capsules before sleep, or 0.3 to 1.0 milliliter liquid extract or 4 to 8 milliliter of a tincture.

Progesterone creams: The 2% natural progesterone creams sold over-the-counter under the brand names FemGest and ProGest, and available through compounding pharmacies, are used by some women in an effort to control hot flashes. A recent study found that 83% of women who tried a natural progesterone cream (versus 14% who used a placebo) felt that it improved their hot flashes. But claims that the product protects against osteoporosis are not sufficiently substantiated. If you want to try one of these creams, start with a 20- to 40-milligram daily dose.

Don't confuse this cream with stronger, pharmacologic doses of natural progesterone that are prescribed to protect the endometrium during estrogen replacement therapy. Like other doctors, I've had patients who developed endometrial precancer and cancer because they relied on an over-the-counter progesterone cream when they should have been taking a prescription product.

Another warning: Yam creams are promoted as a natural source of progesterone. While derivatives of inedible Mexican wild yams (unrelated to our sweet potato or edible yams) are used to produce natural progesterone in the lab, your skin can't convert yam products to progesterone on its own. So these yam-only creams are no more than an expensive moisturizer. Many of these so-called yam creams actually contain no yam extract. Some reportedly even contain synthetic progestins.

DHEA: Another hormone is available over-the-counter, and because it is sold as a dietary supplement, it is not subject to FDA supervision. Dihydroepiandrosterone is a weak male hormone that has been touted as an antiager—something many menopausal women will find appealing. But most of the acclaimed studies on its youthening effects were done on rodents, whose bodies barely produce DHEA in the first place.

DHEA doesn't affect hot flashes; its chief claim when it comes to menopausal symptoms is that it theoretically, in its capacity as a male hormone, might improve libido. But there are no data to show that it does. I do give very low doses (10 to 25 mg daily) of a formula specially prepared by a compounding pharmacy to my patients who have documented low DHEA-sulfate levels on blood tests and who complain of low energy and fatigue. Roughly half of them report that it helps. You'll notice I send my patients to a compounding pharmacy for their DHEA—not to their local drugstore/deli/airport or any of the other variety of places this product is sold. This is because the purity and levels of DHEA in pills you might pull off a store shelf can vary tremendously.

My Herbal Concerns

In listing the products above, I've implied that some of them may help. But as a physician looking at a woman's overall health, I also have to address whether they can cause harm. Megadoses of anything certainly can. Ginseng, for example, can cause ovarian cysts if taken in large amounts. So consult with an expert before you use herbal products—and I don't mean the 23-year-old behind the counter at the health food store. There is also mounting concern about the quality and purity of the herbal products on store shelves, particularly those imported from Asia and South America, where production standards may not be up to U.S. snuff. Contaminants in these products may be hazardous, even potentially fatal. Look for herbal products that meet United States Pharmacopeia (USP) standards for safety and purity. If at all possible, purchase pills and extracts produced in the United States from U.S.-grown herbs.

Acupuncture

Some studies have shown that acupuncture can decrease the frequency and severity of hot flashes. We know that it does raise levels of endorphins, the body's feel-good chemicals. Whether this is what's making women's symptoms improve or whether there is a more specific explanation is unknown. The Chinese originators of acupuncture would say that its success has to do with the way it alters the flow of the body's life energy, called *chi* or *qi*. Whatever the explanation, it shouldn't hurt (literally). Studies have allowed the National Institutes of Health to state that "promising" results have emerged showing its efficacy for use in surgically or chemotherapy-produced nausea or certain types of pain (including menstrual), but further research is needed to uncover additional areas where acupuncture will be useful. We're back to looking for a message on the head of a pin!

I'VE BEEN DIAGNOSED WITH DUCTAL CARCINOMA IN SITU. IS IT CANCER? AND HOW SHOULD IT BE TREATED?

Yes, it's the first diagnosable form of very early stage cancer. So early, in fact, that the cancer cells, which are in the lining of the milk duct, have not spread into the surrounding breast tissue; nor have they migrated to the lymph glands. Ductal carcinoma in situ (DCIS) typically occurs in postmenopausal women and is usually detected as a characteristic cluster of microcalcifications visible on a mammogram. Occasionally it can be felt as a mass during a breast exam. There has been a remarkable increase in the incidence of DCIS in recent years, probably due to improved pickup with mammogram.

If DCIS is left alone, it will become an invasive cancer over the next 15 to 20 years in about one in four women who have it. That's why once the diagnosis is made from a biopsy, it is crucial that your doctor make sure that the entire tissue sample is examined and that there is a cancer-free border around its edges. This may mean that after a needle or punch biopsy, further excision, in the form of a lumpectomy, is necessary. This margin will also help ensure that the surgeon isn't missing an adjacent invasive cancer.

In the past it was felt that most women with DCIS would benefit from radiation therapy following lumpectomy. This was based on a study that found that after 12 years, the recurrence rate of the cancer in the same breast was higher (27%) among women who did not have radiation than among those who did (12%). The newest data suggest that some women may be able to forgo radiation, provided that there is a cancer-free margin of at least 1 centimeter around the DCIS-containing tissue. This option can be considered provided that the surgeon has removed an adequate sample of tissue for a very thorough examination by the pathologist.

Once you've been diagnosed with DCIS, you are at higher than average risk of developing cancer in your other, unaffected breast, and you'll need to make sure you are compulsive about yearly mammograms and monthly self-exams. Because of this increased risk, the question arises: Would you benefit from taking tamoxifen, which has been shown to cut breast cancer rates by half in high-risk women? Unfortunately, the American studies of this drug did not include women with DCIS, while European studies that did include these women failed to show that the drug lessened their risk. Oncologists are divided on the subject and are awaiting further studies. This is a decision you'll have to talk over carefully with your doctor.

I'VE JUST BEEN DIAGNOSED WITH BREAST CANCER— WHAT'S THE NEXT STEP?

First let me give you some numbers: Localized breast cancer has a 98% five-year survival rate and an overall survival rate (if all stages are considered) of 87% in Caucasian women. Unfortunately, these statistics are not as good as in African-American women who have an 89% five-year survival with local disease and an overall 71% survival for all stages. (For unknown reasons, this cancer appears to spread more aggressively in this group of women.) Yes, this is a very serious diagnosis, but with early diagnosis and the right therapy odds are that you can beat this disease.

It would take an entire book to give you all of the surgical, radiation and chemotherapy options currently available. This is not that book. But I am going to walk you through the steps I go through with my own patients once they've received this diagnosis.

1. Find Out What Kind of Breast Cancer You Have
If your diagnosis was made by needle, stereotactic or core biopsy—in other words, if only a very small amount of tissue was removed—a larger excision by a surgeon will be necessary. This tissue can then be analyzed microscopically by a pathologist to determine whether or not the cancer is localized (in situ) or invasive and in what part of the breast tissue it originated (the ducts or lobular tissue). Within each type of cancer (ductal or lobular), there are subtypes, and it's important to know this because they have different rates of growth or spread. The tumor's size is also important in the staging of the disease. Pathology studies will determine whether the cancer cells are estrogen-receptor positive (meaning sensitive to the hormone) or estrogen-receptor negative (not sensitive). A similar test is done to determine their progesterone receptor status. Additional tests are done on the nuclear material of the cancer cells to assess the aggressiveness of the malignancy.

2. Find Out the Cancer's Stage
If the pathology report shows you have invasive cancer, the surgeon will also remove lymph nodes from the underarm to see if the cancer has reached them. In the past, multiple nodes were excised, but many surgeons now prefer to use sentinel node biopsy to ascertain this spread. This involves injecting dye into the area around the tumor to determine which node it spreads to first. This "sentinel" node is then removed and examined. If it is found to be cancer-free, the other nodes are assumed to be free of tumor cells as well, and no further node removal is necessary. If the sentinel node has been invaded by the cancer, then it and other lymph nodes will be removed.

The size of the tumor and extent of its spread will determine the cancer's stage, which will help determine your therapy. The stages are as follows:

Stage I: Localized tumor no larger than 2 centimeters (about 1 inch).

Stage II: Tumor no larger than 2 centimeters that has spread to the underarm lymph nodes or to tissues near the breast such as the chest muscles or ribs.

Stage III: Tumor larger than 5 centimeters that has spread to underarm lymph nodes *or* tumor smaller than 5 centimeters and the underarm lymph nodes have grown into each other or into other tissues *or* the tumor has spread to tissues near the breast (such as the chest muscles and ribs) or to lymph nodes near the collarbone, or it is inflammatory breast cancer, an invasive ductal form of breast cancer.

Stage IV: The cancer has spread to other organs, usually the lungs, liver, bone or brain.

3. Choose an Oncologist and Set a Treatment Course

The stage of the cancer will largely determine your therapy. But it's important to explore all the options available as well as who will provide them. I tell my patients to make sure they are comfortable with their oncologist and feel that the doctor will be there for them when it comes to knowledge, expertise *and* emotional support. The oncologist you choose should discuss with you the possibility of breast-conserving surgery (lumpectomy) versus mastectomy and the need for radiation and/or chemotherapy. Our new understanding of this disease is that, very early on, breast cancer cells can spread through the blood and lymph glands. These micrometastases may be so small that they are not detected. This is why even in certain Stage I cancers, some oncologists recommend that you have both radiation and chemotherapy after lumpectomy. For those women who have a Stage III or IV cancer, I recommend seeking out a center that provides some of the more aggressive forms of therapy, which might include new drugs and treatment protocols. Some of these treatments will certainly be controversial. For example, study results on bone marrow transplant, which we'd hoped would increase survival in women with advanced breast cancer, have to date been disappointing.

4. Get Referrals to a Radiologist and, If Necessary, a Reconstructive Surgeon

If you require a mastectomy, you may choose to undergo breast reconstruction during the same surgery or (especially if you've had radiation therapy) three to six months later. You'll also need to decide whether you want to have a breast implant put in place or a new breast reconstructed from your own tissue.

5. Consider Tamoxifen Therapy

Once you're through treatment, use of this drug for five years will decrease the risk of recurrent cancer by 42% over the next decade, and will reduce the risk of new cancer in the opposite breast by almost half. This brings the death rate from breast cancer among tamoxifen users down by 26%. Until recently, it was thought that this therapy benefited only women whose tumors were estrogen-receptor positive. But even in women whose estrogen-receptor status is unknown, a benefit has been noted. And many oncologists now feel that all breast cancers, at any age, should be treated with tamoxifen.

MY DOCTOR SUGGESTED SIGMOIDOSCOPY. IS THERE AN ALTERNATIVE?

If you are like most women, you're asking this question because you're hoping there's a way to avoid having any type of colon examination. It's amazing how we have become inured to annual pelvic exams but are still so overwhelmingly reticent about an examination that, in this decade and beyond, may be far more important in saving our lives. Colorectal cancer is the third leading cause of cancer death in women. Most colorectal cancers develop over a period of 10 to 15 years from benign growths called polyps, giving you a wonderful window of opportunity to take advantage of an examination that can discover these growths so that they be removed before they become malignant.

There are only two alternatives to sigmoidoscopy, neither of which is easier. In sigmoidoscopy, a thin, flexible, lighted viewing scope (it's dark in there!) is inserted through the rectum into the lower colon for a distance of about two feet. One alternative is colonoscopy, in which a much longer scope is threaded through the complete length of the colon. The other option is a barium enema, which allows viewing of the entire colon wall by X-ray.

Sigmoidoscopy can be performed in a doctor's office without anesthesia. Many of my patients are more worried about the prep for this exam (an enema or medication to cleanse the bowel) than the procedure itself. I can personally attest to the fact that it's no big deal. Neither is the exam. You simply lie on your side (more elegant than your positioning for a gynecological exam) and experience mild pressure and a gassy sensation. Five minutes later, it's all over. If polyps are found, they can sometimes be removed at the time of the procedure, but you'll subsequently need a more complete exam, in the form of colonoscopy, to ensure that other growths aren't present.

Colonoscopy is done on an outpatient basis and requires mild sedation (so you won't feel much, if anything). You'll need to consume only clear liquids for 24 hours before the procedure. That means a lot of apple juice and Jell-O. The afternoon before the test, you'll begin taking a bowel-cleansing medication.

A barium enema X-ray requires no sedation and is much less expensive than a colonoscopy. It will show almost two-thirds of tumors, provided they are larger than one centimeter. But if this test is positive, colonoscopy will be necessary to better visualize and remove the growth.

The fact is, if you're at average risk for colorectal cancer, you should eventually get both sigmoidoscopy and either a barium X-ray or colonoscopy. Although sigmoidoscopy can prevent up to half of colorectal cancer deaths, results are even better with colonoscopy, which finds 95% of growths. The current recommendation of the American Cancer Society is that you begin screening by age 50 with one of these exams, then have an annual fecal occult blood test (which screens for blood in the stool), plus sigmoidoscopy (every five years), barium X-ray (every five to 10 years) or colonoscopy (every 10 years). You also should have a rectal exam every time you have a pelvic exam. If at any point blood is discovered in your stool, you should follow up with a colonoscopy or barium enema. If these don't reveal why you're bleeding, your doctor will want to run tests on your upper gastrointestinal tract.

If you've had polyps in the past, you should have a barium X-ray or colonoscopy within three years of polyp removal. If you have a history of inflammatory bowel disease, you need a colonoscopy every one to two years.

As with most cancers, some of us are at greater risk than others. Any family history of colon cancer mandates a colonoscopy every three years. And if you have a parent or sibling and two or more relatives in successive generations with a history of colon cancer before age 50, as well as ancestors who had endometrial, stomach, small intestine, urinary tract, breast, pancreas or ovarian cancer, you may carry the gene for hereditary non-polyposis (no prior polyps) colon cancer, or Lynch syndrome. You and your family members can be tested for this gene. Anyone who tests positive should begin colonoscopy tests at puberty and even consider removal of the colon to prevent cancer. If you choose not to be tested, at the very least you should set up a schedule for frequent colonoscopies with a gastrointestinal specialist.

By now I'm sure I've scared the s— out of you. You started out asking about a sigmoidoscopy and ended up reading about removal of the colon. But if you don't do the former, you might wind up undergoing the latter for colorectal cancer. (The other preventive actions you can take are to get at least 25 grams of fiber per day, eat a low-fat, fruit- and vegetable-rich diet, minimize consumption of red meat, exercise regularly and possibly consider taking four to six aspirins a week. I personally gave up red meat when the Harvard nurses' study found that it could more than double the risk of colon cancer.) One in every 18 women will develop this cancer in her lifetime, and 25% of those who get it will die from it. In fact, we are far more prone to this cancer than we are to any malignancy of our reproductive tract. If the tumor is detected in its early stages, there is a 90% cure rate, but that number drops to 6% if the cancer has had time to metastasize.

I am amazed at the excuses my patients use to indefinitely postpone colorectal testing. I know the idea of an enema followed by a scope invading the bowel is discomforting. But it is nothing like the discomfort and invasive procedures you will go through if you develop colorectal cancer.

HOW CAN I TELL IF I'M AT RISK FOR OSTEOPOROSIS?

I'm going to give you a litany of risk factors. You, like most of us, will probably find several that fit you. Some of these risks are beyond your control; others are due to lack of due bone diligence in childhood or even in recent years. The wonderful news is that there is much you can do to alter your bone-destroying behavior, and you can also build back some of this lost bone mass and prevent future fractures.

Risk Factors Beyond Your Control
Race/ethnicity: Being Caucasian or Asian ups your risk, especially if you are very light-skinned, with blond or red hair and blue eyes.

Family history: If your mother, sister or grandmother has had osteoporosis and a resultant hip fracture, especially before age 80, your own risk of hip fracture more than doubles. Also be on the alert if any of your female relatives have developed severe curvature of the spine, also known by the sexist term "dowager's hump." Even though women are three to five times more likely to have an osteoporotic fracture than men, don't forget the men in the family: If they fractured a hip, wrist or spine after age 50, they may have passed on a gene that predisposes to osteoporosis.

Body type: Being svelte may make sense for models, but not for bones. Thin, petite, small-boned women are at greater risk.

Age: The older you get, the more you're at risk. Twenty percent of women in their fifties already have osteoporosis, most without even knowing it; by age 60 this number rises to 45%.

Early menopause or missed periods: Because estrogen is crucial to building and maintaining healthy bones, entering menopause (or having your ovaries removed) before age 45 or skipping your periods for more than six months at a time during your reproductive years places you at increased risk.

Personal history of eating disorders or excessive exercise: Having anorexia or bulimia or exercising to the point that you stop menstruating undermines bone health. Once more, you have done yourself an estrogen injustice.

History of poor diet: Your critical bone building is done in childhood and young adulthood, so too little calcium and too much protein (which impairs calcium absorption) during this time can leave you with low bone mass.

History of smoking: Even if you've quit, damage has been done to your bones. While you were puffing away, you were literally poisoning your ovaries and reducing the amount of estrogen they were able to produce, and even caused them to stop working altogether at a younger than expected age. The longer you smoked, the greater the probability that your current lower bone mass is low.

Risk Factors Within Your Control
Sedentary lifestyle: Lack of exercise, particularly weight-bearing exercise such as walking, running, climbing stairs or lifting weights, means you lack the physical stress and stimulation necessary to get bone-building cells to do their thing. Doing some form of this exercise for an hour three times a week can boost a menopausal woman's bone mass by 5.2% in just

one year. A sedentary woman, on the other hand, will *lose* bone mass at a rate of 1.2% in the same year.

Poor diet: You need 1,200 milligrams of calcium per day from food or supplements if you're menopausal and taking estrogen; that need increases to 1,500 mg if you are not taking estrogen or once you reach age 65. You also need magnesium (300 mg to 500 mg) to absorb your calcium. If you eat a lot of protein—perhaps because you are trying a high-protein weight-loss diet—you may be impairing your ability to absorb calcium.

Too little sunshine: You need at least 400 international units of vitamin D each day to help your body absorb calcium; after age 65, this should be increased to 800 IU. Ten to 15 minutes of exposure to sunlight each day will generally give you adequate vitamin D because your skin manufactures the vitamin in response to UV rays. But these days we're all wearing sunscreen (I am and I hope you are). Because no one knows for sure if sunscreens impair vitamin D production, I tell my patients to get vitamin D from fortified foods such as milk or from a supplement.

Heavy caffeine intake: Drinking more than four cups of coffee a day may triple the risk of hip fracture. If you must have some coffee to get (or keep) going, two cups a day is probably fine provided you get enough calcium. You can even "express" deliver some calcium to your bones by drinking café au lait.

Excessive alcohol intake: Alcohol inhibits absorption of calcium and vitamin D and may also decrease your liver's ability to activate vitamin D. More than seven drinks per week is linked with low bone mass, heightened bone loss and an increased risk of fracture.

Smoking: Current smokers lose bone mass at a faster rate than nonsmokers, so even if you've smoked for a long time, it will help to quit now. If you continue to smoke, your risk of hip fracture is more than double that of a nonsmoker.

Being menopausal and not taking estrogen: Once you lose your estrogen, you lose bone mass at a rate of 2% to 3% per year. If you started out with low bone mass or if you're several years postmenopause and haven't taken ERT, you're at risk for osteoporosis.

Other Risk Factors

Certain medical conditions: There are many diseases that can affect
your absorption of calcium or contribute to bone breakdown. Moreover,
the therapies used for some of these conditions can themselves have
bone-damaging effects.

DISEASES THAT AFFECT THE ENDOCRINE SYSTEM

Hyperparathyroidism. Parathyroid hormone is responsible for maintaining a steady level of calcium in your blood. One of the ways it does this
is by taking calcium from your bones, where it's stored. If too much
parathyroid hormone is produced, bone is rapidly demineralized.

Hyperthyroidism. Overproduction of thyroid hormone leads to bone loss.

Cushing's syndrome. Excessive production of corticosteroid hormones
erodes bone mass.

DISEASES OF THE BLOOD

Multiple myeloma

Lymphoma

Leukemia

Pernicious anemia

JOINT DISEASES

Rheumatoid arthritis

Ankylosing spondylitis

GASTROINT\ESTINAL DISEASES

These conditions impair our absorption of nutrients, including calcium.

Celiac disease

Crohn's disease

Chronic liver disease

Use of certain medications: Some drugs inhibit calcium absorption,
while others actually trigger bone breakdown.

GLUCOCORTICOIDS

These steroids are prescribed for many diseases, including asthma and
arthritis. A major side effect is that they prevent bone-building cells from
doing their job, while also diminishing calcium absorption. If you have
taken a glucocorticoid for just six months, you may have developed significant bone loss. Ideally, you should have a bone density scan before begin-

ning this therapy; if you're found to have low bone mass, you should begin taking a biphosphonate (alendronate or etidronate) if you will be on glucocorticoids for more than a few months.

ANTIEPILEPTIC DRUGS

LITHIUM

ANTICOAGULANTS
These include heparin.

DIURETICS
One type of diuretic, the furosemides (Lasix, Furoside), increases urinary loss of calcium.

Long-term overuse or overdosage of thyroid hormone or hydrocortisone: If you've been diagnosed with hypothyroidism or goiter in the past, your doctor may have given you thyroid hormone—indeed, many women take it for decades. Slight overdosing of thyroid hormone may cause no outward problems, but bone loss may insidiously occur. That is why you should be taking the lowest possible dose of this hormone. Your doctor can help ensure this by periodically testing your thyroid stimulating hormone (TSH) level. If it is below normal, you're taking too much thyroid hormone and should be checked for osteoporosis. The same principal holds true for replacement of hydrocortisone; overdosage can be checked with adrenal-specific blood tests.

Long-term or excessive use of certain nonprescription products: Fiber diminishes calcium absorption, so overusing fiber preparations such as Metamucil may increase osteoporosis risk. Antacids containing aluminum will likewise inhibit calcium absorption.

In general, the more of these risk factors you have, the greater your chance of being afflicted with osteoporosis. That's why I feel that baseline bone density exams are essential for all women with risk factors for osteoporosis who are beginning menopause. But even if you're one of those perfect people who have no risk factors, you may not be able to rest (or stand) on your laurels. I think it's prudent for you to be tested as well, especially if you're not planning to take ERT.

SEX HURTS. WHAT SHOULD I DO?

Since you're over 50, I have to assume that most of your discomfort is due to inadequate lubrication and to thinning of the vulvar skin and vaginal wall, which occur as a result of estrogen deprivation. You may have a "sandpaper" sensation when friction during intercourse makes you feel as though the vaginal walls are tearing. Indeed, sometimes the skin on the bottom part of the vaginal opening does tear.

It stands to reason that if these atrophic vaginal changes are due to lack of estrogen, replacing estrogen will reverse them. But if the atrophy has been allowed to become severe, you may not get immediate relief from estrogen pills or patches. The blood vessels leading to this area may have degenerated and will fail to carry adequate estrogen to the receptors in the tissue where it's needed. The receptors themselves may become dormant. So a local stimulus to reach them and wake them up may be called for, even if you are taking ERT. This site-specific therapy can be given as an estrogen cream or in the form of an estrogen-releasing ring inserted into the vagina (Estring). Initially, 2 grams of cream (Premarin, Estrace or Ogen) should be inserted every other night; after four weeks or when you start to notice an improvement in symptoms, the dose can be decreased to 1 gram twice weekly. If you are on ERT, you may be able to discontinue the cream after several months. But if you choose not to take ERT, you should continue the vaginal therapy as long as you want to maintain its effect. Don't be concerned if perchance this cream gets on your partner's penis—he will not have any hormonal side effects. (Believe it or not, this has been studied.)

Some of my patients object to the cream's messiness or the need to take such an active role in the maintenance of their vaginal health. The ring is an ideal alternative. You can put it in and remove it yourself, and it can be left in place for three months, even worn comfortably during intercourse. For those women who want as little estrogen absorption as possible, the ring is probably the therapy of choice.

If you need additional lubrication when friction occurs, there are lubricants that will help you glide through sex. Available brands include Astroglide, K-Y Liquid and Lubrin (I love these names). The substance should be applied to the labia, clitoris or vagina, or to your partner's penis during foreplay. Petroleum jelly is not a good lubricant; it can cake or dry and may also weaken condoms. Nor should you use perfumed lotions or oils, which can result in irritation to you and your partner.

Women who can't or won't use hormones shouldn't feel that they're destined for uncomfortable sex (or no sex at all). Just as you moisturize your skin, you can moisturize the vagina—but obviously not with the same products. Vaginal moisturizers (such as Replens and Vagisil Intimate Moisturizer) are helpful, but need to be used regularly—every one to four days. They don't build up the vaginal lining or restore blood flow the way estrogen does, but they're better than nothing.

MY SKIN IS AGING FASTER THAN I AM. WHAT CAN I DO?

The skin has its natural aging process, which includes thinning, drying and loss of elasticity. But this is very gradual, and in fact the skin is one of the organs that matures particularly well. What is not well is what you've done to your skin over the years, primarily through sun exposure, but also perhaps with smoking. At least half of your uncomely wrinkles, spots and dryness are due to your attempts at a younger age to get a "healthy" tan or your current failure to adequately protect against UV rays. If you want to see how well your skin really has aged, look at a part of your body that has not been exposed to sun, such as the upper, inner arm or your tush. While some of the damage to your skin is irreversible, you can give your skin a chance to recover by protecting yourself from exposure to these environmental toxins.

Although this is not a gynecologic issue, it's a concern for many of my patients. So here are the most common conditions associated with aging skin and what you can do about them.

Dry Skin

This is due to a reduction of oil production. Dryness tends to be worse on the back and ankles, and to especially plague women in dry climates during the winter months. To minimize dryness, avoid long hot showers or baths. (I hate giving this advice. My favorite evening relaxation is a don't-interrupt-me-for-anything 20-minute hot bath before dinner. So I'm constantly forced to choose between my de-stress routine and dehydrated skin.) After you bathe, apply a bath oil or a heavy lotion that does not contain alcohol. Moisture doesn't have to be expensive—petroleum jelly and baby oil work just fine.

Wrinkling

We have to contend with coarse wrinkles and fine wrinkles. The coarse ones come from years of laughing, frowning, squinting and other facial expressions—they're your frown lines, crow's feet and the lines on either side of your nose. The fine wrinkles are the way your skin pays for sun exposure and smoking; the latter is worse than the former because it breaks down the elastin in your skin. The first and perhaps most effective therapy is one that requires no prescription: Use a moisturizer and a sunscreen (or a single product that contains both) daily.

We don't consider our skin to be a sex organ, but it is chock-full of estrogen receptors, and loss of estrogen causes thinning and fine wrinkles. This is why estrogen replacement with a pill or patch has been shown to help the skin retain moisture, maintain thickness and wrinkle less. I think it's possible that if estrogen is applied to the affected skin in a cream it may also plump it up, helping it to appear younger. I'll now reveal a personal secret for which I can offer no substantial scientific support: I resorted to using very small amounts of a vaginal cream (Premarin) on my face after observing what a dramatic effect regular use had on the skin of the labia (and this has been properly, scientifically documented). But remember: If this cream is absorbed into your skin, it will also be absorbed into the rest of your body. Uncontrolled slathering-on of estrogen may cause your blood levels to rise. So, especially if you're also taking estrogen replacement therapy, it should be used cautiously and sparingly and of course with your doctor's knowledge. This is definitely an "off the cuff" and "off the usual skin area" use.

The onslaught of advertising has made it impossible to remain ignorant of the following "cosmeceutical" products available for wrinkle relief.

Retinoids: These plant-derived substances, found in the prescription creams Retin-A and Renova, cause plumping of the skin, which decreases fine wrinkles and helps correct uneven pigmentation. Initially we were told not to use retinoids over long periods of time, but current data suggests doing so is safe. The downside: Retinoids work gradually, taking several months to have an effect. They can also be drying and increase sun sensitivity.

Alpha-hydroxy acids: There are myriad AHA-containing products on the market, most nonprescription. Their effect is similar to that of the retinoids, though they have less impact on skin pigment. They may also thicken the skin. Their strength and ability to be absorbed by the skin vary according to the type of acid and the cream's pH. You may want to ask your dermatologist, or experiment to see which gives you the best results.

Antioxidants: Oxidation ages all organs, including your skin, and it makes theoretical sense that antioxidant vitamins such as C and E will help combat this. Nonprescription products containing these vitamins are widely available, but good, controlled studies of absorption and effectiveness are scarce.

All of the above are do-it-yourself (sometimes with a prescription) anti-wrinkle therapies. For some women, this not enough, and they elect to undergo one of these cosmetic procedures performed by a dermatologist or a plastic surgeon.

Collagen injection: This substance, which supports our skin and bones, is purified from animal or human collagen and injected into the crevices of deep wrinkles. Its effect lasts from three to six months, so maintenance involves follow-up injections.

Autologous fat transplantation: Fat is taken from one area of your body and injected under wrinkled (even finely wrinkled) skin in your face. This may last longer than collagen but does require repeated treatments.

Botox: Injections of botulinum toxin (the same one that causes food poisoning—yuck!) can be used to temporarily paralyze muscles that cause deep wrinkles. It works best for deep frown lines. Despite its toxic name, it's considered remarkably safe for your general health, but on rare occasion the wrong muscles around the eye may be temporarily weakened.

Laser skin resurfacing: This can produce up to a 70% reduction in fine and even deep wrinkles and pigment problems. But it requires several weeks of recovery and can, in some cases, cause long-term skin redness or, very rarely, permanent scarring.

Chemical peels: These resurface the skin much like lasers do, reducing fine wrinkles and pigment problems and generally smoothing the skin. They won't abolish deep wrinkles. Concentrated peels can require a long recovery period; light ones leave skin pink for just a few days, and of course have less dramatic results.

Dermabrasion: This is done with a small spinning wheel or wire brush that literally sands down the outer surface of the skin. Its ability to smooth the skin of the face (with the exception of the eyes) is similar to that of the laser, but subsequent redness may be less. Unlike laser, the results are quite dependent on the skill of the operator.

These techniques will not correct the sagging and bagging of our skin that is also related to age. The plastic surgery options to help correct these are beyond the scope of this section and comprise a book unto themselves. When my patients ask my opinion about face lifts, brow lifts, chin tucks, eye "jobs" and other procedures, I advise them to first analyse whether these will truly make them feel better about themselves. If the answer is yes, I suggest they consult with several board certified plastic surgeons and explore their surgical options (and of course results, cost and possible complications) as thoroughly as possible.

Benign Growths

Brown spots and red bumps seem to sprout from nowhere as our skin ages. Of course, any new growth that fits the A, B, C, D description of potential skin cancer (see page 116) should be checked by your dermatologist. These are the most common benign conditions:

Cherry angiomas: These pinhead-sized red dots are due to overgrowth of very small blood vessels. They can sometimes grow to be quite large and turn black. They tend to develop in clusters during pregancy and then don't go away. They do not need to be treated, unless they are cosmetically unacceptable.

Seborrheic keratoses: These brownish, waxy-looking patches can be flat or raised and are often found on the face, back and under the breasts. Their borders are clearly demarcated (this helps distinguish them from melanoma). They do not need to be removed unless they become red or irritated or bleed.

Acrochordons: Commonly known as skin tags because they project out from the skin, these wrinkled, reddish growths most often occur around the neck, under the arm, near the breast or in the groin area. If they are constantly being rubbed and become irritated, or if you find them annoying, they can be removed by your dermatologist.

After answering this question I've looked at myself from head to toe and have self-diagnosed just about everything on the list. So take comfort in the fact that you're not alone.

WHAT TESTS SHOULD I HAVE?

These are the examinations, tests and procedures I recommend for my patients in their fifties.

Examination/test/procedure	How often
Blood pressure	At least every two years
Cholesterol test	Nonfasting total and HDL test every five years
Fasting plasma glucose test	Every three years
Thyroid hormone test	Every five years
Pelvic exam & Pap smear	Annually; Pap at doctor's discretion after three negative tests
Rectal exam	Annually
STD testing	At your/your doctor's discretion
Clinical (physician) breast exam	Annually
Breast self-exam	Monthly
Mammogram	Annually
Electrocardiogram	Every five years
Bone mineral density	Once
Fecal occult testing	Annually
Colorectal cancer screen	Every five to 10 years, depending on screening method used
Immunizations	Tetanus booster every 10 years
Eye exam	Every three years
Skin exam by dermatologist	Every two years
Skin self-exam	Annually

WHAT CAN GO WRONG AT MY AGE?

Type 2 Diabetes

This is the most common form of diabetes, accounting for 90% of cases. Roughly one in 12 American adults will get it, most after age 40. Type 1 diabetes usually occurs in childhood and young adults. In this condition the pancreas stops making insulin. In Type 2 diabetes the pancreas produces some insulin, but the body's tissues don't respond very well to it, or are *insulin resistant*. Because the pancreatic cells can still be coaxed to make insulin and insulin therapy is not usually necessary, this form of diabetes is also known as non-insulin-dependent diabetes mellitus (NIDDM). Most Type 2 diabetes is preceded by a symptom-free period in which insulin production is unable to keep blood glucose levels steady and at normal range after a sugar consumption "challenge." This is called *glucose intolerance* and can be measured by testing blood glucose levels before and after a special drink with a known amount of glucose is given. Obesity contributes to insulin resistance, as does polycystic ovarian syndrome and long-term use of corticosteroid drugs.

After coping with insulin resistance over a period of time, the pancreas becomes so fatigued that the inevitable happens: It becomes ineffective and fasting blood sugar rises to more than 126 mg/dl. This is now considered diabetes. Symptoms can include fatigue, excessive thirst, unexplained weight loss, frequent urination or recurrent yeast and bladder infections. But for many women, prior insulin resistance acts as a ticking time bomb. Present 7 to 10 years before symptoms of diabetes develop, it is already causing fat to accumulate at the waistline as well as abnormal cholesterol and triglyceride levels; retinal, kidney and nervous system damage; plaque deposits in the arteries; heart disease and cerebrovascular disease. These complications make diabetes the fourth most common cause of death. Four out of five people with Type 2 diabetes will die of cardiovascular disease. Women are hardest hit. Diabetes erases our female cardiac superiority, and we are more likely than men to develop heart disease if we have diabetes.

So how do we reverse this poor prognosis? Step one is to recognize that you have the disease, which means testing your fasting blood sugar level once every three years after age 45, and yearly if you had diabetes during pregnancy, if you have a family history of Type 2 diabetes or are obese, have polycystic ovary syndrome, hypertension or any symptoms of diabetes.

Once the diagnosis is made, you have to embark on a lifetime course of therapy. Since the major complications of this disease are due to insulin resistance, it's probably best to focus on improving insulin sensitivity rather than lowering blood glucose levels. Therapy doesn't necessarily mean a pill or a shot. Regular physical exercise and weight loss will improve insulin sensitivity. The ideal exercise regimen combines an aerobic workout (walking, biking or swimming, for example) with strength training to build lean body mass and decrease body fat. A diet high in fiber, low in saturated fat and low in simple carbohydrates (from starchy, sugary foods) is best. There's no need to be extreme in the restriction of dietary fat; this will only prompt you to eat more carbs, which are quickly converted to sugar by the body, causing subsequent increase in insulin and triglyceride. It's probably better to make sure you get the right fats—i.e., the monounsaturated or unhydrogenated (no trans fats) polyunsaturated fats. If you institute these three lifestyle changes—exercise, proper diet and weight control—you may also be able to gain appreciably more control over your cardiovascular destiny.

If your blood sugar level is very high at the time you are diagnosed or if, despite your best efforts (and I hope you've really made an effort), you are unable to regulate it, better glucose and lipid control through chemistry may be in order. There are two traditional groups of drugs that, when used alone, are very effective at lowering blood sugar. The first group is known as sulfonylureas (current brand names include Glucotrol and DiaBeta). Except for one particularly long-acting formulation of Glucotrol, these drugs have been associated with weight gain and may not be the preferred therapy if you are obese. There were some concerns that because insulin levels are raised by this type of drug, cardiovascular risk might also be raised. But the drugs appear to cause a modest fall in triglycerides, and recent clinical trials have not shown an increase in heart-related deaths in people with diabetes who were treated with the sulfonylureas.

The second type of effective therapy is metformin (Glucophage). It works by suppressing glucose output by the liver and enhances insulin action in the muscles. So it actually decreases rather than increases insulin levels. It reduces triglycerides and LDL (bad) cholesterol levels. It also curbs appetite and may help some people lose weight. Other classes of medications have been approved for use in the United States. One of them, troglitazone (Rezulin), lowers blood sugar by improving insulin sensitivity; this in turn allows insulin levels to decline. This increases HDL ("good") cholesterol levels and cuts triglycerides by one-fifth. Because of this, Rezulin was initially considered the optimal first-line drug therapy for Type 2 diabetes.

But everything wonderful has a price: Approximately 1% to 2% of patients who use it develop liver damage, and there have been reports of almost 30 deaths from liver disease. Because of this, the FDA has restricted the use of this drug and recommended it be used only in patients whose diabetes is not adequately controlled by other drugs, and extensive liver enzyme tests should be used to detect early warning signs of liver damage. Two new medications in this same class of drugs have also been approved. They are rosiglitazone (Avandia) and pioglitazone (Xenicol). Their longer-term safety and efficacy are also being determined.

To complicate therapy options (and that's why you need a diabetes expert for your ongoing care) there are two additional classes of drugs that have been introduced in recent years. The first includes acarbose (Precose) and miglitol (Glyset), which inhibit enzymes in the small intestines that break down complex sugars into simple sugars. They also slow digestion and absorption, and thus diminish glucose entry into the circulation. So the pancreas has more time to effectively increase insulin when needed.

The other new drug is repaglinide (Prandin), which, like the sulfony-lureas, works by stimulating insulin secretion. However, it is more expensive and has no direct effect on lipids.

Orlistat, a weight-loss drug recently approved by the FDA, is also being studied for its effect on Type 2 diabetes. Because it causes significant decreases in glucose and insulin, as well as in cholesterol levels, researchers are optimistic about its ability to help people minimize the complications of Type 2 diabetes.

Because Type 2 diabetes is associated with abnormal cholesterol levels, cholesterol-lowering drugs may be necessary if, after six to nine months of the therapies listed above, you still flunk your cholesterol test. Aggressive high blood pressure control is also crucial because even mild hypertension significantly magnifies the heart attack, stroke and kidney failure risks associated with this disorder. Because insulin resistance can impair the body's ability to break down clots, the American Diabetes Association has endorsed the use of a daily dose of enteric-coated aspirin (81 to 325 mg) to reduce the risk of heart attack for all people with diabetes who are over age 30 and have either a history of heart problems or risk factors such as high blood pressure or high cholesterol. Finally, if you have diabetes, consider taking estrogen replacement therapy, which in and of itself can significantly lower your risk of heart attack and death from heart disease.

Autoimmune Diseases

One in 10 women will develop one of these diseases in her lifetime. They all seem to share a similar immunologic defect: The fighter cells of the immune system fail to recognize the body's own tissues and go into attack mode, treating the tissues as a foreign invader. Just being a woman places us at a higher risk than men, and unless we recognize the symptoms that accompany these diseases, we will delay proper diagnosis and therapy. The fifties is a peak time for the development of some of these diseases and for experiencing the consequences of others.

Systemic lupus erythematosus: This disease occurs when antinuclear antibodies (ANAs) attack the nuclei of our cells, potentially affecting almost any organ or tissue in the body. For more details about it, see page 113.

Rheumatoid arthritis: The chief autoimmune attack here is on our joints. The tissues become inflamed and can be destroyed, resulting in permanent deformity. A common symptom of RA is morning stiffness that lasts for hours. RA peaks in our forties and fifties as our hormones ebb, and we are four times more likely to develop RA if we have a first-degree relative with it.

RA can begin with fatigue, poor appetite and weakness, followed, months later, by joint swelling, redness, severe tenderness and, eventually, deformities. Bumps called rheumatoid nodules can appear under the skin and near the joints. One way RA is diagnosed is with a blood test that checks for the presence of special antibodies that appear in 75% of women with this disease. As with lupus, the heart, lungs and blood vessels can rarely become inflamed. Women with RA are also at very high risk for osteoporosis, due both to the disease's effect on bone mass and to steroid treatment.

There is no standard progression of this disease. One in five women will have little or no serious joint deformities. If complications occur, they usually do so within the first six years. Treatment involves controlling joint pain, inflammation and stiffening with aspirin and other anti-inflammatory drugs as well as low-dose steroids. If these fail, immunosuppressants, antimalarial drugs, chemotherapy and even surgery or joint replacement will be considered. Early aggressive therapy can make a huge difference.

Scleroderma: Collagen is an important component of our bones and skin, and we bemoan its loss as we enter menopause because it heralds the development of osteoporosis and wrinkles. But too much collagen can be as dire as too little. Scleroderma occurs when there is a disordered, accelerated laying down of collagen that goes on to scar our skin, blood vessels and internal organs, especially the gastrointestinal tract, lungs, heart and kidneys. The disease is four times more common in women than men; it usually begins between our thirties and fifties. As the body's connective tissue is attacked, fluid accumulates under the skin, which thickens and hardens as it becomes bound to the underlying layers of fat. Facial and body movement can become limited. If internal organs are affected, digestion is impaired and pneumonia as well as heart or kidney failure can ensue. The diagnosis is made when characteristic skin changes are accompanied by the presence of antinuclear antibodies in the blood. Treatment focuses on relieving symptoms and improving functioning. Immunosuppressants may reduce scarring, low-dose aspirin may prevent clots from forming in damaged vessels and steroids are called into action to treat inflammation. Although this disease can be fatal, in some cases it spontaneously disappears after a number of years. This is the one time we celebrate loss of collagen.

Sjögren's syndrome: The weapon of attack in this disease is the autoimmune lymphocyte, which first infiltrates mucous membranes and glands throughout the body and then can go on to attack internal organs. The hallmark of this disease is extreme dryness of the eyes, mouth, nose, throat and/or vagina. The stomach, pancreas, gallbladder, heart, brain, blood vessels, muscles and joints can eventually be affected. There is no single diagnostic blood test for SS, but many women may test positive for specific antinuclear antibodies and rheumatoid factors. The most medical therapy can do to treat this disease is relieve symptoms. Artificial tears and saliva as well as vaginal lubricants and estrogen creams can rehydrate dry tissues, and NSAIDs can ease muscle and joint pain, while steroids, antimalarials and other immunosuppressive medications help combat complications.

Multiple sclerosis: Scientists disagree as to whether this is a true autoimmune disease. But what is clear is that T-cells attack the myelin sheath that covers the nerves, causing inflammation and subsequent degeneration (demyelinization). The damaged nerves can no longer properly conduct impulses. Nerve cells in the brain scar, and protein deposits called plaques build up. Women are twice as likely to develop this disease. Early-onset MS peaks in our teens, late-onset after age 45. MS appears to have a genetic link, and having a first- or second-degree relative with this disorder gives you a 2% to 5% lifetime chance of developing the disease.

Initial symptoms of MS are weakness and fatigue with exertion, lack of dexterity, feelings of tingling or numbness in one or both legs, dizziness and blurred vision and partial visual loss. Once these symptoms occur, they can stop or they can slowly or rapidly progress. The older you are when you get MS, the more likely it is to follow a rapid, disabling course. This can result in memory loss and impaired judgment; trouble walking and swallowing; and bladder and bowel problems, including incontinence.

MS is diagnosed through an evaluation of symptoms, brain MRI and spinal tap. Therapy focuses on managing symptoms and preventing progression of the disease. Rest, stress reduction and proper diet are important. Steroid drugs can reduce nerve inflammation, and immunosuppressants may also help. Immune-system-modulator therapies (Betaseron, Avonex, Copaxone) can lessen the frequency and severity of attacks in people with relapsing-remitting MS (the most common kind), and the MS Society now recommends taking one of these medications even if the disease is not currently causing symptoms because silent damage to the nerves may be taking place.

Myasthenia gravis: In this case, the autoimmune attack is on receptors located between our nerves and muscles. Because the number of functioning receptors are depleted, fewer signals get through to the muscles, and they fatigue and fail to contract. The eyelids may begin to droop, and eye muscles function poorly, causing double vision. Chewing and swallowing—even smiling—may be difficult. Eventually, movement requires tremendous effort, and weakness of the diaphragm and respiratory muscles can prevent normal breathing. The thymus, a gland below the neck that produces immune cells, may become enlarged and even develop malignant tumors.

Messages are normally carried from the nerve to the muscle through a substance called *acetylcholine*. Diagnosing MG involves administering a substance that inhibits breakdown of acetylcholine and finding that muscle action dramatically improves. Another test in which small, harmless electric shocks are given every few seconds will show that MG is present when stimulated muscle contraction quickly diminishes with successive shocks. Finally, a blood test can detect antiacetylcholinestrase receptor antibodies, which are found in 80% of those with MG.

The chief therapy for MG is anticholinestrase, which prevents breakdown of acetylcholine. It's not a cure, but it allows people with MG to lead full, productive lives. Additional therapy includes removal of the thymus, even if a tumor isn't present. Eighty-five percent of those with MG improve with this surgery. Finally, the usual autoimmune medications, such as steroids and immunosuppressants, can help prevent this condition from progressing.

Fibromyalgia: This pain syndrome (see page 100) is primarily a female illness and peaks between the ages of 40 and 60. It may be related to autoimmune problems, but in truth the underlying cause is uncertain. It is correlated with sleep disorders, general diminishment of health and well-being and chronic fatigue syndrome. The diagnosis and therapies I've previously discussed are often given by a rheumatologist.

Thyroid Nodules and Cancer

Thyroid cancer, which peaks during the fifties and sixties, is, fortunately, one of our most benign cancers. Its hallmark is a nodule that can be felt with careful examination by you or your doctor. The thyroid is a soft, butterfly-shaped gland above your collarbone and below your Adam's apple in the lower portion of the neck. Most of us can't feel our thyroid unless there is something wrong. The "wrong" (a thickening or nodule) can be found in as many as 50% to 60% of women, but only if we were all to be examined by ultrasound. Without special testing, truly palpable nodules are picked up in only about 6% of women. They are five times more common in women than in men, but the vast majority—up to 95%—are benign. Of course, whenever a mass is found there is concern that it might be malignant, and a workup is in order. You are at greater risk for a malignancy if as a child you underwent radiation therapy to the head and neck for an enlarged thymus gland or for acne, or if you have a family history of thyroid cancer.

Any workup should start with a blood test to detect over- or underproduction of thyroid hormone. Both conditions can be associated with benign enlargement of the gland (goiter). Another blood test should be done for levels of serum calcitonin (high levels may indicate that a certain type of thyroid cancer is present).

There are three ways to determine whether or not a nodule is benign. Ultrasound of the thyroid is obviously noninvasive and will demonstrate if the nodule is solid or fluid-filled (cystic), and can also determine whether there is a single nodule or multiple nodules. But it won't definitively establish whether a mass is benign or malignant. So the next possible step is a radionuclear scan of the thyroid, in which a radioactive substance is injected into the veins to reveal a malignancy. (If the nodule is malignant,

the radioactive substance won't show up there. This is called a "cold nodule.") The third method of diagnosis is a fine-needle aspiration (FNA)
biopsy of the nodule. Some doctors go directly to FNA when a nodule is
discovered.

If a nodule turns out to be malignant, surgery is required. Depending on
the size and presence of other nodules, part or, in most cases, all of the thyroid gland is removed. In the latter instance, replacement thyroid hormone
therapy will be necessary for life. If there is no spread to adjacent lymph
nodes, this surgery should be a cure, and even with early spread, radio-
iodine therapy combined with careful monitoring gives a better than 90%
five-year survival rate.

Even though the majority of thyroid nodules are not malignant, they
often need to be treated once they're properly diagnosed. Taking extra thyroid hormone will keep the gland from working too hard (which may have
caused the mass in the first place) and usually will shrink the nodule. If this
doesn't succeed and the nodule continues to enlarge or to produce excess
thyroid hormone, removal of the nodule or radioactive iodine therapy to
destroy the gland may be necessary.

Lung Cancer

This has become the number one cancer killer of American women; a little
more than a decade ago, its fatality rate surpassed that of breast cancer. I
despairingly agree with those disgusting ads: Smoking and lung cancer truly
have become "a woman's thing." In 1998, lung cancer took 67,000
women's lives (as compared to 43,500 deaths from breast cancer). It
amazes me that this disease does not strike the same chord of fear in
women as breast cancer.

Early detection of lung cancer is infrequent. There is no simple routine
screening test for lung cancer, and its classic symptoms of coughing, shortness of breath and fatigue (all of which may feel routine to a smoker) tend
to occur when the disease has progressed. By the time lung cancer shows
up on an X-ray, it has probably spread. Survival rates are dreadful, although
surgery, radiation and chemotherapy are all employed in an effort to combat the disease. The overall five-year survival rate is 14%, and even when
lung cancer is detected early, this rate is only 49%.

Eighty-five percent of lung cancers are caused by smoking. The toxins in
cigarette smoke damage cells in the airways, and over time this damage
results in cancer. Even if you stopped smoking 15 years ago, the residual

YOUR FIFTIES / 255

damage means you have twice the risk of lung cancer of a lifetime non-smoker. Still, this is better than the 35-fold increased risk faced by a current long-term smoker.

Nonsmokers can get lung cancer too, frequently because of exposure to secondhand smoke. Nonsmoking women married to smokers have a 1.5-fold increased risk of all cancers when compared with women married to non-smokers. It's also estimated that 17% of lung cancers in nonsmokers are due to passive exposure in childhood or adolescence.

Chronic lung diseases such as tuberculosis, bronchitis, emphysema and asthma can also lead to lung cancer, as can exposure to environmental pollutants such as asbestos and radon. Air pollution alone may not significantly increase risk, but when combined with smoking it can be deadly.

I'm always amazed when women who smoke ask me what vitamins they can take to protect their lungs. Unfortunately, there is no magic pill to reverse the effects of cigarettes. In fact, one study found that smokers given high doses of beta-carotene in pill form actually had an increased risk of death. But there does seem to be some advantage (for both smokers and nonsmokers) to eating lots of fruits and vegetables and decreasing saturated fat consumption.

My patients who have smoked (or—God forbid—who continue to smoke) also ask me if they should have annual chest X-rays. There is no current official recommendation to do so. A recent study from Cornell and New York University found that special CT scans could detect some lung cancers early enough for them to be successfully treated. The problem was that a quarter of the patients scanned had abnormal nodules. These nodules were followed for several months, and only those that grew were biopsied. Fewer than 40% of the nodules turned out to be cancer. Once this scan becomes more widely available, doctors will have to ensure that just to make sure of a diagnosis, they don't put patients through unnecessary and risky biopsies and surgery. In the meantime, the best therapy I can offer my patients who continue to smoke is avid encouragement to stop; I offer prescriptions for Zyban, Xanax, the Nicorette inhaler or anything else that will help.

MY TOP 10 LIST FOR STAYING HEALTHY IN YOUR FIFTIES

1. Consider hormone replacement therapy; if you decide it's not for you, explore all other avenues of symptom control and heart and bone maintenance.
2. Stop smoking.
3. Exercise regularly (30 minutes of moderate activity almost every day). If you're not already doing some form of resistance training with weights, add this to your routine.
4. Make sure you get the checkups and screening tests recommended for your age group, including mammography and sigmoidoscopy or colonoscopy.
5. Take a multivitamin and consume 1,500 milligrams of calcium from foods or supplements daily.
6. Don't assume that vaginal dryness and diminished libido are inevitable in this decade. Take steps to address these problems.
7. Maintain a healthy weight with a diet low in fat (especially saturated and trans fats) and high in fruits, vegetables and fiber.
8. Limit alcohol intake to one drink a day or less.
9. Explore your family's medical history to look for clues to your genetic risks. Take any additional screening or prevention steps necessary.
10. Allow yourself leisure time—you deserve it—and cultivate interests outside of home and work.

YOUR SIXTIES

CONGRATULATIONS—YOU'RE OUT of the "F" decades (forties and fifties) and into the "S's." At this point in your life, "S" stands for more than your age. You're self-assured, you have succeeded in reaching many of your goals, and should finally be savoring the rewards of decades of hard work. But society has programmed us (with its Medicare and Social Security programs) to think that 65 is a turning point when we automatically convert from being vital, contributing and independent (think: Madeleine Albright) to ailing, inactive and dependent (think: nursing home resident). Why women face this devastating ageism that negates our value, potential and sexuality, while men in their sixties still run for president, become CEOs of corporations and date younger women, is a sociological dilemma that I can't begin to address in this book. I'll leave that to Betty Friedan. But this belittling concept of who we have become should not become who we are. Let's not diminish our achievements. We've come a long way, women, and we should make a health commitment to go farther as we proudly enter our sixties and declare this the "I deserve to feel good" decade.

The transition of menopause is behind you, and many of your symptoms have abated. If you began hormone replacement therapy in the mid- to late 1980s, you now have new and sometimes better treatment options. If you have not started HRT, you have the opportunity to evaluate your bones, your heart and your sense of well-being and to reevaluate your decision if warranted. What you did (or didn't do) for your health in the previous decade has not set an immutable course for your future. You can make a huge difference in the quality and quantity of your years to come by what you do now.

Although hormonal depletion is the chief topic of conversation when it comes to gynecologic health in women over fifty, there are other reproductive organ changes that can accompany the sixties. Years of standing, combined with the stress of carrying and delivering a baby (or babies), possibly exacerbated by weight gain, may have weakened your pelvic support system. As a result, the bladder, uterus, vaginal walls and rectum may drop, or prolapse, causing multiple symptoms. (And while we're on the subject of drooping . . . No matter what you do, your skin has continued to lose collagen, and those sags and wrinkles have inexorably worsened.)

The other more health-threatening concern for this decade is, of course, cancer—chiefly endometrial and ovarian. We know what causes the former—unopposed estrogen (either from production by fat cells or from estrogen replacement without adequate progesterone). Thankfully, this is not a silent cancer; it is usually heralded by unexplained vaginal bleeding. But ovarian cancer is silent and is increasingly common as women age. Because we have no established screening test for this disease, regular pelvic exams are in order but won't guarantee early diagnosis.

Changes in your fat-to-muscle ratio that began in your late forties continue in this decade, and exercise still has its powerful protective effect, as does estrogen replacement.

The good news is that you aren't experiencing the very rapid loss of bone mass that occurred in the years immediately following menopause. However, if you did not prevent that loss, you may be at significant risk for fracture. If you've never had a bone density scan, now's the time. Calcium, exercise, vitamins and medications can help make fragile bones more sturdy at any age.

Hypertension, diabetes and cholesterol abnormalities all increase with age, making coronary artery disease the number one health concern for women in their sixties. Other heart disorders may also increase in this decade. Heart rhythm disturbances such as atrial fibrillation may develop, and this may increase risk of clot formation. It's not just the vessels of the heart that we're worried about. Those that feed our brain can also become blocked by plaque or weakened by incessant high blood pressure, resulting in stroke. Vigilance in diagnosing and treating any of these problems will vastly improve wellness and the duration of your life.

The wear and tear on the gastrointestinal system that began in your fifties can worsen in this decade, a time when many women complain of heartburn and constipation. I know these seem like minor annoyances, but if you find yourself paying an inordinate amount of attention to commercials for antacids and constipation remedies (or if you're paying an inordinate sum of money for these products), you shouldn't hesitate to discuss these digestive issues with your doctor. They are not an inevitable part of growing older, and on occasion they may be symptoms of a more serious disorder.

It's common to forget, but if you're forgetting the common to the point that friends and family have started to comment on it, you may want to investigate whether you are at risk for Alzheimer's disease. Early diagnosis can allow for the use of new therapies that can slow the progress of this disease. But don't think that every time you forget your keys or some inconsequential fact or name, your brain is in serious trouble. Information overload, fatigue, lack of stimulation and certain medications can all contribute to memory lapses.

Yes, this is the decade of Medicare, when we become eligible for an insurance we associate with illness. But there we go again—bestowing a negative connotation. The strides medicine has made have allowed us to live longer and better, and by our mid-sixties we're finally entitled to avail ourselves of these benefits without painful concerns about personal affordability. This is a decade of health in which all women can profit from what medicine has to offer. What a shame if we ignore or are not informed about these offerings and don't take an active role in their pursuit!

DO I STILL NEED PAP SMEARS?

Don't think that because you've remained cervical-cancer-free thus far that you're out of the woods. One-fourth of the cases of cervical cancer and 41% of the deaths from this disease occur in women older than 64. An awful lot of women and their physicians have ignored this fact: Surveys have shown that half of all women age 60 and older have not had a Pap smear for more than three years.

Assuming you still have a cervix (in other words, you have not had a total hysterectomy, in which the uterus and cervix are removed), you still need Paps. The same recommendations for Pap smear screening apply at this age as when you were younger. You need a Pap smear once a year. If you have three consecutive negative tests and if you are *truly* low-risk for cervical cancer (i.e., you've had no more than two sexual partners in your lifetime and your partner has had no more than two sexual partners in a lifetime, or if you've never had a sexually transmitted disease, an abnormal Pap, or smoked), then you can be screened less frequently—every two to three years. But if you don't fall into the low-risk category, you need to continue to have annual screenings.

I'VE HAD A HYSTERECTOMY. DO I STILL NEED A PELVIC EXAM?

Yes. First of all, if your uterus was removed and your ovaries left in place, it's imperative that they be examined to be sure you have no cysts or cancer. And even if your ovaries were removed, the pelvic exam is an entrance to more than your reproductive organs. It's a way of checking your bladder, rectum, vagina and colon. Because you've had a hysterectomy, you may be at higher risk for certain types of pelvic prolapse, in which the top of the vagina is no longer adequately supported and pushes downward toward the opening of the vagina. Bladder and rectal support also may be compromised by a hysterectomy, causing symptoms of incontinence or urgency. A simple examination of the vagina will also reveal the health and welfare of the tissue lining it. Having a pelvic exam will help you start a dialogue about these problems and their correction. Furthermore, most women won't have a rectal exam that might reveal rectal cancer unless they are already up in the stirrups for a gynecologic exam.

When you're in the doctor's office, you can use the opportunity to discuss hormone replacement therapy. Even though you're in your sixties, you may still have symptoms of estrogen deficiency such as hot flashes, sleep disturbances, short-term memory loss and diminished sense of well-being. The fact that you are among the one-third of women whose uterus has been removed means you're at an advantage: You can take estrogen without the hassle of taking progesterone. You should also discuss with your "pelvic examiner"—whether it's a gynecologist or an internist well versed in women's health—issues of coronary artery disease and osteoporosis.

The final question is whether because you have had a hysterectomy, you still need a Pap smear. The answer depends on what kind of hysterectomy you've had. If your cervix was removed with the uterus (total hysterectomy), Pap smears are probably not necessary. However (there are an awful lot of "howevers" in medicine), there is a minuscule chance of developing cancer in the top of the vagina if you've had a history of human papillomavirus (HPV). So many doctors continue to do a Pap smear, using cells scraped from the vaginal cuff. You're also at higher than average risk for vulvar and anal cancer if you've had HPV, so these areas should be carefully checked during your gynecologic exam.

IS IT TOO LATE TO START TAKING HORMONES?

It's never too late to hormon-ate. The positive effects of estrogen replacement therapy can begin at any time and will continue for as long as you take it. The majority of postmenopausal women don't take hormones. Many chose to "wait and see," deciding that if they weren't having significant symptoms, then distant health problems were just that—distant. If your cholesterol levels are creeping in the wrong direction, your blood pressure is ominously rising, your vaginal lining is shriveling and your bones are thinning, you can begin to rectify the situation. Once you start ERT, you will get all the cardiovascular benefits of estrogen listed on page 199; however, they may not be as extensive as they would be if you had started estrogen at the onset of menopause. Artery protection starting in our early fifties might have put you in better vascular shape, but you *can* shape up.

Your bone situation is more encouraging: It appears that beginning estrogen in your sixties may be almost as efficacious as starting in your fifties. Beginning ERT at 65 will enable you to increase your bone density by an initial 5% to 10%, and ultimately to halve your annual risk of future bone loss. This translates into a lifetime total fracture risk reduction of as much as 69%, very close to the 73% risk reduction derived by women who start taking estrogen at the onset of menopause.

Vaginal atrophy and dryness may not initially respond to oral estrogen as quickly as they would have if you'd started taking the hormone a decade ago. This is because you've lost many of the hormone receptors that supply the vagina, as well as thickness of the walls, blood supply and supporting fat in the vaginal lips. In order to get a satisfactory response to estrogen, it may be necessary to jump-start the process with a local estrogen cream or vaginal ring in addition to using systemic estrogen.

For many women in their sixties, the fear of memory loss or Alzheimer's disease looms ominously. Although I can't promise that estrogen will make you sharper, there are several studies indicating that it has an effect on short-term memory and perhaps delay the onset or diminish the severity of Alzheimer's disease.

Please note: This is one of the shortest answers in this book. That's because I don't have to waffle—if you need it, it will help.

I'VE BEEN TAKING PREMARIN AND PROVERA FOR A DECADE. SHOULD I SWITCH TO SOMETHING NEWER?

There is an adage that has been expressed by our medical sages (and our grandmothers): If it ain't broke, don't fix it. If Premarin and Provera have kept you free of menopausal symptoms and provided you with the cardio-vascular and bone protection you so richly deserve, there are very few reasons to abandon these medications. My first piece of advice: Check your lipid profile and make sure it's as good as you and your doctor would like. Since the Postmenopausal Estrogen-Progestin Intervention (PEPI) study has shown that natural progesterone may have less of a dampening effect on estrogen's lipid benefits (raising HDL and lowering LDL), you might want to consider switching to this natural progesterone (Prometrium) if your levels are significantly off. And if your triglycerides are high, you may benefit by switching from oral estrogen to the patch.

Another potential progesterone-related side effect you may have noticed with this standard HRT regimen is bloating and/or PMS-like symptoms. Natural progesterone, in pill or vaginal gel form (Crinone) might help to minimize some of these problems (see page 217).

If your libido has now decreased appreciably, you might benefit from adding testosterone. Instead of Premarin, consider taking Estratest (the half-strength dosage usually suffices). Or you can add testosterone with lozenges, ointments or creams (see page 219).

Finally, if you're developing hot flashes 18 hours after taking Premarin (or any oral estrogen) or if you tend to get headaches, you might want to try applying an estrogen patch, which can ensure a more steady supply of the hormone and reduce these symptoms. The encouraging news is that no matter what form of HRT you use, you will continue to obtain its benefits as long as you continue taking it.

MY DOCTOR FOUND AN OVARIAN CYST. SHOULD I WORRY?

Unfortunately, yes. But having said this, I want to let you know that as we're doing more vaginal ultrasounds to assess the uterine lining in women on hormone replacement therapy, we're finding that 17% of post-menopausal women have small, nonworrisome ovarian cysts. The worry increases if cysts appear in both ovaries, or if a single cyst is large, has a thickened wall, jagged indentations, thick septums (dividing walls) within it or solid components. Obviously, all this has to be diagnosed with ultrasound. At the same time, your doctor will look for evidence of free fluid in the pelvis, another ominous sign that the cyst could be malignant. Numerous papers have been written on the subject of whether ultrasound can sufficiently assuage concern about a single ovarian cyst in a menopausal woman. Some researchers feel that a cyst of less than 5 centimeters that has thin walls and clear fluid is benign, but once this declaration has been made, someone invariably writes a paper on a series of seemingly benign cysts that were not.

There is another diagnostic test that might help reassure you and your doctor: the color Doppler ultrasound, which measures blood flow to the cyst. Malignant tumors are characterized by enhanced blood supply, which helps them to grow and take over. So if greater than normal blood flow is detected, this may indicate a malignancy. On the other hand, if the Doppler reveals no abnormal blood flow and the cyst appears simple (thin-walled and containing clear fluid), and especially if it is relatively small, it might be sufficient to simply reexamine you in two to three months to see if there has been any change. I have patients whom I've followed for years who have an unchanging 3-centimeter cyst. We know it's there, but it isn't growing, so we're not concerned.

Having given you this diagnostic scenario, let's return to your particular cyst. Usually you won't know it's present unless it twists on itself or ruptures (see page 96). This, however, is very unusual in postmenopausal women. What's more likely is that your cyst was detected during a routine office visit or an ultrasound. Once your doctor has looked for the suspicious changes I've listed above, she will also want to get a blood test for cancer antigen 125 (CA-125), which is elevated in 80% of women with the most common form of ovarian cancer. If the CA-125 level is greater than 65 in a postmenopausal woman with a pelvic mass, it is predictive of a malignancy 75% of the time. But remember, that means that 25% of the time an elevated CA-125 together with a cyst does not mean a malignancy. And not all malignant cysts produce CA-125, which is why a suspicious cyst should be evaluated even in the absence of this tumor marker. Also note: There are other malignancies that can cause CA-125 to rise, as well as nonmalignant conditions such as uterine fibroids, pelvic inflammatory disease, endometriosis, hepatitis, congestive heart failure and liver failure.

If your ultrasound and/or Doppler testing is suspicious, and especially if your CA-125 level is elevated, your cyst must be removed and a definitive diagnosis made. The question is whether you can start with a less invasive laparoscopy to "see what's going on in there" rather than the more extensive laparotomy. This is very controversial. Most oncologists would prefer to err on the side of caution and choose laparotomy because it is an "open" surgery that allows direct assessment and removal of the cyst, ideally without rupturing it. (If the cyst is malignant and rupture occurs, there is a slight chance that spilled cancerous cells will take hold in the pelvis.) Having said that, I know that I and some of the oncologists I work with have performed laparoscopies on postmenopausal women whose cysts appear less worrisome (they're smaller than 5 centimeters in diameter and have few, if any, solid components, and the woman's CA-125 level is only minimally elevated). It's a gut call. Once I insert the scope, I try to prevent spillage either by carefully aspirating the fluid from the cyst with a needle, or by putting a plastic bag through the laparoscope and placing it around the cyst during removal so that any spilled cells are prevented from entering the pelvic cavity.

If there is high suspicion that the cyst is malignant, laparotomy (open surgery) should be performed. It's also essential that two medical professionals be present at the surgery. The first is a gynecologic oncologist, who is experienced in staging the tumor if a malignancy is found and is skilled in the surgical procedure necessary to remove as much of the malignant tissue as possible. (The more malignant cells that can be removed at this initial surgery, the better the prognosis.) A pathologist also must be in the O.R. in order to examine the growth and do a test called a frozen section to confirm microscopically whether it is malignant.

Let's look at the two possible scenarios that can ensue once surgery is undertaken. The first is that the cyst is benign, and in your age group, this usually means that it is either a cystadenoma, mucinous cystadenoma, dermoid cyst or hydrosalpinx (see page 140). In the case of the first two diagnoses, because of the chance that these cysts will later recur in the other ovary, the recommendation for postmenopausal women is to remove both ovaries. However, your uterus, if it's normal, can stay put. That means that if the initial procedure was a laparoscopic one, your doctor will be able to perform a bilateral oopherectomy (removal of both ovaries) through the scope and you can go home a few hours later. Since you're already menopausal, additional loss of estrogen will not be an issue. If you were on estrogen therapy, you can continue it. But remember: You still have a uterus and will need to continue taking progesterone. Your postmenopausal ovaries, however, may not have been completely defunct and may have been quietly producing small amounts of male hormone. So after this surgery, if you feel your libido has taken a dive, you might benefit from the addition of testosterone. If your initial surgical procedure was a laparotomy and both ovaries need to come out, it could be argued that a hysterectomy is not a bad idea. This is something you have to discuss with your doctor before you go into the O.R. (see page 143).

The second possible scenario is that, unfortunately, a diagnosis of ovarian cancer is made. If the initial procedure was a laparoscopic one, you will remain under anesthesia while your doctor performs a laparotomy in order to remove both ovaries, the fallopian tubes, the uterus and cervix (a total abdominal hysterectomy and bilateral salpingoopherectomy), together with the removal of the pelvic lymph glands and omentum (the apron of fat that covers the bowel), and exploration for and removal of any cancer implants throughout the pelvis and abdomen. Depending on the type and extent of the cancer, chemotherapy and/or radiation will follow.

Because these scenarios are so radically different and the final diagnosis will be made during surgery when you're asleep, it's paramount that you discuss all possibilities with your surgeon before you enter the O.R. This is especially true if you're interested in saving your uterus in the event the cyst is benign. And once more, make sure that at least one of your surgeons is experienced in performing cancer surgery.

CAN I BE SCREENED FOR OVARIAN CANCER?

We have put men and women on the moon and have been very successful in screening for prostate cancer in men. But science has failed thus far to come up with a way to screen all women for ovarian cancer. And to add insult to significant cancer mortality, ovarian malignancies do not give early warning signs. In 70% of cases, the cancer has spread outside the pelvis by the time it is discovered. This is why fewer than 40% of women who are diagnosed will survive five years. This metastasic spread, rather than the initial cancer, is what causes symptoms that include abdominal discomfort, upper abdominal fullness and early satiety (feeling full after eating only a little food). Other symptoms—which many of us experience without any dire disease—include fatigue, increasing abdominal girth, urinary frequency and shortness of breath. If we have no significant risk factors we each have a one in 70 chance of developing ovarian cancer in our lifetime. The median age of diagnosis is 61. Ovarian cancer is the fifth leading cause of cancer deaths in women.

The only tests that can detect ovarian cancer before these late symptoms occur are pelvic exam, abdominal and transvaginal ultrasound and analysis of CA-125 levels in the blood. But these have all been deemed either inadequate or not cost-effective. Let me explain: By the time your doctor feels something in a pelvic exam, that something may have advanced and spread throughout the abdomen. Although CA-125 is elevated in the bloodstream in 80% of late-stage ovarian cancers, only half of women with early-stage disease have what's considered an abnormal level. Because of this, the American College of Obstetricians and Gynecologists does not recommend routine CA-125 screening in menopausal women who have no known risk factors. Changes in CA-125 from year to year, however, may be more accurate predictors of ovarian cancer than a simple elevation in the CA-125 level above 35. For that reason, some doctors are now testing baseline CA-125 levels when a woman becomes menopausal and repeating the test on a yearly basis to see if there is a slight elevation, in which case further screening with ultrasound might be necessary. But this is not a universally accepted recommendation.

Ultrasound is expensive and has a high false-positive rate. If we were to perform vaginal probe ultrasound on every woman over age 40, we would pick up a lot of cysts, benign tumors and fibroids. Once we have run the test and have an abnormal result, we're stuck: If we can't be sure our findings are benign, we have to explore further. Roughly 67 women would have to undergo surgery in order for a single case of ovarian cancer to be diagnosed. Color-flow Doppler ultrasound measuring blood flow to the ovaries allows us to be more precise, and if this more costly test is combined with a test of CA-125 levels, we can positively predict ovarian cancer in postmenopausal women 94% of the time.

So why shouldn't we all undergo these two tests? The answer is a matter of simple economics. If over 40 million women have both tests annually (and is annually even enough?), the cost would be nearly $14 billion. But if you have a known risk factor, forget about cost-benefit ratios. You should be screened. The most significant risk factor is genetic; 10% of ovarian cancer are gene-linked. Women who because of family history are high risk for this cancer, or who test positive for BRCA1 and BRCA2 mutations (see page 344) should have early (beginning in their thirties or 10 years earlier than the onset of the cancer in a relative) and aggressive screening. So although I don't want to negate the need for your personal testing, I would be negligent if I didn't point that if you are at genetic risk, your children are also, and you should make sure they get checked.

I'M BLEEDING. COULD IT BE UTERINE CANCER?

Yes. Ninety percent of women who develop this cancer have vaginal bleeding or bloody discharge as their only initial symptom, and you're in the right age group—the average age of diagnosis is 60. Uterine cancer develops as the result of overactivity and chaotic growth of the endometrial glands that line our uterus. During our reproductive years these glands should have led a very organized life, growing and shedding each month. If at any point their hormonal directives went awry and they either got too much estrogen over too long a period of time (causing growth) and/or too little progesterone (so they failed to shed), they became confused. Precancerous, and then cancerous, changes ensued. Your glands are more likely to have undergone this transformation if you:

- never had children (a two- to threefold increase in risk)
- went into menopause after 55 (which roughly doubles risk)
- are obese (if you're 21 to 50 pounds overweight, your risk triples; it rises to 10 times normal if you're more than 50 pounds overweight. Obesity is such an important risk factor for this cancer that I routinely screen my very overweight patients who are not on HRT with ultrasound, or check to see if the uterine lining is overstimulated by giving them progestins.)
- have diabetes (a 2.8-fold increase in risk)
- have taken estrogen therapy without progesterone (a four- to eightfold increase in risk)
- took or are taking tamoxifen (which doubles or triples risk)
- have previously been diagnosed with atypical endometrial hyperplasia and have not received therapy (which makes your risk up to 30 times the norm)

This multitude of factors makes endometrial cancer the fourth most common cancer in women, after lung, breast and colorectal cancer. Two percent to three percent of women will develop this cancer during their lifetime.

Having given you all these statistics, I don't want you to think that finding blood on your underwear is synonymous with a diagnosis of endometrial cancer. Don't panic. There are a lot of other reasons for vaginal bleeding, especially if you're taking hormone replacement therapy.

Women who take their hormones cyclically (see page 218) know to expect a "period" each month, in the days after they finish taking their progestin or progesterone. I often find that my patients have the opposite concern, worrying if they don't get this expected bleeding. Not bleeding simply indicates that your uterine lining has become less reactive to hormonal stimulation and ceased to shed. This, like bleeding at the "right" time, is okay.

There should be some concern, however, if you bleed when you're not supposed to on cyclical hormones or if you bleed when taking continuous hormones. (Remember: The whole point of continuous HRT is not to bleed.) This is especially the case if you've been taking this therapy for more than a year. Before you frantically run to the telephone to make an appointment with your doctor, you should know that if you've been a good girl and have been taking the right amount of progestin at least 12 days a month or continuously, the chance that you've developed uterine cancer is slim. So your first step should be to do a little sleuthing on your own: Did you forget to take a dose of estrogen or, if you're on the patch, to change it at the right time? Did you skip a dose of progestin (missing this hormone is more likely than missing estrogen to lead to bleeding)? Have you been taking antibiotics, which can affect the absorption or action of your hormones? Or have you suddenly started a new medication, especially a steroid (pills or shots)? Have you recently traveled across time zones, which can play havoc with your body's hormonal balance by upsetting melatonin and cortisol levels? Or have you been under severe stress (another cortisol disruptor)? If your answer to any of the above is "yes," relax and simply go back to your usual routine and see if the bleeding stops. However, when you next see your doctor, make sure you inform her of this incident.

If your attempts at self-discovery do not yield any clues and/or your bleeding continues, get to your doctor. At this point you need a more anatomically based explanation, and that can be achieved with vaginal probe ultrasound. This noninvasive test allows your doctor to view the endometrium and judge whether it is abnormally thickened or uneven. If its total thickness is less than 4 millimeters, it's highly unlikely that uterine cancer or precancer is present and causing your bleeding. So a negative ultrasound finding means that you can stop worrying, though you won't necessarily get an explanation as to why you bled in the first place. Should you continue to bleed, there are several medical solutions. The first is to double your dosage of whatever progestational agent you're taking for one or two cycles. The second option is to lower your dose of estrogen. The third possible solution is to stop both hormones for a week and let whatever tissue is left in the endometrial cavity shed. Then you can restart the hormones and see if you no longer bleed.

If none of these very logical options works, your uterus may be reacting in an illogical way. At this point I would suggest that you return to your doctor for a closer look via hysteroscopy and sampling of cells from the uterine lining. It's possible that the original ultrasound may have missed a small polyp or even a fibroid that's projecting into the uterine lining. But often there's still no visible cause and the pathologist can't find anything wrong with the endometrial cells. Chances are, if you stop your hormones altogether, you'll also stop bleeding. But then you'd be forgoing all the benefits of HRT. So you might want to consider undergoing a procedure that scars (or ablates) the endometrium (see page 127). This should permanently halt the bleeding. You'll still need to take a progestational agent with your estrogen to protect the tissue under the endometrial scar from becoming malignant.

The other possible scenario that can play out if you're taking hormones and develop abnormal bleeding is that the endometrium, when measured, is abnormally thickened and is greater than 4 millimeters. This could be caused by precancerous cell changes or cancer, but more likely is due to a polyp or fibroid. Injecting saline into the uterine cavity during the ultrasound will help your doctor to make this diagnosis. If a malignancy is suspected, your doctor will need to obtain cells from the endometrium and send them to the pathologist. In the bad old days, you would have been booked for a D&C (dilation and curettage). This procedure was usually performed under general anesthesia in a hospital. But neither the general nor the hospital is required today. An adequate cell sample can usually be obtained with an office procedure called endometrial aspiration biopsy (or endometrial sampling) and a local anesthetic. A thin cannula is inserted through the cervix and suction is applied while it's gently moved back and forth so that cells from the entire wall are obtained. This is a quick, easy way to achieve a diagnosis and is up to 98% accurate; however, if ultrasound shows a suspiciously thickened endometrium, your doctor may opt to get a better look while doing the sampling with a hysteroscopy. If an endometrial sampling done via a cannula reveals no abnormal changes but bleeding continues, you'll also need a hysteroscopy.

This intricate tale of investigation is based on the premise that you are taking HRT. But what if you aren't? It's most probable that your bleeding is a result of irritation to a severely thinned vagina or uterine lining. In fact, endometrial atrophy is found in 60% to 80% of women with post-menopausal bleeding. Endometrial polyps and fibroids account for another 2% to 12%. Potentially precancerous endometrial hyperplasia is responsible for another 5% to 10%, while endometrial cancer is found in 10% of postmenopausal women who bleed. But even if there's only a one in 10 chance that your bleeding is due to cancer, it should be investigated promptly.

Now on to what happens if these cells are indeed abnormal. Hyperplasia, an overgrowth of glands, can range from completely benign (simple); to more extensive but still without abnormal cells (complex hyperplasia); to a true precancer (atypical hyperplasia); and finally to a very localized cancer (carcinoma in situ). Not every diagnosis of hyperplasia portends a future cancer. Left untreated, simple hyperplasia progresses to cancer in only 1% of women, complex in 3%, and if atypical cells are found, cancer can develop up to 29% of the time. But once hyperplasia is diagnosed, we don't leave it untreated. Initial therapy, especially for simple or complex hyperplasias without atypia (abnormal cells), does not involve a hysterectomy; high-dose progestin therapy can usually reverse these changes. Some physicians will treat atypical hyperplasia or even carcinoma in situ this way. However, many (myself included) are more cautious and feel that a vaginal hysterectomy is a better choice. This is in part because 25% of women with atypical hyperplasia are found to have additional areas of cancer when the uterus is removed.

Clearly, if endometrial cancer is diagnosed, a hysterectomy is the treatment of choice. However, before this is performed, a scraping of the cervical canal (endocervical curettage, or ECC) should be done. This will allow your doctor to assess the stage of the cancer. If the cervix is not involved, it might be possible to undergo a laparoscopic-assisted vaginal hysterectomy (see page 149) and biopsy of the lymph nodes instead of a more invasive abdominal surgery. The need for radiation therapy will depend on the final staging of the cancer and whether the cancer cells appear more or less aggressive. This can only be determined after hysterectomy. Final staging is based on how deeply cancer has invaded the uterine wall (myometrium), whether it has spread to the cervix and/or pelvic lymph nodes and whether it has metastasized further within the pelvis or abdomen. If cancer cells are found in the fluid surrounding the organs in the pelvis and abdomen, high-dose progestin therapy, in the form of Megace, may be added.

No one wants to hear the diagnosis of cancer, but if you're going to get a gynecologic cancer, this has the best prognosis. It's slow-growing, gives a vivid early warning sign (bleeding), and the surgery, although major, is not outwardly disfiguring. The overall five-year survival rate is 73%; women diagnosed at a very early stage have a five-year survival rate as high as 96%, while those diagnosed after the cancer has spread but while it is still contained within the pelvis have a survival rate of 66%. Once a woman is adequately treated, she should be followed carefully with frequent pelvic exams and chest X-rays. Since there is no evidence that after proper treatment estrogen increases the risk of recurrence, if you had early stage cancer and your surgeon feels that you got a complete cure, you can start (or resume) estrogen therapy immediately after surgery if you want to. If your disease was more advanced, most doctors will want you to wait one to three years after surgery to ensure that there is no recurrence before starting estrogen. Make sure you and your doctor take other steps to relieve menopausal symptoms and protect your heart and bones during this waiting period.

THE LIPS OF MY VAGINA ARE ITCHING. COULD IT BE MORE THAN A YEAST INFECTION?

The same bacteria, yeast and other unwanted microbes that cause vulvar itching throughout your reproductive life unfortunately continue to be an issue in this decade. However, your normal flora may have changed as a result of years of estrogen depletion if you have not used HRT. That means you're less likely to develop yeast infections but more likely to develop bacterial vaginal infections. The vulvar skin has become thin and is more easily irritated. In order to cure this problem you may need to use a local estrogen cream or an estrogen ring to build up the vaginal lining and skin and restore a normal pH level, which encourages the return of normal flora.

There are other vulvar disorders that can cause itching and irritation in your sixties but that are not infectious. One of them has a particularly serious-sounding name: lichen sclerosis. Although this disorder can occur at any age, it is most common in postmenopausal women. The skin of the inner and outer lips of the vagina becomes white, thin and paperlike. The lips may grow together, hiding the clitoris and closing off part of the vaginal opening. These changes often extend up to the pubic hairline and down to the rectum and may be accompanied by severe itching. Because of the scarring, sex is painful, even impossible. A diagnosis of lichen sclerosis can be made by your doctor with a biopsy, and fortunately its symptoms can be lessened or even completely reversed with medication. A powerful steroid cream (0.05% clobetasol proprionate or 0.05% halobetasol) is the therapy of choice. With proper use of one of these creams, close to 80% of women can get complete relief of symptoms. Most women will have to continue to use the cream one to three times a week to remain symptom free. Once treated with a steroid cream, vaginal dilators may need to be used to restore the vaginal opening. If your clitoris has been buried by fusion of the labia, it can be exposed with minor surgery. Even if the therapy works, if you have been diagnosed with lichen sclerosis, you should be carefully monitored by your doctor with a visual examination for signs of vulvar cancer. A persistent ulcer or nodule requires biopsy or excision.

Although I want to reassure you that you don't have to think cancer every time you experience itching, there is a possibility that skin changes accompanying vulvar cancer can make you feel irritated or itchy. You are in the right age group for developing this cancer—the average age of diagnosis is 65—and the most frequent symptom is a long history of itching. Vulvar cancer accounts for 5% of all gynecologic malignancies.

We're all very used to examining our faces in a mirror—we're probably not adept at doing the same with our vulva. But the most common sign of this cancer is a visible mass. Any lesion that is raised and fleshy or ulcerated, white or wartlike should be examined by your doctor. Many of us self-medicate for vulvar itching, so if you've tried over-the-counter medications and they don't work, or if your doctor has prescribed other medication that was also ineffective, don't assume that itching is a part of getting older or is normal; insist that your doctor take a closer look at the problem. Because both the patient and physician tend to be nonchalant about itching, many vulvar cancers aren't picked up until after they have spread. If the cancer is discovered while the abnormal cells are still localized or the tumor has invaded less than 1 millimeter of tissue, a local incision is all that is needed for cure. But a malignancy that has grown deeper will require a more extensive—and thus more disfiguring—excision, possibly including removal of lymph nodes in the groin. If the cancer has spread to these lymph nodes, radiation therapy may also be needed. The difference between complete cure and genital disfigurement and even death is determined by time and neglect. (If the lymph nodes are negative, there is a 90% five-year survival rate; this number falls below 50% for women with positive lymph nodes.) There is no excuse for accepting or ignoring a seven-year, or even a seven-week, itch.

I'M RUNNING TO THE BATHROOM ALL THE TIME—AND SOMETIMES I DON'T MAKE IT. WHAT CAN I DO?

Your bladder muscle is supposed to contract and expel urine from the urethra only when you consciously tell it to (in other words, when you're perched on—or hovering over—a toilet seat). Unfortunately, nearly 40% of women over age 60 experience loss of bladder muscle control. The sensation you're describing has several components. First there is urgency—the sudden, uncontrollable need to void. Then there is frequency—you may be going to the bathroom more than eight times a day. Finally, there are the times when you don't make it to the bathroom: This is known as urge incontinence and may lead to accidents in which you lose a lot of urine at once. All of this is the result of unstable bladder contractions (detrusor overactivity) or diminished bladder capacity.

I'm so glad you're asking me what you can do about this problem. Too many women assume that this condition is a natural result of aging. Add to this a sense of embarrassment, and we have the embarrassing statistic that the average woman waits eight damp years before she seeks help for this problem. And help there is, from behavioral to pharmaceutical and even surgical. The first thing to do is to keep a two-week bladder diary. On the next page, I've provided a sample page based on the diary recommended by the American Foundation for Urologic Disease's Bladder Health Council. You might want to photocopy it, fill it out and share it with your doctor.

Looking at the diary will help you and your doctor to determine the type of bladder problem you're experiencing. There are three main types of incontinence, and you may find that, like 40% of women with bladder problems, you're suffering from a combination of these types.

Stress incontinence: This is the loss of urine with any increase in abdominal pressure, such as during coughing, sneezing or intercourse.

Urge incontinence: This is the condition I've described above, and the one you probably have. Sometimes the detrusor overactivity is due to irritation of the lower urinary tract, which can be caused by bladder infection or inflammation. It can also result from neurologic diseases that affect the bladder, such as diabetes, multiple sclerosis and stroke.

Overflow incontinence: This condition, which causes frequent or constant leakage of small amounts of urine, is the result of a chronically full

Bladder Diary

Time of Day	Type and Amount of Fluid Intake	Amount Voided (in ounces)	Amount of Leakage (small, medium, large)	Activity Engaged in When Leakage Occurred	Was Urge to Urinate Present?
6 to 8 A.M.					
8 to 10 A.M.					
10 A.M. to noon					
noon to 2 P.M.					
2 to 4 P.M.					
4 to 6 P.M.					
6 to 8 P.M.					
8 to 10 P.M.					
10 P.M. to midnight					
Overnight					
Other					
Comments					

bladder that is not properly emptying. It's especially common in women with prolapse of the bladder (cystocele) and those with diabetes or other neurologic problems.

Once you and your doctor have looked at your diary, you'll also need to undergo some basic testing. This should include a urinalysis to check for infection, and a pelvic exam to determine whether the uterus, bladder or vagina has lost its support and has dropped or prolapsed. The size of your uterus and whether you have fibroids or any pelvic tumors pressing on the bladder will be checked. You'll also be asked to empty your bladder. Then the doctor will insert a catheter or use a vaginal probe ultrasound to see if there is an unusually large amount of urine left behind, a sign that your bladder is not emptying fully and a hallmark of overflow incontinence.

All of this can be done by your regular doctor, and depending on the results you may be referred to a urologist or urogynecologist for what's called urodynamic testing. The length, angle and sphincter control of the urethra are tested, as are the bladder's capacity and contraction pattern. When all this is completed, a decision can be made about therapy. I'm sure you'll prefer the least invasive cure possible, so I'll start there.

Behavioral modification: Your bladder is smarter than you are, and if you ignore it and let it overfill, it protests by contracting. If you're one of those people who's purchased a designer bag to hold your designer bottled water, and you're drinking more than eight glasses a day, you probably need to cut back. But don't cut back too far — concentrated urine will only further irritate the bladder. Avoid overdosing on caffeine, spicy or acidic foods, alcohol, sugar, artificial sweeteners and chocolate. Although these taste terrific going down, they irritate coming out.

The next step is to set a schedule for going to the bathroom and to stick to it whether you have to go or not. If you get the urge to urinate in between scheduled bathroom visits, don't rush to the toilet. Stop what you're doing, sit down if possible and relax your entire body. Breathe deeply as you contract your pelvic muscles repeatedly. This should diminish the urgency. When it has subsided, see if you can wait until your next scheduled bathroom visit. Then, when it's time, proceed to the toilet at a normal pace. Note: If accidents happen in the beginning, don't be discouraged. Start with hourly bathroom trips during waking hours; then, each week, increase the length of time between visits in 15-minute increments until a normal voiding interval of every two and a half to three hours is established.

Behavioral training: We all know about muscle training and what we need to do to keep our arms and abs toned and defined. But there are special training methods that allow us to do the same for muscles we can't see: those surrounding the urogenital tract. Biofeedback can help you identify these muscles and teach you how to contract and relax them selectively. A gauge that measures vaginal and anal sphincter activity can show you whether you're contracting the right muscle. Once you know which muscles to use and how to use them, you can practice at home with Kegel exercises (see page 106). As part of this muscle training, some doctors apply painless electrical stimulation to encourage the muscle to contract and build strength. You may also be taught to insert and support a weighted vaginal cone for the same reason. Finally, you should also practice slowing or stopping the urinary stream at least once a day.

These simple solutions have been shown to reduce incontinence episodes by 80% and for most women are more effective than drug therapy. But in some women, behavioral treatment alone isn't enough, and drug therapy or surgery becomes the next step.

Drug treatment: The drugs that are currently used for detrusor muscle overactivity are designed to relax that muscle by blocking the receptors to certain neurotransmitters. The two most commonly used drugs are oxybutynin chloride (Ditropan) and tolterodine (Detrol). They're similarly effective, reducing frequency of urination by up to 20% when compared to placebo. They are roughly twice as effective as a placebo pill at diminishing incontinence episodes. The major drawback is that these drugs affect receptors in other parts of the body, triggering side effects such as dry mouth, constipation, headache, dizziness, blurred vision and gastric upset. Initially, studies showed that Detrol caused fewer of these side effects that Ditropan. But a new slow-release Ditropan XL has been released to the market and appears almost equally tolerated.

Other medications can be used to help relieve bladder irritation and unwanted contraction. These include tricyclic antidepressants, bladder analgesics such as flavoxate hydrochloride (Urispas) and pyridium, smooth-muscle antispasmodics (Levsin) and calcium channel blockers. These are prescribed alone or in combination. Estrogen replacement therapy, including local vaginal therapy, has been shown to be helpful for postmenopausal women with overactive bladder and two-thirds of women with stress incontinence report improvement in symptoms when they take estrogen.

Surgery: The usual cause for urge incontinence is inappropriate muscle contraction, and surgery will not correct this problem. However, 40% of women with incontinence have a combination of urge and stress incontinence, and surgery to remove any pelvic tumor or resupport a prolapsed bladder or poorly angled urethra may relieve the latter. The combination of pelvic prolapse and incontinence is so common that 11% of women will undergo corrective surgery in their lifetimes. There are approximately 200 fix-and-support procedures, ranging from invasive intra-abdominal surgeries to less drastic vaginal ones using special sutures and slings. The important thing is to make sure that some part of your incontinence is the result of a lack of internal support. Otherwise the surgery won't work—and it may make your symptoms of urgency and frequency worse.

MY DOCTOR RECOMMENDED SURGERY TO LIFT MY BLADDER. WHAT DOES THIS ENTAIL, AND SHOULD I GO THROUGH WITH IT?

I assume that if surgery is being performed to lift your bladder, it's because your bladder has dropped from its normal position at the top of the vagina and is now protruding down into the vagina and perhaps even out of the opening of the labia. This is called *cystocele.* Doctors can grade the degree of prolapse according to how far down into the vagina the bladder has come. First- and second-degree prolapse means the bladder is still within the vaginal cavity, even when you apply pressure such as that exerted during a bowel movement. If the bladder descends past the vagina with pressure, the prolapse is considered third degree. And if the bladder is always protruding out, the prolapse is fourth degree. Because the pelvic support system for your bladder is also the support system for your uterus and rectum, cystocele is most commonly accompanied by uterine prolapse, *rectocele* (the bulging of the rectum into and out of the lower posterior portion of the vagina), and even *enterocele* (the bulging of the small bowel into the upper posterior portion of the vagina). This general fallen state is termed *pelvic organ prolapse* and occurs to some extent in half of all women over age 65. Your pelvic support and integrity are determined by the inherent strength of the collagen in your pelvis, your muscle tone, your estrogen status and previous insults to your pelvic support system (pregnancies, large babies and difficult vaginal deliveries). Of course, the ultimate insult is the fact that human beings have evolved into upright bipeds. All those years of standing put a tremendous strain on the sling of pelvic tissue supporting your organs.

Surgery to resupport your bladder can usually be performed using a vaginal approach. The surgeon opens the vaginal tissue stretching over the bulging cystocele, pushes the bladder up and uses sutures to tuck it inward and tighten the support tissue on both sides. After this, the excess vaginal tissue is trimmed and closed. This is called an anterior colporrhaphy. If presurgery testing shows that there are changes in the angle of the bladder or if stress incontinence is your major symptom, there are other procedures that can be performed to tack up or support the bladder neck. Some of these are abdominal procedures such as the traditional Marshall-Marchetti-Krantz procedure, in which sutures are placed on either side of the bladder neck and anchored to the pubic bone. This is considered the gold standard for the treatment of stress urinary incontinence and has a success rate of 80% to 95%.

Other therapies involve abdominal surgery using a sling made either of your own tissue or a synthetic material to support the bladder, as well as a vaginal procedure that requires using a special needle to help attach the tissue supporting the urethra to the pubic bone. These methods have a success rate ranging from 30% to 72%.

The initial procedure may not work, especially if it was not the appropriate one, and need for reoperation is fairly common, occurring in as many as 29% of women. A possible complication after vaginal (or total abdominal) hysterectomy for pelvic prolapse is the prolapse of what's left, the top of the vagina. Another serious complication is scarring that prevents normal urethral sphincter function and leads to an inability to void or to further incontinence. Overcorrection—lifting the bladder too high or altering the angle of the urethra too much—can also cause postsurgery problems and the need for long-term use of catheters. And, of course, an injury to the bladder or urethra can occur at the time of surgery. This can result in bleeding, infection and the formation of a fistula, an open channel between the bladder and vagina that causes constant urine leakage and infection. Fortunately, the latter is relatively rare.

I know this sounds worrisome and confusing. That's why the treatment of pelvic organ prolapse and urinary incontinence has evolved into a subspecialty called urogynecology. You'll want to talk over your options with either a urogynecologist or a gynecologist or urologist who routinely treats and does surgery on women with prolapse and continence problems. In addition to bladder repair, you may need to consider a vaginal hysterectomy, as well as repair of rectocele and/or enterocele. Whatever procedure(s) you and your doctor choose, make sure it's going to correct everything that has prolapsed—not just your bladder.

After giving you this extensive lesson in Pelvic Support Surgery 101, I want to provide you with a short course on mechanical treatment options. If you don't want surgery or your doctor has ruled it out because of other health problems, support devices can help keep your organs in place and prevent urine loss. A silicone, rubber or plastic pessary can be inserted into the vagina and used to elevate a sagging bladder, cervix, uterus and rectum. Pessaries come in all shapes and sizes and should be custom-fitted much like a diaphragm (most of them have to be removed, however, before intercourse). Four to six weeks prior to being fitted, you should begin using a vaginal estrogen cream and continue using it when the pessary is in place. This will help prevent irritation and bleeding. Some pessaries, such as the silicone doughnut, can be left in place for months at a time without removal or inspection; others, including the cube-shaped pessary, should be removed at bedtime each night and replaced in the morning. Pessaries can cause irritation and discharge, and have complications of their own. If you have a cystocele, they can make your problem worse because of constant pressure and change in urethral angle. A pessary specially designed for women with stress incontinence, the Introl device, consists of a ring with two prongs that support either side of the urethra.

If pelvic prolapse isn't causing you discomfort and your only problem is loss of urine, you may want to try Impress, a small foam shield worn externally over the opening of the urethra and held in place by a special gel that sticks to wet skin for up to five hours. You have to take it off and replace it every time you void. The other option is Reliance, a bulb-shaped insert placed into the urethra and inflated with air, blocking the opening and preventing leakage. A string deflates the balloon so that it can be removed when you urinate.

Pelvic prolapse and accompanying urinary incontinence have enormous personal, social and medical consequences for women. It can cause us to withdraw from life, becoming virtual prisoners in our homes. It restricts our intimate contact and sexual activities. And if it progresses, it becomes one of the chief reasons women are admitted to nursing homes.

Adult protection, in the form of diapers, is not an inevitable part of growing older. So if you have a significant bladder problem, do something about it. It doesn't always have to be surgery—there are many ways to help. You can depend on it.

DO OTHER WOMEN MY AGE ENJOY SEX?

Of course they do. But to quantify (and even qualify) sex in the sixties, we have to look at existing surveys of frequency of intercourse, orgasm and masturbation. And guess what? Many of the major surveyors never bothered to survey women over age 64! So when I give you numbers, I'm relying solely on the Janus Report on Sexual Behavior, a poll of more than 1,400 women of all ages published in 1994. It showed that 41% of women 65-plus years of age had intercourse a few times weekly, 33% had sex weekly and 22% had intercourse rarely. But having sex doesn't necessarily mean you're enjoying it, so let's look at the "orgasm with a partner" table, which shows that half of women over age 65 experience orgasm frequently, while another 37% have orgasms sometimes. And 13% rarely or never achieve this stage of sexual response. Not too bad, considering that the numbers for those pert, hardly-out-of-adolescence women in their early twenties showed that as many as 21% rarely or never have orgasms.

Unfortunately, many women in their sixties don't have a partner, while others have partners who are no longer sexually partnering because of erectile dysfunction. (Unless, that is, they've discovered Viagra.) The stats on how many women in their sixties (who were taught that nice girls don't touch themselves "down there") masturbate are woefully slim and may not be accurate because of reservations about owning up to this form of sexual activity. The Janus study reported that just 4% of women over age 65 masturbated once a week or more, 61% did so rarely and 35% never masturbated.

Whether these numbers reflect our true sexuality and ability to enjoy being sexual beings as we age is doubtful. What I can tell you is that many of my patients want to be sexual no matter what their age and resent being told by society, their doctors and men that this isn't possible.

It's unfortunate that we have been conditioned to compare ourselves to the norm. As we get older, society implies that the norm is "none." This certainly dampens our enthusiasm about keeping up with the Joneses! The only way to achieve a healthy sexuality is to instead keep up with whatever level of frequency, quality and intimacy fulfills your individual physical and emotional needs. This means that you have to want to maintain your libido and genital health. Having delivered this sermon on sexual aspirations, I'll review the hormonal and medical problems that can sabotage your sexual health.

Libido: You've gotten through menopause and made your decision about replacing the hormone that is associated with this change: estrogen. But there is another hormone that has been silently slipping away since your forties: testosterone. This is the hormone that governs your libido. You may have been blissfully unaware of this hormonal decline even with the onset of menopause. While your ovaries stopped producing estrogen, they continued to produce some testosterone, and this hormone's actions were less inhibited. But this relative male hormone ascendancy often plummets off about six years after you hit menopause or when you start taking estrogen therapy (estrogen binds up testosterone, rendering it less potent).

So when all is said and done, most women in their sixties have a testosterone deficiency—and as a result many have a libido deficiency. Adding testosterone, especially if you're on HRT, may give your libido a boost (see page 219).

Genital health: This is mainly an estrogen issue. Deprivation of this hormone is what's depriving you of your ability to comfortably have intercourse. I've already explained how to remedy this on page 241. The longer you've waited to address this problem, the more aggressive your therapy will need to be. In addition to using estrogen creams or rings and taking HRT, your genital renewal may require use of a local testosterone ointment to build up the labia. If the vaginal walls have atrophied, the vaginal cavity may have become smaller and inflexible. Your doctor may need to prescribe dilators that you can insert into your vagina to help reopen and expand it.

Medications: As most of us get older, we find ourselves buying pill boxes to organize our medications and communicating frequently with either our friendly pharmacist or our not-so-friendly mail-order service. As we pop both over-the-counter and prescription medications, we may be sabotaging the brain centers, neurotransmitters, hormones and blood supply needed for our sexual response. The following medications are the most common culprits in women your age:

- blood pressure–lowering medications
- diuretics
- cholesterol-lowering drugs
- antidepressants
- tranquilizers and sleeping pills
- antacids
- antihistamines
- anti-inflammatory drugs

Obviously, many of these medications are important to the quality of your life (not to mention your life), and I'm not suggesting that you stop them in order to improve your sexual response. But you can play drug detective and try to determine whether a new therapy has altered this response. Or ask your doctor if you can change medications or lower your dosage to see if it makes a difference. For example, if you're on Prozac or another selective serotonin reuptake inhibitor, your libido might benefit if you switch to Wellbutrin or add this drug to your current therapy.

Medical problems: It's not fair: Not only do we deal with increasing medications as we get older, but the conditions we're taking these medications for may make sex uncomfortable or difficult. The top offenders in your age group are:

DIABETES
One-third of women with this disease develop vaginal dryness and irritation and decreased genital sensitivity and libido. Much of this can be treated with HRT as well as a local estrogen cream or ring.

HEART DISEASE
These chronic illnesses may make it difficult to muster the strength for intercourse or cause you to fear that having sex will have dire consequences, such as a heart attack. But if you've been through cardiac testing or rehabilitation and your doctor has told you that you are fit enough to climb two flights of stairs, you're also fit enough for sex. (Somewhere, someone has done the study necessary to prove that the former equals the latter in energy units.)

CANCER
Chemotherapy causes fatigue, lethargy, depression, nausea, vomiting, hair loss and weight gain, all of which make sex the last thing you want to consider. But this is temporary, and as your sense of well-being returns,

know that from a physiologic point of view there's no reason that your ability to engage in and enjoy sexual intimacy should be impaired. Because many cancers are treated with body-altering surgery, the real challenge to your sex life may be a change in your self-image. When it comes to breast cancer, taking an active role in making the choice between lumpectomy and mastectomy has been shown to help women better deal with postsurgery body image issues. But we're very resilient, and no matter what surgery a woman undergoes, the most important factor is that she continues to nurture the bonds of her relationship. Because a diagnosis of breast cancer usually means stopping HRT and possibly beginning tamoxifen, you may be dealing with vaginal dryness. Make sure you use a lubricant during intercourse, and try one of the over-the-counter vaginal moisturizers (see page 241). If sex is still uncomfortable, talk to your doctor about using a vaginal estrogen ring for local relief; many physicians feel that the very small amount of estrogen absorbed through this ring is acceptable even for women with breast cancer. Local testosterone may also help.

AUTOIMMUNE DISEASES

All of these diseases can exacerbate vaginal dryness and decrease genital sensitivity. This can be treated with the usual: local estrogen and testosterone.

PELVIC PROLAPSE

This can be a physical barrier to intercourse. Surgery to lift the pelvic organs (see page 277) may be the answer, since most pessaries block the vaginal canal.

INCONTINENCE

Empty your bladder before intercourse. If involuntary loss of urine still impedes your ability to enjoy this form of sexual expression, get appropriate bladder testing. There's much that can be done to remedy this problem (see page 273).

In our new Viagrally stimulated society, I would be remiss if I didn't respond to the plea that arises so frequently in my practice: "My husband got a prescription for that little blue pill. Help!" Thirty million men in the United States suffer from erectile dysfunction, and thanks to Bob Dole, the acronym E.D. has entered our living rooms (not to mention our bedrooms). Two-thirds of the men who take Viagra will be able to have successful intercourse. But that's defining success from the male point of view. If you are not used to having intercourse and suddenly attempt to resume it, you may find that you're uncomfortable—either emotionally or physically. Many relationships become platonic when sex is not possible. Reintroducing intercourse to the picture requires more than a pill—it requires passion. It's helpful to start slow, talking before touching and exploring ways to rekindle fantasies and arousal. If necessary, try using books and videos as erotic aids. You may also need to reconsider your hormonal status and improve your genital health with estrogen and possibly testosterone.

I'VE NEVER BEEN A REGULAR EXERCISER. IS IT TOO LATE TO START?

It's about time you asked. I've exercised my right to recommend exercise from the beginning of this book, and let me reassure you that it's never too late to start. Too many women think that once they hit midlife they can give up on exercise or that it's too much of a hassle to begin. And when I say too many, I'm referring to an astounding four-fifths of the population in your age group who do not engage in regular, sustained vigorous exercise. To enhance your momentum, let me give you some facts about what exercise can do for your health:

Protect you from cardiovascular disease. Exercise cuts your risk of heart attack and stroke in half.

Help you lose or maintain weight. An example that I like to use comes from the American Heart Association: A 200-pound person who does not change her diet but who begins walking briskly 1.5 miles every day will lose 14 pounds in a year.

Reduces the risk of osteoporosis. Menopausal women who walk, jog or climb stairs three times a week have been found to increase bone mass 5.2% in just one year. Those who regularly engage in weight training can do even better, increasing bone density by as much as 8%.

Decrease your risk of developing diabetes. Exercise decreases insulin resistance, which may help prevent or control this disease.

Curb your cancer risk. Exercise lowers the chance of developing colon and endometrial cancer, and some studies have shown that it reduces the risk of breast cancer. (The Harvard nurses' study failed to validate the breast cancer connection, but epidemiologists are still investigating.) There is at least a sixfold decrease in overall cancer death rates for women who exercise and are physically fit.

Sharpens your mind. Exercise increases blood flow to the brain, improves reaction times and has been shown to help us perform better on tests of mental agility. And while I'm on the subject of the mind: Exercise also decreases depression and anxiety, and helps women fall asleep more readily and sleep longer.

Helps control arthritis pain. You have to be careful not to overdo it, but regularly stretching and moving the joints will often ease pain.

Strengthens the immune system. Studies show that people who are physically fit get fewer colds, probably because exercise increases the circulation of immune cells.

Now that you're convinced of exercise's benefits, let me reassure you that you don't have to put on a skimpy leotard and start prancing around to loud music in a mirrored studio. We used to bombard you with charts and target heart-rate zones and dictums of vigorous activity that had to be performed for at least 30 minutes. Frankly, this was overwhelming for most of us and didn't fit into our schedules. So the inevitable happened: We joined gyms, bought machines and swore we would become exercisers, but the pressures of our daily lives made this difficult if not impossible. But lo and behold, the Surgeon General, Centers for Disease Control and Prevention, National Institutes of Health and American College of Sports Medicine have decided that 30 minutes of daily, moderate physical activity—as opposed to more vigorous workouts—yields almost the same substantial health benefits.

Let me be more specific: We're talking about physical activity that fits into your lifestyle. The activity doesn't have to be intense, or even for a full 30 minutes at once. Three 10-minute sessions per day are just as good as one 30-minute session. The end goal is to expend about 200 calories altogether. So if you don't want to engage in a formal exercise program, walk up stairs rather than take an elevator; walk short distances (such as a mile) instead of driving; do calisthenics while watching the morning news (hopefully the *Today* show). When you do housework, remember that you have more than a clean house to gain from the exertion. Rake leaves in the fall, play actively with your grandchildren. As long as these activities are performed at an intensity that corresponds to that of a brisk walk, you'll get the benefits of exercise. The greatest drop in your mortality risk comes when you go from being sedentary to being a moderate exerciser. However, I don't want to discourage you: If you choose to do more and become highly fit, you'll improve on this percentage.

In addition to your daily half-hour of cardiovascular exercise, you should be doing some form of strength-training exercise for a minimum of 15 minutes, three times a week. This includes weight lifting, resistance training with specially made rubber bands or even doing sit-ups, squats and other moves that involve lifting your own body weight.

You'll also need to add on flexibility exercises—ideally you'll do this right after your cardiovascular and strength-training sessions, when you're particularly limber and muscles are easy to stretch. This will help to prevent future injuries. As you get older, certain activities that we now take for granted—getting up from a chair or bending down to retrieve something from the floor—can become more difficult. Remaining flexible can help you perform these activities in the decades to come.

Exercise has to become a priority in your life—perhaps not as great a priority as getting to work or making sure that you and your family eat—but a priority nonetheless. I always tell my patients (and myself) that if exercise isn't one of our top four priorities for the day, we won't get to it. So put it on your daily to-do list and get going.

WHAT TESTS DO I NEED?

These are the examinations, tests and procedures I recommend to my patients in their sixties.

Examination/test/procedure	How often
Blood pressure	Every two years
Cholesterol test	Every five years
Fasting plasma glucose	Every three years
Thyroid hormone test	Every two years
Urinalysis	Annually
STD testing	At your/your doctor's discretion
Pelvic exam & Pap smear	Annually; Pap at doctor's discretion after three negative tests
Rectal exam	Annually

Examination/test/procedure	How often
Clinical (physician) breast exam	Annually
Mammogram	Annually
Electrocardiogram	Every five years
Bone mineral density	Once at age 65
Fecal occult testing	Annually
Colorectal cancer screen	Every five to 10 years, depending on screening method used
Immunizations	Tetanus booster every 10 years
Pneumococcal vaccine	Once at age 65
Influenza vaccine	Annually after age 65
Eye exam	Every three years until age 65; annually or every other year after that
Skin exam by dermatologist	Every two years
Skin self-exam	Annually

WHAT CAN GO WRONG AT MY AGE?

Osteoporosis

Bone awareness campaigns have become effective, perhaps because calcium makers are vying to market their products, and women in their sixties and beyond are aware of the fact that their bones may silently become less than supportive. But awareness doesn't necessarily translate into action. We are still undercalciumed, under-weight-bearing-exercised, underscreened and undertreated. Because of the emphasis placed on osteoporosis prevention (which, I have already stressed, should begin in childhood), many of us, physicians included, do not realize how extremely treatable this disease is. The earlier you are at diagnosis, the more aggressively you should be treated; the results can be truly bone- and life-affirming.

First, I'll state the gruesome statistics. Osteoporosis affects 23 million

Americans and is the underlying cause of 1.5 million fractures every year. One-half of all women will break their weakened bones after the age of 65. It gets worse. Within a year following such fractures, the likelihood of death is increased by up to 20%. One in three women will fracture their hips by the age of 90. This is much more than our chance of developing breast, uterine and ovarian cancer combined. Once this type of fracture occurs, 20% of women will die either from surgery (hip pinning and hip replacement) or from the complications resulting from prolonged bed rest and convalescence. Half of those who survive will no longer be able to walk unassisted and will require long-term nursing care, 25% of them for the rest of their lives!

Our spines are even more vulnerable than our hips. One-half of all fractures due to osteoporosis occur in our upper spine. The vertebrae literally collapse under the weight of the head and neck they support. Once these crushed vertebrae no longer stack up evenly, they curve outward and produce the characteristic dowager hump, causing loss of height that is usually 1.5 inches or more.

Little is coupled so dismissively with the word *old* (again, a very subjective term) in describing women that this term is not taken seriously. But the nerve damage, pain, limited mobility and even paralysis associated with compression fractures of our vertebrae are extremely serious. This deformity can also cause other serious health problems. The rib cage is pushed down into the abdomen, and this constricts the internal organs so that the digestive tract, heart and lungs can't function properly.

There is much that can be done before all of these dire consequences of osteoporosis really compromise your health. If your height has decreased by 1.5 inches or more, or if you've noticed increased curvature of your upper spine, consider the fact that you do have osteoporosis. Also, if you've fractured your wrist from a minor trauma, or if you've had a chest or back X-ray that reported what appears to be a vertebral fracture, the diagnosis has been made. Finally, if you break your leg, ankle or even your pelvis with minimal trauma, or crack a rib with coughing (again, a diagnosis that is often made after a chest X-ray to determine why you are coughing), you should have a more complete bone evaluation. In fact, you probably should have been screened earlier before these features occurred. But this is no time to quibble, and you can still benefit from therapy.

The state of the art for testing bone density is the Dual Energy X-ray Absorbtiometry, or DEXA, which measures the density of the spine and hip and can calculate total body bone density with an accuracy within

2%. It's quick, taking about ten minutes, and safe, using less radiation than most simple X-rays. Unfortunately, the machine is rather large, and testing costs between $175 and $275. Some insurance plans will cover it only if you have a diagnosis of osteoporosis, or if your doctor writes that you have considerable risk for this disease. Your test results are compared to those of an ideal average woman (a puzzling term) of similar race who is 30 years old and has reached her peak bone density. The assumption is that this should also have been yours at 30, and that whatever it is currently represents a loss. But, of course, you may not have reached this "bone best" at any point in your life, and the number reported as a standard deviation may not reflect your postmenopausal life. What really counts is whether you've reached or plummeted to 2.5 standard deviations below that elusive mean. A decrease of 1 standard deviation roughly corresponds to 10% bone loss, doubling your fracture risk. If you are 2.5 standard deviations below the mean, you have significant osteoporosis. This number was chosen because more than half of patients with fragility fractures have a bone mass that is below this value. It doesn't mean that tomorrow you'll break something, but as you get older, it signifies considerable risk, and a lifetime risk can approach 100% if you've lost 30% of your bone mass.

Before I go further, let me just mention another more portable and less expensive method for bone screening: The Heel Ultrasound Densitometer. This "put your foot in and see what your bones are like" machine measures how easily ultrasound waves pass through the heel bone. The more porous this bone, the more easily the waves pass through. The results have been shown to correlate quite well with the overall status of your bones, so a low reading constitutes a warning sign of osteoporosis. But a word of warning: Your heel will not be the cause of major disability or death. Your hip and spine can be, so an abnormal heel density should mandate that you have a more precise DEXA scan.

Bone density shows us what our bones have done. But there are also tests that can demonstrate what our bones are currently doing. Deciding whether bone loss is active and ongoing can help your doctor determine how aggressively it should be treated. For example, if you have a low bone density but you don't qualify for a diagnosis of osteoporosis and you are not actively losing additional bone, it might suffice for you to take calcium and vitamin D and exercise. But if there are signs of current breakdown of bone, an antiresorbtive medication such as estrogen, raloxifene (Evista), biphosphonate or calcitonin (Miacalcin) should be considered. Several tests can be used to confirm ongoing bone loss. A 24-hour urine collection can be done to check the amount of calcium excreted in your urine and will help to determine if you are absorbing calcium in the first place (remember, it won't come out in your urine if it didn't get into your body through your GI tract). Certain collagen products that are released when bone is broken down or resorbed are also secreted in the urine, and the levels of these can be measured. (These include tests for pyridinium crosslinks and C- and N-tellopeptides of collagen.) Another biochemical marker for breakdown is urine excretion of a substance called hydroxyproline. Not only will these chemical markers reflect your current risk, but a decrease in their levels will predict the success of therapy.

All of these tests are of little value (except to the manufacturers and labs) if you don't follow up with appropriate therapy, and there are lots to choose from. Even low-dose estrogen (Premarin 0.3 mg, Climara 0.025 mg or Vivelle 0.0375 mg) helps prevent bone loss and can increase bone density. But the more possibly the merrier, and if you're fighting true osteoporosis, higher doses of estrogen are probably better at building bone mass. Another alternative is to add alendronate sodium (Fosamax), which has been shown to work synergistically with estrogen. In other words, the two are better than one. If you are not on estrogen and won't or can't take it, Fosamax on its own can decrease your future fracture risk by up to 50%. This latter medication is poorly absorbed and needs to be taken on an empty stomach with 8 ounces of water (I've found that cold water is best), and you must be up and about and not eating or drinking anything else for at least 30 minutes.

If you have a history of acid reflux or ulcers or develop symptoms of heartburn with this medication, don't give up. There are excellent alternatives. Raloxifene (Evista) both increases bone mass up to 2.5% a year and decreases spinal fracture risk by as much as 50% in three years if you already have osteoporosis (the results are less clear or may take longer if your bone density is low, but not in the osteoporotic range). It also reduces cholesterol and the bad LDL, but does not raise good HDL (as estrogen does). Preliminary data show that at least in postmenopausal women who have established osteoporosis, breast cancer risk is diminished by 70%, although there is no current recommendation to use this therapy as a breast cancer preventive drug. (Right now, the manufacturers of tamoxifen are in a legal battle with those of raloxifene to make sure they don't make this claim as part of their promotional campaign.) If you are already on ERT, however, I would not advise adding raloxifene to hedge your bone or breast bets. There are no established data on whether the combination of these drugs augments them. Finally, since you are at least five years postmenopausal, you are also a candidate for calcitonin nasal spray. This seems to build bone mass more slowly (less than 2% a year), but has been shown to decrease spinal fractures by nearly 36%. I have to say this now, even if the manufacturers didn't: "Just a puff a day can keep fractures away." There are some preliminary data indicating that when calcitonin is combined with estrogen, the two work better together than each alone, but as yet there is no official recommendation for this double therapy.

We may have come a long way in developing drugs to help prevent or stop bone loss, or even to help build up bone, but reliance on pills, patches or sprays alone will not reverse this disease. Osteoporosis is, to some extent, a lazy woman's disease, and to combat it, as the verb implies, you have to stop being lazy. That means making sure that you engage in weight-bearing exercise (walking or jogging does this; unfortunately, swimming and most stationary bikes don't) and weight resistance exercise (15 minutes of lightweight calisthenics three times a week), and, of course, you should stop "de-boning" medications and activities. That means you should make sure that if you take thyroid hormone, you are not taking excessive doses (this can be checked with a TSH test). If at all possible, limit or stay away from steroid medications, don't smoke and cut down on caffeine and alcohol consumption. And finally, and perhaps most important, get enough calcium and vitamin D.

That "enough" has increased since the last decade. As you traverse your sixties, there is a decrease in absorption of calcium from your GI tract, as well as a decrease in vitamin D production from your skin and kidneys. Your parathyroid hormone levels increase and this, in turn, causes calcium resorption from bones, perhaps in order to maintain steady levels of calcium in your bloodstream as you absorb less. To compensate for these changes, you need 1,500 milligrams of calcium and 800 units of vitamin D a day. You obviously can get your calcium from food, and milk products are some of the best sources. A glass of milk gives you 300 milligrams, and a cup of nonfat yogurt gives you a bountiful 400 milligrams. Unfortunately, cottage cheese is not a good calcium source (only 80 mg a cup). You can get some calcium in green vegetables, but not as much as you think. One cup of broccoli gives you 170 milligrams. Collards and dry black beans are better, supplying 270 milligrams. Some soy milks give you almost as much calcium as cow's milk, and four ounces of tofu have 150 milligrams of calcium. Three ounces of canned sardines in oil with the bones are great if you like them and supply 370 milligrams of calcium. We now have calcium-fortified orange juice and cereals, which may give you as much of this mineral as a glass of milk, but when all is said and done, you would need the equivalent of about three glasses of milk and one cup of yogurt to get your daily calcium. Most of us don't ingest or even digest this, so you will probably have to resort to supplements.

Are there good, better and best calciums that have my seal of approval? My answer is that I approve of any type that you tolerate and will take in a consistent fashion. The formulation that gives you the biggest calcium bang per tablet or per chew is *calcium carbonate,* which consists of 40% elemental calcium. Some of the better-known commercial products include Tums, calcium-rich Rolaids, Caltrate and Viactiv. These should be taken with meals and no more than 500 or 600 milligrams at a time (so don't try to take all 1,500 mg at once; it won't get absorbed and may also cause stomach upset). Calcium carbonate can, in some women, cause constipation and bloating. You also need sufficient stomach acid to allow for its absorption, so if you take medications to reduce stomach acid, or you can't take this with meals, you might want to switch to *calcium citrate,* found in Citracal and other products. This doesn't require high levels of gastric acid to be broken down and absorbed (and we tend to lose gastric acidity after the age of 65). This is a more dilute form of calcium containing only 24% elemental calcium per tablet, so you will need twice as many tablets as in the carbonate form. It should be taken in divided doses between meals and at bedtime (and one of the best times for absorption and uptake by bones may be at night before sleep). It also has been relatively cleared as far as kidney stones are concerned and may actually prevent them. I take two Citracal tablets at mid-morning and then wait to see if I have a good calcium day and get another 600 to 800 milligrams from foods. If I don't, I take a Viactiv chocolate chew, which contains calcium carbonate, as a kind of second dessert (it tastes like a Tootsie Roll). It's easy and allows me to adjust my dose on a daily, as-needed basis.

I also want to home in on the source of calcium in these supplements. Synthetic may be better than natural. Products made from bone meal and oyster shell can contain lead, and this is not an element we want to add to our diets.

Some calciums are prepared in formulations that contain magnesium.

Yes, we need this second mineral to help our calcium absorption. Our bodies probably need 250 to 300 milligrams a day, and we absorb only half of the magnesium we ingest. The RDA of 300 milligrams may be too low. Fortunately, many foods, including milk, fresh green vegetables, whole grains, wheat germ, seeds, nuts and even seafood, are excellent sources of magnesium. If your diet does not include these magnesium-rich foods, it's okay to add it, but there is no reason to supplement more than 500 milligrams a day.

Sticks and stones and falls, and even gravity, can indeed break your bones if you have osteoporosis, but the current available therapies can help you break out (and not break down) from the encumbrances of this disease.

Heart Disease

Each year, twice as many women die from heart disease and stroke as from *all* forms of cancer combined. By our mid-sixties, one-third of us will have some type of heart or blood vessel disease. Traditionally we've been told to worry about the hearts of the men in our lives, not our own. The fact is that being a woman is one of the best things we can do for our heart, at least when we're younger: Our estrogen production postpones the onset of cardiovascular disease by 10 to 15 years when compared to men. So guess what? By the age of 60, we're catching up. And once we reach our mid-seventies, we've caught up. Heart attack accounts for 60% of sudden deaths in women. Nearly one in three of us will die of heart disease, making it by far the number one killer of American women. Yet we erroneously continue to view this as a male disorder and ignore prevention, early diagnosis and aggressive therapy. In a recent survey, only 8% of women considered heart disease to be our top health threat!

All women need to know we're at risk for heart disease. But you're especially at risk if you:

Have a family history of cardiovascular disease: "Family history" is defined as having a first-degree male relative who died from coronary heart disease before age 55, or a first-degree female relative who died from it before age 65. This is one of the strongest—if not the strongest—risk factors for heart disease, increasing your risk anywhere from two- to sixfold.

Smoke: The more you smoke, the greater your risk. A pack-a-day smoker faces a more than fivefold increase in her risk for heart attack. And don't kid yourself into thinking that low-tar or low-nicotine brands are safe. There's no such thing as an acceptable level of smoking. Just one to four cigarettes a day doubles your risk of coronary artery disease. The cigarette may look long, white and clean. But your arteries will be thickened, jagged and blocked. The good news is that two to four years after you've stopped smoking, your heart attack risk will be similar to that of women in your age group who never smoked.

Have high cholesterol: Your cholesterol level in and of itself is not a good indicator of risk—you have to examine each of its components. When it comes to women in your age group, an HDL (high-density lipoprotein) level below 35 mg/dl is the strongest lipid predictor of risk. Your risk is borderline-high if your HDL is between 35 and 50 mg/dl. HDL is the good cholesterol that has a Teflon-like effect on artery walls, preventing plaque from forming. The most common causes for low HDL (all these risk factors are interrelated) are smoking, being overweight, being sedentary and not taking ERT. A high level of the plaque-forming low-density lipoprotein (LDL) may be less important in determining your risk, but it's not good if it's above 160 mg/dl. It's considered borderline-high when between 130 mg/dl and 159 mg/dl.

The final lipid you have to consider is triglyceride, which, if high, has an important predictive value in women, especially if HDL is low. This is the only lipid that must be tested when you're fasting (the other blood tests are reliable even if you've eaten). A level over 400 mg/dl is high; 200 to 400 mg/dl is considered borderline high, although frankly if you approach this 400 mark, you'll need treatment.

Have high blood pressure: Half of all women in their sixties are hypertensive, and a third of us don't even know it. Yet women with high blood pressure are six times more likely than those with normal pressure to have a fatal heart attack.

Are overweight: Where your heart's concerned, weight gain shouldn't be taken lightly. Gaining just 11 to 17 pounds after the age of 18 increases your risk of heart disease by 50%, and if you gained more than 45 pounds, your risk is increased by 300%. And it's not just what you put on, but where it settled. If the weight accumulated like a spare tire around your middle, it's especially threatening (see page 173).

Have diabetes: This is a stronger risk factor for women than it is for men. Eighty percent of women with Type 2 diabetes will die from heart disease.

Are sedentary: Being inactive nearly doubles your risk of cardiovascular disease. Exercise conditions all of your muscles and this in turn decreases the work load on your heart; it also reduces clot formation, may increase your HDL and mitigates risk factors such as obesity and high blood pressure.

Don't take estrogen: This hormone is what gave you your cardiac gender advantage before menopause, and taking postmenopausal ERT probably reduces your risk of heart disease by 50%.

You may have committed heart abuse in the past, but there's much you can do now to decrease the chance that you'll become just another cardiac statistic.

What to do:

KNOW YOUR FAMILY HISTORY
It's the first step toward getting the right cardiac testing at the right time.

STOP SMOKING
Prevention should start with smoking cessation (if, despite everything you know, you're still smoking). Quitting will reduce your risk of cardiovascular disease by 60%. For advice, see page 119.

EXERCISE
For advice on how much and what kind, see page 176.

CONTROL DIABETES AND/OR HIGH BLOOD PRESSURE
I've explained how to manage the former on page 247. The latter is covered on page 183.

IF YOU DRINK ALCOHOL, DO SO IN MODERATION
That means no more than one drink a day. If you have risk factors for heart disease, one to three drinks a week can reduce your chance of fatal heart attack by up to 41%. Alcohol helps raise HDL cholesterol; it also relaxes smooth muscles in the cardiac vessels and reduces clot formation. Wine (and grape juice) contains flavonoids that diminish the effects of LDL on plaque formation.

What to eat

IF YOUR CURRENT CHOLESTEROL PROFILE IS ABNORMAL
You need to eat a diet that derives less than 30% of its calories from fat—less than 7% from the saturated fat found in meat and dairy products—and that contains fewer than 200 milligrams of cholesterol. This is called a Step 2 diet.

IF YOU HAVE NORMAL CHOLESTEROL
Follow the Step 1 diet, which allows 300 milligrams of dietary cholesterol and up to 10% of calories from saturated fat (although, frankly, a Step 2 diet won't hurt).

NO MATTER WHAT YOUR CHOLESTEROL LEVEL
Avoid trans-fatty acids (the hydrogenated oils found in packaged snacks such as chips and crackers, as well as in stick margarine and shortening). Butter substitutes made with soybean oil or others that are trans-fat free are a healthier alternative. Or use one of the new margarines that contain cholesterol-lowering compounds called sterol and stanol esters. Brand names include Benecol and Take Control. High-carb, very low fat diets may do more harm than good. Processed, starchy foods can increase insulin production, which further throws off your cholesterol equation. You may not be eating the fats, but your body is still making them. What fat you eat should be whenever possible the monounsaturated type found in olive and canola oil.

Also concentrate on a high-fiber diet. Some studies have shown that the soluble fiber in some breakfast cereals, especially oatmeal, reduces risk of cardiovascular disease in women by as much as 23%. Cold-water fish such as salmon, which contain heart-healthy omega-3 fatty acids, is a great source of protein. If you eat meat, make sure it is very lean; trim the skin from poultry. And of course you'll want to eat at least five servings of fruits and vegetables every day, especially dark green leafy vegetables and citrus fruits and juices. These contain folic acid, a natural controller of homocysteine, an amino acid that may be toxic to the lining of the arteries. They're also a good source of antioxidant nutrients that are thought to protect against heart disease.

What to take

VITAMINS
Antioxidant vitamins act like a sponge, sopping up and neutralizing marauding free radical molecules that are formed as your body metabo-

lizes oxygen. These radicals' only political goal is to steal back the electrons they lost during oxidation. But in the process they attack LDL cholesterol, causing it to form artery-clogging plaque. Of all the antioxidants, vitamin E has the best-established heart-protecting effect. The Harvard nurses' study showed that taking more than 100 international units of E (separately and not as part of a multivitamin) decreased the risk of major coronary disease by 40%. My recommendation takes into account E's other possible protective effects. I tell my patients to take 400 I.U. daily because it's practically impossible to get protective levels of E from food alone. The other antioxidants, vitamin C and beta-carotene, have not been shown to have a strong effect against heart disease, although you may want to take them for other reasons.

FOLIC ACID

This is a proven heart-friendly nutrient thanks to its lowering effect on homocysteine levels. The dose of 400 micrograms per day found in most multivitamins could be expected to reduce your risk of heart disease. It's also thought that folic acid enables us to derive heart-healthy benefits from modest alcohol intake (or even grape juice). So if you're counting on a drink a day to keep the cardiologist away, make sure you're also taking your multivitamin. Your multivitamin should also contain B_6, which appears to help folic acid to lower homocysteine levels. However, if your homocysteine level is found on a blood test to be high, you'll need higher doses of both folic acid and B_6 as prescribed by your physician.

ASPIRIN

The men in our lives are popping their aspirin. Based on a 1983 study of its protective effects on male physicians, they know this will decrease their future risk of heart attack by as much as 44%. The dose recommended for them is 325 milligrams every other day. We don't have a similar study detailing dosage for women (I guess at the time there were too few women physicians, and those who were around were not felt to require heart protection; we were more interested in career protection). But we do have data from the nurses' study (which consisted of all women), and this allows us to predict that one to seven aspirins a week (a full dose or 325 mg) decrease the relative risk of our first heart attack by 32%. The way aspirin works is by inhibiting the aggregation, or stickiness, of platelets to existing plaque so clots can't begin to form. But since this anticlotting punch can be delivered with the equivalent of just one baby aspirin a day (81 mg), this may suffice. Recently, the American College of Chest Physicians came to the consensus that all women over 50 with one or more cardiovascular risk factors, which include diabetes, hypertension, cigarette smoking, lack of exercise and abnormal lipids, should begin taking a baby aspirin a day (the FDA, however, only recommends it if you've had a previous heart attack or angina, or have undergone cardiac vessel surgery). But, if you don't fall into these high-risk categories, I and many cardiologists feel you would still benefit from anticlotting protection. However, since the effect of baby aspirin on platelets can last for 8 to 10 days, taking it 3 times a week will probably suffice, and most of us should begin doing that "male aspirin thing" by the age of 55. The aspirin can be enteric-coated, so it's less likely to upset your stomach. But if you've had a history of ulcers or bleeding problems, already take anticoagulation therapy or have an aspirin allergy, obviously you must check with your doctor before starting this long-term regimen.

And remember aspirin may increase bruisibility of the small blood vessels anywhere in your body; you might notice you get black and blue with just slight mishaps. Whether this bruising significantly increases your risk for certain types of brain hemorrhage is still debatable, and most doctors feel the cardiac benefits outweigh this concern. For once, I'll tell you to be influenced by those commercials. If you have any symptoms of a developing heart attack, pop at least a low-dose aspirin of 325 milligrams on your way to the hospital.

CHOLESTEROL-LOWERING DRUGS

The lipid-lowering drugs called *statins* include lovastatin (Mevacor), atorvastatin calcium (Lipitor), pravastatin (Pravachol), simvastatin (Zocor) and cerivastatin (Baycol). These drugs inhibit the last step in the production of cholesterol so that total cholesterol and, very specifically, LDL, are lowered. Another benefit of these drugs is that there is some degree of triglyceride reduction and HDL elevation. Atherosclerotic plaque formation is diminished, and in some cases, the plaque that's already there may shrink. There is no question that if your cholesterol levels are abnormally high, you should be taking one of these drugs. They reduce risk of cardiovascular disease by 25% to 60% and deaths from heart attack and stroke by 30%. Even if you have normal cholesterol levels, if cardiovascular disease is diagnosed, the *statin* therapy is also justified. It will lower your risk of heart attack by 29% and stroke by 19% after five years of use. One study even suggested that in women there can be as much as a 40% decrease in risk of these events after just six months of therapy. This leads to the currently much pondered question of whether all of us, regardless of whether or not we have documented coronary vascular disease, should take one of these *statins* for cardiovascular peace of heart (and mind). A recent study showed that many of us should. A daily dose of 20 to 40 milligrams of Mevacor for five years decreased first heart attack by 40% in men and women with average total cholesterol and LDL levels but with below-average HDLs. So at this point, I would carefully review your risk factors and your lipids with your doctor. If you have one of the risk factors, or even if you don't have clear risk factors but your HDL is low, consider *statins*.

DIABETES AND ANTIHYPERTENSIVE MEDICATIONS
If you have either or both of these disorders, aggressive therapy will significantly reduce your chance of heart attack and stroke (see pages 183 and 248).

What tests you should have: By now, you've probably had one or more electrocardiograms (ECGs), either as part of your physical or before you had any type of surgical procedure (most hospitals require them after age 45 or 50). This test can reveal many things: an irregular heartbeat, abnormal propagation of the electric wave causing your heart's contraction and any past damage to a portion of your heart muscle. But, in and of itself, it is not an adequate test for detection of developing heart vessel blockage or impending risk of heart attack in women. Only 1.1% of women between the ages of 45 and 74 have abnormal ECGs, so most women can't rely on this test as the final word for their coronary vascular assessment. That being the case, the next logical step (at least for men) in the cascade of cardiac testing would be to have a stress ECG (an ECG performed while exercising on a treadmill). Unfortunately, this test is falsely abnormal in as many as half of the women tested. You'll get much more valid results if you exercise within your capabilities while your heart is imaged with cardiac ultrasound (a stress echocardiogram). Perhaps the most accurate assessment is a thallium exercise stress test, in which blood flow to the heart is imaged during exercise with radio tracers injected into a vein. Our only gender problem with this test is that adjustments have to be made for breast tissue, which can obscure the radioactive signals emitting from heart arteries. The last test is more time-consuming for both you and the technical team performing it, and it is obviously more expensive. You generally need to be referred for this. It's appropriate, however, for you to request this referral if you have any of the risk factors I've listed above. Once you've had these tests, if they are abnormal, your doctor should refer you for the next most accurate and complete assessment of your coronary arteries. This is the angiogram, in which dye is injected via catheter into the coronary vessels. If this is very abnormal, the invasive procedures I talked about earlier might need to be performed.

There is a new, controversial "lie down and do nothing" test that will allow you and your doctor to detect calcium buildup in your coronary vessels. This is called an electron-beam CT (EBCT) or a coronary calcium scan. Because most plaque contains calcium or gets calcified, measuring this allows for evaluation of the degree of plaque deposit and coronary heart disease. These calcium deposits are quickly measured with the ultra-fast CT scanner, which is seven times faster than conventional machines. It generates pictures that aren't blurred by the motion of the heart and blood. After taking into account your age, gender and cardiac risk factors, a calcium score is given and may give you and your doctor some idea about your risk for coronary artery disease. The test takes about 10 minutes. It costs approximately $400, and most insurance carriers do not cover it. The proponents of this CT scan (especially the radiologist and cardiologist who developed it) feel that it will pick up disease in individuals who are not aware they had a problem or who had "passed" their simple stress testing. They themselves admit, however, that 2% of those whose CT tests are fine then go on to have heart attacks. The detractors feel that 50% of middle-aged and older adults have some plaque and calcification, that the stability of this plaque (the fact that it doesn't break off or break into pieces that clog the vessel) is more important than the presence of the plaque itself, and that this test cannot predict stability. Moreover, even though it may only cost you the out-of-pocket sum of money, in many cases it will lead to huge bills for the insurance companies as they pay for tests ranging from thallium stress ECGs to potentially invasive tests such as angiography. The latter is invasive, and the results of these tests may show that you are not in cardiac risk. And, finally, if you pass the CT scan with flying colors (or, more precisely, your vessels are not overwhelmingly white), will this lead to complacency and a failure on your part to change to a cardiac-healthy lifestyle or, more seriously, not seek attention for symptoms of heart attack because you presume you are in good cardiac health? Right now, the American Heart Association has discouraged both the use of the electronic beam CT as a screening procedure in low-risk, nonsymptomatic patients and the "widespread proliferation of screening programs for coronary calcium as a single isolated diagnostic modality" until more data are available. Currently, I'm informing my patients about the test, encouraging them to have it if their other physicians can derive additional valuable information, especially if they are at risk. I also make sure they know that if it's positive, they will need additional work-up and if it's negative, they still need careful follow-up.

Signs and symptoms of a heart attack: Prevention is never too late, but you also need to recognize the symptoms of coronary heart disease and be aware of the warning signs of heart attack. Women under the age of 74 may be twice as likely to die as men once they have a heart attack (this twofold risk gradually decreases from age 50 to 74). This is due to several causes. The underlying disease causing the heart attack may be different. In men, atherosclerosis slowly but surely develops, but while this is happening, reserve arteries may sprout to compensate for the diseased vessels and nourish the heart muscle. But women develop atherosclerosis later than men because they had estrogen before menopause. If a vessel becomes blocked in our sixties or early seventies, it's more likely due to the fact that platelets have abnormally clumped together and caused clots to form, closing the vessel, or that the artery underwent prolonged spasm. Since this is a sudden process, there is no backup supply of blood, and the damage to the heart muscle can be more complete than in a male who has ongoing atherosclerosis. The good news, however, is that before a heart attack, many women have something called *unstable angina,* and if this is treated quickly and aggressively, their outcomes are better than those of men. So don't wait until you have a crushing pain in your chest that radiates to your left arm. Notice and seek attention for any recurrent discomfort, pressure or tingling feeling from your waist up to your neck or any shortness of breath or nausea, especially if it occurs with exertion or strong emotion. Don't write this off as simple indigestion, anxiety or stress. You could be making a fatal mistake. Women routinely delay seeking care, and when they see their physicians, they are often sicker and more likely to have other conditions, such as diabetes, hypertension, elevated cholesterol and stroke, than men. There is, unfortunately, also a gender gap when it comes to prompt or aggressive therapy, so when you get to your doctor or the emergency room, make sure that you are not dismissed without minimal testing, which should include a thorough history and physical and an electrocardiogram. Often your doctor will also order blood tests that can detect cardiac muscle damage. Once a diagnosis of cardiac mishap has been made, you should be receiving intensive cardiac care, usually in a special cardiac unit. The degree of heart damage should be assessed, medications for any rhythm abnormalities given and assessment of the status of your coronary vessels should be quickly done. If necessary, more invasive procedures to correct a blocked coronary artery are in order. These include:

- *Angioplasty:* A catheter with a collapsed balloon at its tip is threaded into the vessel, and the balloon is then distended to break up the clot.
- *Stent placement:* A hollow tube made of metal mesh is left in the artery to keep the walls apart and prevent recurrent closure.
- *Coronary bypass:* Veins or arteries from under the breast bone or from other parts of the body are used to replace clogged cardiac vessels.

Unfortunately, because we have smaller vessels than men, these procedures tend to be more technically difficult and fraught with higher complication rates for women. No matter what course of therapy is appropriate, the faster we are properly diagnosed and the quicker we are treated, the more likely we will survive.

Diverticulosis

You've had more than 60 years to eat the processed, refined foods that distinguish our Western diet from that of Third World countries. In other words, you grew up eating white bread instead of whole grain, french fries instead of brown rice, beef instead of legumes and frosted cereals instead of bran. These choices may have been considered more modern and civilized, but your gut's preference is for a more primitive, fibrous diet. Without fiber, the muscle walls of your large intestine may weaken over time, allowing small pouches (or herniations) to form. Each pouch is a diverticula, and several of these constitute a condition called diverticulosis. Stool can become lodged in these sacs, causing infection, bleeding or even rupture. This is diverticulitis ("-itis" is what happens when your "-osis" gets infected). Think appendicitis, but with scores, if not hundreds, of miniature appendices that become inflamed. Although this is not a female disorder—as a matter of fact, it's more common in men—I've included it here because it is so common, and many women see their gynecologist first when they feel any type of discomfort below the waist. And because half of all people develop this condition by their sixties, I often have to diagnose it or distinguish it from true gynecologic conditions such as ovarian cysts or tumors.

Aside from occasional rectal bleeding, diverticulosis is a silent condition. But if you have followed my advice and had your screening sigmoidoscopy, colonoscopy or barium enema in your fifties, you may have been informed that you have this condition. Unfortunately, many women are not screened, and their first warning may be the dire symptoms of an acute infection. These include pain and local tenderness in the left lower abdomen, as well as fever and constipation. If an infected sac ruptures, these symptoms may worsen and the abdomen may become distended, hard and exquisitely sensitive to pressure or motion. Nausea, vomiting and heavy rectal bleeding can ensue. This is an emergency. Don't wait until you're this sick to see your doctor. If the inflammation is caught early when you're not very ill, you can be treated at home with rest, a liquid diet and oral antibiotics. Your symptoms should subside within 24 hours. (I tell my patients with diverticulosis that the minute they feel abdominal discomfort—especially if they're constipated—they should begin a liquid diet. This may help prevent the next stage.) If you're too sick to be treated at home, you should be hospitalized, fed nothing by mouth and given intravenous fluids and antibiotics. You'll slowly begin eating solid food again and adding fiber, in the form of a psyllium preparation. Two weeks after you recover from the infection, you'll need a barium enema to confirm that it was in fact diverticulosis that caused your symptoms, and that it hasn't gotten worse. One month after your recovery, you should be back on a high-fiber diet.

In 20% of those with diverticulitis, surgery may be needed to remove a portion of the infected bowel and/or drain abscesses. You're more likely to be in this 20% if you've had two or more previous attacks of inflammation or if you are taking Prednisone. This disease can have long-term complications. A channel, or fistula, can develop between the bowel and the bladder, causing continual bladder infections. This is more common in women who've had a hysterectomy. Fistulas can form between other internal organs, and bowel obstruction can also occur.

Even if you already have diverticulosis, you can avoid a worsening of your condition with a fiber-rich diet. Aim for 30 milligrams of fiber per day; use a powdered fiber supplement if necessary. Make sure you're drinking eight glasses of water each day. Although this is not a universal recommendation, many physicians feel you should not consume foods whose tiny particles can block the entrance to the diverticulae. This includes seeds, nuts and popcorn. Chew everything you eat thoroughly.

MY TOP 10 LIST FOR STAYING HEALTHY IN YOUR SIXTIES

1. Continue (or start) doing regular, moderate physical activity.
2. If you have diabetes, hypertension or abnormal lipids, make sure they are treated aggressively.
3. Increase your calcium to 1,500 milligrams at age 65; increase your vitamin D to 800 international units and take a multivitamin with at least 400 micrograms of folic acid. Also consider taking cardioprotective vitamin E.
4. If you have not taken estrogen, have tests to see if your bones and heart would benefit from this or some other therapy.
5. Talk to your doctor about the possible benefits of taking baby aspirin.
6. Know what tests are recommended for your age group and demand them from your doctor and your insurance carrier.
7. Insist on referrals to specialists when necessary.
8. Consider getting medigap insurance to cover what Medicare won't; also determine whether you might want long-term care insurance.
9. Consider ways to maintain intimacy and your sexuality.
10. Continue to develop new interests—read good books, take up a new hobby, go out of your way to meet interesting people and do interesting things that will stimulate your brain.

YOUR SEVENTIES AND BEYOND

CONGRATULATIONS, YOU'VE ACHIEVED your golden years. The sages (a mature group of individuals) who linked a precious element to these decades of our lives knew a thing or two. *Precious* should also be the adjective that applies to your health during these years. You have to treat your body and soul as carefully as you would a valuable jewel. By handling your health with care—getting screening tests, not being afraid to approach your doctor with any symptoms or problems, eating right, exercising and following the appropriate therapies for any chronic diseases—you may be able to impact not only your longevity but your quality of life. Staying healthy in your seventies and beyond is about more than just remaining disease-free or being able to get around on your own. It's about controlling any illnesses you do have (the average woman in your age group has two chronic conditions and an even greater number of daily medications to manage) and continuing to engage in activities that you enjoy. It's also about making a contribution to your family, friends and the world around you, despite the regretful fact that our society so often devalues and rejects elderly people. (I debated the use of the term "elderly" here, but considering the fact that my daughters feel that anyone over age 50 is elderly, I decided it was fine.)

Too many women dismiss new symptoms as simply a consequence of aging. Yes, there are changes in the body after 70, and some of them may cause pain and disability. But you don't have to accept them as inevitable—you can often not only relieve the symptom, but also stop the progression of whatever condition is causing it. Rather than become depressingly repetitious, I'll start with a blanket statement: Everything that was happening in your sixties is continuing to occur. However, there are some new issues to deal with as well.

By now, you've outlived your ovaries by about two decades, and if you haven't taken estrogen (or if you took it and stopped), you may have severe vaginal atrophy and associated bladder problems. Estrogen deprivation may also have contributed to significant osteoporosis and increased your risk of cardiovascular events and possibly Alzheimer's and even colon cancer. Even if you did take estrogen, you can't assume that you're completely protected from these disorders, with perhaps the exception of vaginal atrophy.

Unfortunately, chronic diseases are very much a fact of life as we get older, and by this decade, almost a third of you will be diagnosed with some form of coronary artery disease. One in five of you will experience peripheral vascular disease due to plaque-clogged vessels; this can lead to calf pain and, left untreated, muscle wasting and ulcers on the legs and feet. All of this is made worse if you have hypertension or diabetes. Heart rhythm irregularities are also common in your age group; if not treated with anticoagulants, one type, atrial fibrillation, can result in stroke.

Transient ischemic attack (TIA), a form of early stroke or "prestroke," is often poorly diagnosed. When these episodes of impaired blood flow to the brain happen repeatedly, brain function can be impaired, and dementia can result. Sometimes it's difficult to differentiate this from Alzheimer's disease, which also becomes increasingly prevalent as we age. Up to 1 in 10 women over age 65 have this disease, but that number increases to as many as 1 in 2 by the age of 85. Another neurological disease that becomes more common with age is Parkinson's, which peaks at age 75. Your lifetime risk of developing this movement disorder is 2.5%. Although the first sign of this illness is often a tremor, not every tremor equals Parkinson's. Some tremors are hereditary and will not progress any further.

Probably one of the scariest diseases in any age group is cancer. Because the aging immune system loses its ability to cancel out mutations and halt the growth of resulting abnormal cells, the longer you live, the more likely you are to develop cancer. Approximately half of all cancers occur between the ages of 65 and 90. Breast, colorectal, stomach, ovarian and bladder cancers all increase in prevalence after age seventy. But the good news is that when it comes to lung and breast cancer, age may result in less aggressive tumors that are more responsive to therapy. Despite this, there is a tendency on the part of some doctors—and even some patients—to think that older people don't warrant diligent cancer screening and, once diagnosed, don't need to be treated aggressively. Age should not be the decisive factor in choice of therapy. Even in the case of advanced cancer, rigorous treatment can delay progression, minimize disability and improve chances of survival. There is a similar tendency to dismiss the need for a thorough search for the possible causes of anemia. Advanced age alone is not a reason for anemia; there may be an underlying malignancy, a nutritional deficiency, a bone marrow disorder or internal bleeding that's to blame.

Chronic joint disease is far less likely than cancer to be fatal, but it is one of the chief causes of pain and disability in your age group. Because of joint disease, many women think they can't or shouldn't exercise. This leads to an even greater risk of disability. Currently there are many strategies for treating the pain that will allow you to lead a more normal life—and, yes, even exercise.

Other major, treatable causes of disability include cataracts (half of us will have them after age 65; by age 75, the prevalence reaches 70%) and glaucoma, the second most prevalent cause of blindness in the United States. One in 50 older adults have glaucoma and half of them don't even know it. The most common cause of blindness, age-related macular degeneration, can sometimes be treated with laser surgery, particularly if it's diagnosed early.

Another vital sense that is often lost with advancing age is hearing. About one-third of women have some degree of hearing loss by age 70; that proportion rises to one-half by age 75. Other ear-related problems such as dizziness and vertigo occur just as frequently. All these vision and ear problems, combined with an unsteady gait, are prime factors behind the increased tendency toward the falls we so fear—those that result in serious fractures, particularly of the hip.

Age also diminishes our immune response to infections, and we are more likely to become ill. And because our natural defenses can't mount a forceful attack, the signs and symptoms of infection such as fever and elevated white blood cell count may be delayed or never develop. As a result, diagnosis can be made late, with dire consequences. More than 90% of deaths attributable to influenza occur among those age 65 or older. Pneumonia, skin infections and kidney infections can likewise become increasingly serious.

I don't want to create a sense of gloom and doom for those of you who are traversing these decades. One of the reasons I'm writing this chapter is to show you what medical science has to offer so that you can embark on what is now known as "successful aging." Successful aging isn't necessarily disease-free aging. It's defined as having high cognitive and physical function that allows you to maintain many of the activities you've become accustomed to and to be actively engaged with life. Perceiving yourself as in control of your own life is also an important factor. This is not a time to passively sit back and say, "I am at the mercy of my genes." In fact, by the time you hit your seventies, genetic risk factors become far less important to your health than environmental ones over which you can exert some control. Successful aging requires us to rethink how we view what was formerly called "old age." A better term might be "the third age"—in other words, we've endured the uncertainties of youth, raised our family in our "second age" and now can continue to pursue personal achievement and self-development in our "third age." I look forward to many activities I was too busy to get to during my overly hectic second age. Let's see . . . right now that includes pottery (my family chuckles at this one), adventure travel (not just back and forth from L.A. to New York), reading the classics, studying comparative religions—and maybe I'll learn to cook. As my husband often reminds me—and by this decade we can allow ourselves to see the point—we should have a chance to smell the roses.

As you prepare for these "wow, I'm here—let's make the most of it" decades, be reassured that from a medical point of view, we've made enormous progress. Were I to write a treatise on the third age at the outset of the twentieth century, the pages would have been blank. Thanks to better nutrition, healthier lifestyles, antibiotics and advances in medical therapies, life expectancy for American women has increased by 31 years since 1900. Today, half of women who reach age 65 will go on to live to age 85. And if you make it to age 85, you stand to live another six years. The older we get, the more likely we are to live longer. So here's how to do it as gracefully and healthfully as possible.

DOES IT PAY TO CONTINUE TAKING ESTROGEN AFTER AGE 70?

Yes. Estrogen works as long as you take it, and when you stop, you lose the cardiovascular and bone protection, not to mention estrogen's benefits to your genitalia and bladder. (The percentage of pages of this book I've already devoted to hormonal issues is roughly equivalent to the percentage of your lifespan you could spend taking estrogen. So I'll spare you further discourse on ERT. For its pros and cons, see page 198.) It's estimated that once you stop estrogen replacement, within five years your risk returns to the same level as that of a person who's never taken estrogen. Although the academic purists do not yet allow the categorical statement that estrogen replacement decreases risk of Alzheimer's disease, the majority of peer-reviewed studies that have examined a connection between the two have found that long-term estrogen use may decrease the risk of Alzheimer's by one- to two-thirds. And a study that emanates from my coast (California) suggested that the longer estrogen was used and the higher the dose, the more effective it was.

I HAVEN'T HAD A MAMMOGRAM IN AT LEAST FIVE YEARS. SHOULD I WORRY?

I don't suggest that you obsess that you have hidden breast cancer, but I do want you to be more obsessive about getting appropriate screening. Breast cancer is a disease of longevity, so the older you are, the more likely you are to develop it. That often quoted and very scary statistic that a woman has a one in eight lifetime risk of developing this cancer is based on the presumption that she will reach the age of 85. But by age 75, your risk is already 1 in 11.

A recent dismaying federal survey found that mammograms were underused in older women. Fewer than a third of women in your age group (or even those in their late sixties) are getting mammograms at least every two years. Unfortunately, some doctors (and women themselves) may not think mammograms are called for as they get older and have other health problems. I don't need a survey to confirm this: I often have to argue with and cajole my 70-plus patients into getting their mammograms and convince them that breast care should remain part of their total health care.

The good news is that because breast cancer in your age group appears to be less aggressive (even if it is more common), it may be reasonable to screen every two years instead of every year as you did when you were younger. Fortunately, mammograms are also more accurate in older women, so your risk of a false-positive finding is low. In the absence of any data showing us when we should stop screening, I recommend that

you get a yearly breast exam by a medical professional and a mammogram at least every two years. You should also continue to do monthly
self-exams.

I KNOW I HAVE OSTEOPOROSIS. ASIDE FROM TAKING
MEDICATION AND CALCIUM, WHAT SHOULD I DO?

The next most important step you can take is to ensure that when you take
steps, you don't fall. Falls are the leading cause of accidental death in people over age 65. And the frequency with which we fall is astounding: One-
third of those in your age group who are up and about and living
independently will fall, and the proportion increases to half by age 80.
Although it seems we're tripping and sprawling all over the place, fortunately, most of these falls don't result in serious injury. About 5% result in fracture or hospitalization, and fewer than 1% cause hip fracture.
The more common fractures of the forearm, wrist and pelvis are not life-
threatening, nor are sprains and dislocations. However, they can restrict
your mobility and make it more likely that you'll fall again. All these are
general statistics for men and women and do not take into account the
fact that women are more likely to have fragile bones. Because you're in
this category, your chance of serious injury is of course higher.

Your likelihood of toppling is greater if in addition to osteoporosis you
have other risk factors. Despite the fact that you mastered the ability to
stand and walk in infancy, it's an extremely complicated feat requiring the
integration of sight, balance, muscle strength, bone support and the work-
ings of centers in your nervous system that give you a sense of where your
body is in space. Your heart's ability to supply blood to your brain when
you rise to a standing position is also key. The following conditions may
disturb your equilibrium: Parkinson's disease, cardiovascular diseases that
cause blood pressure fluctuations or cardiac arrythmias, previous stroke or
TIA, vision problems, gait disturbances (particularly those that require a
walker, cane or leg brace), vertigo, arthritis, diabetes, thyroid disorders,
anemia, dehydration, foot disorders and depression.

Obviously, in order to treat these health conditions, you may be taking
medications. These too can pose a risk. The chief offenders here are
diuretics (which can lead to dizziness or weakness), antihypertensives
(which can cause blood pressure to drop when you stand), antidepressants, sleeping pills and narcotic painkillers (all of which can affect the
central nervous system) and, of course, alcohol (at least a third of older

women are alcohol users and up to 10% are heavy drinkers). It's likely you won't be able to stop taking these medicines, but you can discuss any dizziness or unsteadiness you feel with your doctor, who may be able to lower your dosage or switch you to another medication. When it comes to alcohol, you probably should not be drinking at all—it packs a double bone fracture punch by preventing absorption of calcium and promoting unsteadiness.

Perhaps the most easily preventable cause of falls is environmental hazards. These include:

Lighting. Light may be too dim or too direct, which creates glare. Inaccessible light switches may force you to walk through a dark room in order to turn on the light.

Floors. Torn or slippery carpets or overly polished floors are hazardous to hips and limbs.

Stairs. Handrails may be missing, stairs may be too high, too slippery or poorly lighted, so that an ascent or descent becomes dangerous to your bones.

Furniture. Unstable chairs or tables and chairs that lack armrests or proper back support should be replaced. Furniture should not clutter hallways or other pathways. Cabinets and shelves should not be so high that you have to reach or stand on a chair or ladder in order to reach them.

Bathroom. This is a frequent location for falls. A slippery bathtub or shower, or one with no grab bar installed, is a major hazard. Towel bars should not be used as grab bars. The toilet seat may need to be raised to make getting up easier, and grab bars should be installed next to it. Doors should not lock from the inside; privacy is important, but this would prevent someone from coming to your aid if you should fall.

It's a good idea to have a home health professional with a background in fall prevention evaluate your surroundings and help you decide on necessary changes. Fall prevention does not mean you have to wrap yourself in cotton and not hazard a step into the world around you. But you have to achieve a balance between concern about falls and the need to maintain mobility and independence. Exercise, far from being a no-no, can improve your strength, flexibility and endurance. So take walks, climb stairs (carefully) and do lightweight resistance training, perhaps initially with a physical therapist who will show you what's safe. The more you improve your strength and flexibility, the more balanced you will be—literally and figuratively.

I'M TIRED ALL THE TIME AND HAVE NO ENERGY. WHAT'S WRONG—OR IS THIS JUST A PART OF GETTING OLDER?

Fatigue is so common as we age that many women hesitate to complain about it, and if they do, they may be told it's just "your age, my dear." This is not an acceptable diagnosis. Clearly you may not have the energy or physical ability to do everything you did in decades past, but you should not be overwhelmingly tired. Fatigue is a symptom of many major and minor disorders, and its cause—especially if it comes on suddenly—should always be explored. Just about every chronic illness can cause fatigue, and sometimes the fatigue itself is the first sign of the disorder. I've dealt with many of them, such as heart disease, thyroid problems and autoimmune diseases, in other chapters. So I've decided to focus here on some of the more common and more commonly overlooked reasons for fatigue that occur with age. The cause of your exhaustion should be exhaustively searched for so that you, with your doctor's help, can do something about it.

Anemia

When you don't have enough red blood cells to transport oxygen and nourish tissues, fatigue results. Some form of anemia occurs in more than a third of women in your age group. Although I don't propose that you become a hematologic expert, you should know a thing or two about your blood so that you can make sure you get the proper tests and understand the results. These are the three chief ways that the body's supply of red blood cells is depleted.

Decreased red blood cell production: There are several conditions that can impair your body's ability to make red blood cells. The first is iron deficiency, which leads to a lowered production of hemoglobin, the oxygen-carrying part of the blood cell. This deficiency can occur as a result of malnutrition, blood loss or chronic inflammation. After menopause (and lack of monthly blood loss) most women don't need to increase their iron intake. But in these decades, your absorption of iron may have decreased, especially if you're taking medications that reduce the acidity of your stomach or if you have a health condition that reduces stomach acidity.

The main cause of iron deficiency anemia, though, is blood loss. This can occur as a side effect of bleeding disorders and cancer (anywhere in the body, but especially in the GI tract), as well as ulcers, polyps or hemorrhoids. The most common reason for GI blood loss is use of nonsteroidal anti-inflammatory drugs or steroids. It's mandatory whenever iron deficiency anemia is discovered to do stool tests to check for hidden blood, and usually more in-depth investigation with colonoscopy, endoscopy of the upper GI tract or bowel X-rays is warranted. Identifying the source of blood loss may do more than help your fatigue—it may save your life. Once bleeding is controlled, iron supplements can begin to correct your anemia in just two weeks.

Another common reason that the body does not make enough red blood cells is chronic disease. The list of possible culprits is long but includes autoimmune diseases, cancer and chronic infections. The degree of anemia and your fatigue level are related to the severity of the disease. One type of cancer, multiple myeloma, results in the growth of abnormal cells in the bone marrow and overproduction of certain proteins. A combination of anemia, fatigue and an elevated sedimentation rate (revealed by a blood test) should raise a red flag for this disease in anyone in your age group. Red blood cell production in the bone marrow can also decrease in response to certain medications, including anticonvulsants and drugs used to treat autoimmune diseases.

Finally, myoloproliferative disorders and in the most severe form, leukemia, may cause significant anemia. These impair the bone marrow's ability to make both normal red and white blood cells. The risk of adult-onset leukemia increases with age, and fatigue is a prime symptom. If your white cell count is high or shows abnormal cells, or if you have anemia with decreased red blood cells, normal iron levels and no other clear-cut cause, a bone marrow test is in order.

Abnormal red blood cell production: The most common reason for this type of anemia is a deficiency of vitamin B_{12}. The blood cells that are formed in people with this deficiency are abnormally large and are inefficient oxygen-carriers. Pernicious anemia, a form of B_{12} deficiency, is a genetic autoimmune disorder most commonly affecting persons of northern European descent in which special gastric cells required for vitamin B_{12} absorption are destroyed. Often the neurologic symptoms and dementia triggered by this condition appear long before the symptoms of anemia are recognized—another reason it's important to take anemia seriously.

Weight loss and mouth sores are hallmark signs of pernicious anemia. Monthly vitamin B_{12} injections can cure this condition.

The other B vitamin that is often lacking in older women is folic acid, which may be missing from the diet or inadequately absorbed by the body. The cure for folic acid deficiency is simple—daily 1-gram supplements. But beware: If you also have a B_{12} deficiency and don't get treated, your anemia may improve but neurologic damage can continue. So don't just self-medicate with over-the-counter folic acid. You should have a blood test of your B_{12} levels first. Both types of deficiency can occur even if you're eating well if for some reason your body is not absorbing the nutrients from your food. And the same conditions that cause iron deficiency anemia can cause a B_{12} and folic acid deficiency.

Increased red blood cell destruction: Called *hemolytic anemia*, this is usually due to autoimmune diseases that attack red blood cells and reduce their lifespan. One type of autoimmune reaction is triggered by exposure to cold temperatures. Treatment can include the use of steroids and immune-suppressing drugs as well as removal of the spleen and avoidance of exposure to cold.

Sleep Disorders

I started with the worst possible scenario: the idea that anemia as the result of illness is at the root of your fatigue. But sometimes fatigue is just due to the fact that you're not getting adequate sleep, or that you're getting the wrong kind of sleep. There's a perception that gaining years equates with losing hours of sleep. But it's not the total hours of sleep you're losing—it's the amount of time your brain is in deep sleep. Spending more of your night in the lightest stage of sleep means you're more easily awakened. Moreover, as you get older, your body's internal clock may be thrown off so that you gradually slip into a pattern of falling asleep earlier (and thus awakening earlier) or falling asleep later (and getting up late, thus missing the *Today* show). This may be inconvenient, especially to the rest of your family, but it won't necessarily leave you feeling fatigued.

Another misconception is that the older you are, the longer it naturally takes to fall asleep. The true problem isn't usually falling asleep but staying asleep. Up to one in four elderly people have insomnia, which can take the form of midnight awakenings, early-morning awakenings or, less commonly, difficulty getting to sleep. This doesn't just cause fatigue, it impairs mental and physical function and is a major reason for depression. (Conversely, depression can lead to insomnia.) Despite this, fewer than 15% of those with chronic insomnia get treatment, and when they do get help, it usually comes in the form of the easiest thing to prescribe: a sleeping pill. Short-acting benzodiazepines such as temazepam (Restoril) and the drugs zolpidem (Ambien) and zaleplon (Sonata) are current favorites. They may help you fall asleep faster and should leave you with minimal daytime hangover. Longer-acting benzodiazepines can cause morning-after grogginess. But any sleeping pill can increase the risk of harmful drug interactions and, in general, long-term use of hypnotics is associated with an increased risk of death.

The better solution to your sleep problem is a behavioral approach. We're bombarded with ads about oral hygiene and feminine hygiene. Now it's time for me to sponsor one on sleep hygiene. The first rule of good sleep hygiene is to limit your time in bed to the hours when you're actually sleeping. Don't lie awake looking at the clock, tossing and turning and worrying about falling asleep—the anxiety over insomnia will only serve as a self-fulfilling prophecy. If you can't fall asleep, get out of bed. Read a book, watch a boring movie on TV or do anything else you find calming. When you are in bed and expect to fall asleep, make sure there are no distractions. Your bedroom should be comfortably cool, dark and quiet. During the day, keep yourself occupied with interesting activities (boredom is linked with insomnia). Exercise (no later in the day than midafternoon) and avoid taking naps. Steer clear of caffeine after noon. Don't eat a large evening meal and, most important, don't try to lull yourself to sleep with a nightcap. Alcohol may help you fall asleep, but causes interrupted sleep and wakefulness later on. Also avoid long-term (greater than a couple of weeks) use of over-the-counter antihistamines and other purported sleep inducers.

There are other less common sleep disorders that may be leaving you with daytime fatigue. The first is apnea, in which the upper airway collapses on itself, cutting off the flow of oxygen. In order to resume breathing, you might unknowingly awaken—often with a loud snort—dozens of times a night. Apnea is more common among women who snore, those who are overweight and those with unusually short, thick necks. It is a prime cause of unexplained excessive daytime sleepiness and has also been linked with high blood pressure, heartbeat irregularities, chest pain, heart attack, stroke and sudden death. In other words, apnea needs medical attention, usually in the form of a trip to a sleep clinic, where you can be evaluated. Therapy includes weight loss and a device called a continuous positive airway pressure (CPAP) machine, which forces a steady flow of air into the airway, preventing it from closing. Surgery can also be used to reshape the inside of the throat and upper airway.

I've covered sleep problems related to your head and your airways. Now it's time to move to your lower extremities. Restless leg syndrome and periodic limb movement disorder become more common the older you get. The former is described as a tingling or crawling pain in the legs that is only relieved by movement. It tends to strike at bedtime and can make it difficult to fall asleep. Periodic limb movements—rapid flexing of the toe, ankle, knee or hip in one or both legs—occur during sleep in more than a third of those over age 65. These repetitive limb movements may lead to insomnia and daytime fatigue. Restless legs can be treated with aspirin and a hot bath at bedtime. If the problem persists, your doctor can prescribe bromocriptine or L-dopa. If symptoms are severe, short-acting sleeping pills may be in order. Periodic limb movement disorder is harder to treat. L-dopa helps some people, but if you have this problem, you'll probably need to consult a sleep specialist.

Depression

Fatigue can certainly be depressing, but depression can also lead to fatigue. Depression affects up to 15% of older people who live independently. The risk is roughly double among those who are institutionalized. The first noticeable symptom may be cognitive problems: confusion and inability to process information that can impair the ability to think to such an extent that it can mistakenly be diagnosed as dementia. Another outward sign is complaints about imagined or exaggerated physical problems. (I hesitate to say this because some doctors dismiss women's complaints of headaches, GI problems and body aches as stemming from underlying depression and may not perform appropriate workups. But when testing is complete and nothing is found, depression should be considered and treated.)

The classic signs of depression in an older woman may be different from those I outlined for younger women, but the diagnosis of true clinical depression is warranted if you feel depressed, irritable or anxious, have crying spells, have feelings of hopelessness and helplessness or have suicidal thoughts. One way to tell if you have some degree of depression is to answer yes or no to the following questions:

1. Are you basically satisfied with your life?
2. Have you dropped many of your activities and interests?

3. Do you feel that your life is empty?
4. Do you often get bored?
5. Are you in good spirits most of the time?
6. Are you afraid that something bad will happen to you?
7. Do you feel happy most of the time?
8. Do you feel helpless?
9. Do you prefer to stay home rather than go out and do new things?
10. Do you feel you have more problems with memory than most?
11. Do you think it's wonderful to be alive now?
12. Do you feel pretty worthless the way you are now?
13. Do you feel full of energy?
14. Do you feel that your situation is hopeless?
15. Do you think that most people are better off than you are?

Scoring: Give yourself one point for every "no" answer to questions 1, 5, 7, 11 and 13 and one point for every "yes" to questions 2, 3, 4, 6, 8, 9, 10, 12, 14 and 15. Add up the total number of points. On this scale, you rate normal if you scored between 1 and 5, mildly depressed if you scored between 6 and 10 and very depressed if you score 11 points or more. (Questionnaire courtesy of Haworth Press, Binghamton, New York.)

If you qualify for a diagnosis of depression, you will probably benefit from an antidepressant and should consider seeing a psychotherapist. The choice of drug should be governed by which causes the least side effects in older adults. The SSRIs may have fewer significant adverse reactions, but your starting dosage should be on the low end of what would normally be prescribed to a younger person, and you may have to wait six to eight weeks before you'll know if it's effective. To prevent relapse, you should stay on the therapy for 6 to 12 months.

Your doctor will also want to look at a complete list of the drugs you're taking because many of the medicines given to women in your age group can have depression as a side effect. These include steroids, reserpine, anti-Parkinson's drugs and beta-blockers.

I DON'T HAVE THE APPETITE I USED TO, AND I'M LOSING WEIGHT. SHOULD I BE CONCERNED?

Maybe. There are some naturally occurring processes that decrease appetite with age. The number of taste buds on the edge of the tongue that detect sweet and salt diminish, leaving the central taste buds, which identify sour and bitter taste, to dominate. This means food may not taste as good as it used to. Unfortunately it doesn't smell as good, either, because nerves in your olfactory system have undergone a slow decline since about age 50. (Being a longtime smoker makes taste and smell problems more likely.) These changes in the senses that are so important to anticipation and enjoyment of food occur in up to 40% of older individuals and may prompt unhealthy dietary choices. In order for something to taste good, you may tend to oversalt or oversweeten it, both of which can be detrimental to your health. You may also unconsciously narrow your eating repertoire, leading to a less nutritious diet. Dental problems and decreased salivary flow may also limit your ability to chew and swallow a variety of foods.

Even as you're eating less, you may also be tolerating less. Digestion tends to slow as you age, so you're likely to feel full faster than you used to and to develop reflux, which causes heartburn. With all this going on, it's not surprising that you're also losing weight. It's ironic that so many women spend much of their adult lives trying to keep their weight down, only to find that after the age of 65, they begin to lose weight naturally. There is cause for concern if, without trying, you lose more than 10 pounds or 5% of your previous body weight in one month, or 10% of your total body weight in six months. This intense weight loss may be due to depression, alcohol abuse, recurrence of anorexia nervosa, chronic illness and cancer. It can also be a side effect of certain medications, including digoxin, antidepressants and antibiotics. So your doctor should be made aware of your declining weight and should check for conditions or medications that might cause it.

In order to prevent unhealthy weight loss from happening, you need to consume between 1,600 and 1,900 calories per day, depending on your weight and activity level. Even though you have a decrease in your energy requirement with age, there is no decrease in your need for most nutrients. The RDA of 50 grams of protein per day for the average woman may be low and you may be better off with 60 grams, even more if you have an acute or chronic disease. (Fifteen percent of seniors living independently and up to 85% of those cared for in institutions are getting too little protein.) All of the other recommendations I made regarding fat intake and nutrient needs (see page 175) still apply, but because of the increased incidence of insulin resistance and diabetes with age, it's probably more important than ever to make sure your carbohydrates are complex and not from processed starch and grains. Also make sure you're taking in 20 to 35 grams of fiber daily. The insoluble kind found in wheat bran, whole grain breads and cereals and the skins of fruits and vegetables will help protect against colon cancer, while the soluble kind found in oat bran, fruits, vegetables and legumes will slow intestinal absorption of sugars, helping to control diabetes. So make sure you eat five or more portions of fruits and vegetables a day. To help ensure adequate calorie and nutrient intake, don't skip meals. In fact, try eating more small meals throughout the day rather than three big meals. Never allow more than 16 hours to pass between dinner and breakfast. And if you can't seem to take in adequate calories (16% of older Americans fail to consume 1,000 calories a day), let your doctor know and consider adding calorie-dense liquid nutritional supplements to your daily menu.

ARE THERE ANY SPECIAL VITAMINS AND MINERALS I SHOULD TAKE?

To date, the official Recommended Daily Allowances for most nutrients have not been tailored to people your age. There's no question that the best way to absorb and make use of your vitamins and minerals is with the right foods. But because many women don't obtain some of these important nutrients through diet alone, especially if they're affected by any of the conditions listed above, my general recommendation is to take supplements to protect yourself from disease and help maintain health. Almost all of the following nutrients can be found in a good multivitamin.

Folic acid: Inadequate consumption of this B vitamin, found in green vegetables, orange juice and fortified cereals and breads, is linked with high blood levels of homocysteine, a risk factor for cardiovascular disease. Low levels are associated with anemia, depression and dementia. This vitamin also appears to help regulate mood, and adding it to SSRI antidepressant therapy may improve results. Recommended levels of folic acid intake are still being debated, but many experts would agree that you need at least 400 micrograms. High-dose folic acid (up to 5 milligrams per day) may have a homocysteine-lowering effect but should not be taken without a doctor's supervision.

Vitamin B$_{12}$: The metabolism of folic acid and vitamin B$_{12}$ is interrelated. Both help break down homocysteine. But while too little folic acid is associated with depression, a shortage of B$_{12}$ can result in nerve damage. Vitamin B_{12} deficiency occurs in up to 15% of older adults, especially those with upper gastrointestinal problems. Its potential risks are so significant that many doctors feel routine screening of vitamin B_{12} levels is warranted. Because folic acid supplementation (even the levels added to cereals and breads) may mask a B_{12} deficiency, you should also be sure you're getting at least 2 micrograms of B_{12} in supplement form daily. If you're already B_{12} deficient, the suggested dose is much higher: 100 micrograms per day.

Vitamin B_6: This too should be supplemented because more than half of women in your age group have an inadequate dietary intake. Low levels of B_6 are related to high levels of homocysteine and cardiovascular disease; the vitamin also helps with the synthesis of important neurotransmitters, and a deficiency can lead to nerve damage and convulsions. You should aim for 1.6 milligrams per day, though many multivitamins give as much as 25 milligrams. Megadoses of this vitamin (over 400 mg) can, however, cause neurologic problems.

Antioxidant vitamins (A, C and E): Research has shown that when these vitamins are included in the diet through consumption of large amounts of fruits and vegetables, they are associated with a lower risk of heart disease, stroke, cancer, macular degeneration, cataracts and Alzheimer's disease. It's not clear whether all these effects are obtained solely through food or if supplementation can produce the same results. So aside from my usual advice to take your fruits and vegetables, I'm also going to advise that you take a multivitamin that contains all three of these antioxidants and that you add on an extra 400 international units of vitamin E each day.

Calcium and vitamin D: In the previous chapter I stressed the importance of getting 1,500 milligrams of bone-protecting calcium each day, from foods or supplements if necessary. To aid in calcium absorption you also need vitamin D, and in your age group it's probably wise to aim for 800 international units each day. Most multivitamins don't contain enough calcium, so you'll have to take an additional calcium or calcium-plus-D supplement.

Iron: A lot of multivitamins contain iron, but unless you have been diagnosed with iron-deficiency anemia, you probably don't need to take this in supplement form. In fact, because iron decreases calcium absorption when the two are taken simultaneously, I suggest you take a multivitamin without iron if you want to take your calcium at the same time.

Zinc: Some studies have found that when supplements of this mineral are added to the diet of older adults, there may be an improvement in night vision, immunity and wound healing as well as a decrease in the progression of macular degeneration. Aim for 12 milligrams per day.

Selenium: This trace element received wide attention after a study of 1,300 patients given supplements for 10 years found a significant reduction in their cancer mortality and in the incidence of lung, colon, rectal and prostate cancer. How much of this mineral is present in the grains and vegetables you eat is dependent on the soil where the plant was grown. Since most of us haven't a clue as to the exact geographic origins of our food, believers in selenium's anticancer powers advocate supplementation—200 milligrams per day.

I SEEM TO BE POPPING A LOT OF PILLS. AM I DOING MORE HARM THAN GOOD?

The answer depends on what pills (both prescription and over-the-counter) you're popping, why you're taking them and whether, on their own or together, they're causing any harmful side effects. I have a twofold complaint when it comes to prescribing medications for my patients in your age group. The first is that up until 1993, clinical trials of most of the medications currently on the market did not have to include women. Second, even though this sex bias has been largely remedied, age bias remains, so that we have very little information on the specific effects of new or existing drugs on people over age 70. Any pill that you take has to be absorbed, broken down, accepted by the tissue it's targeting and, finally, removed from your system. At any point in this process, something can go wrong because of changes in your body that occur with age. The more drugs you take, the more likely something will go wrong in this complicated process. And you're probably taking a lot: The average older person is using 4.5 prescription drugs and 2.1 nonprescription drugs and fills 12 to 17 prescriptions per year. That doesn't even account for herbs and vitamins.

Why are you different from a younger person when it comes to the way your body processes drugs? Let's start with the popping of that pill. It needs to be absorbed in your GI tract, and with age there is a decrease in stomach acidity and intestinal motility—the speed with which your pill is pushed through your digestive system. Many medications need acid in order to be absorbed, so less will enter the bloodstream. On the other

322 / RELAX, THIS WON'T HURT

hand, medications that don't rely on acidity might be absorbed in greater quantities. In the small intestine, there is a decrease in the size of the surface of the lining with age. This too decreases absorption. To make matters worse, certain age-related diseases such as congestive heart failure can also contribute to this effect.

Once absorbed, many drugs have to travel through the liver (a process called first bypass), where they are broken down. This reduces the levels of the whole drug in the bloodstream and allows only certain altered by-products to travel to the body's tissues. Once more there can be a decrease of this blood flow to and activity in this detoxing organ with age-related diseases. As a result the drugs are left to circulate in the bloodstream in their more potent form and level.

After a drug is either absorbed directly through the intestine or released through the liver, it has to be distributed to its target organs in the body. With age comes reduced total body water content, reduced lean tissue and an increase in fat. The less water your body contains, the higher the drug's concentration in your tissues. And the more fat your body contains, the more likely certain fat-soluble drugs, such as Valium, will remain in the tissue, prolonging their effect.

Unfortunately, I'm not done. The metabolizing of drugs in the liver depends on certain enzymes that may decrease with age or be altered by other medicines, dietary deficiencies or use of alcohol. And finally, in order to be eliminated from your body, most drugs need to be excreted in urine. Clearance of many drugs through the kidneys declines with age, so that many medicines, including antiarrhythmia drugs, antibiotics, antihypertensives, beta-blockers, calcium channel blockers, ulcer drugs, pain medications and diabetes drugs, accumulate in the body, where they may cause side effects.

To make things more complicated, for a drug to work it has to affect receptors in cells and tissues. And guess what? The receptors' response can either increase or decrease with age. The receptors to some beta-blockers and warfarin (Coumadin), for example, may have increased responsiveness, so lower doses may be in order.

Obviously you can't assess how well your body is processing any of the medications you're taking—unless, that is, the drug causes obvious side effects. Your pharmacist should be able to give you a list of the possible side effects of every drug you're taking. Certain drugs are widely agreed to be inappropriate for elderly people. These include amitriptyline (Elavil), indomethacin (Indocin), diazepam (Valium) and chlorpropramide.

Even if you're on the right drug at the right dosage and it's doing its thing well, you can still develop adverse effects from an interaction between this and another medication that you're taking. Up to 40% of nonhospitalized elderly people are at risk for this "polymed" interaction, and a quarter of these are potentially serious. One drug can cause another drug to become more or less potent by altering absorption, changing its binding to a protein or metabolism, or affecting its excretion. Or the two drugs taken together may worsen mild side effects normally seen with one. Warfarin (Coumadin), for example, can have a heightened effect if it's taken with aspirin, furosemide, cimetidine (Tagamet), sulfa antibiotics or metronidazole (Flagyl). It is less effective, however, if it's combined with barbiturates, rifampin or carbamazepine. Theophylline, a drug used for asthma, can be rendered toxic by cimetidine, erythromycin or ciprofloxacin and made less effective by phenytoin, rifampin or carbamazepine. Digoxin will have a decreased effect if mixed with antacids, cholestyramine and cholestipol, but it can build to dangerous levels if combined with quinidine, verapamil or diuretics. And speaking of diuretics: Combining them with NSAIDs can impair kidney function, while mixing them with ACE inhibitors, tricyclic antidepressants, alpha-blockers, vasodilators or levo-dopa can lead to falls, weakness and fainting. Finally, beta-blockers combined with verapamil or digoxin can lead to slow heartbeat or other rhythm abnormalities.

SO IF I DO HAVE TO TAKE A LOT OF MEDICINES, WHAT'S THE BEST WAY TO MANAGE THEM?

I can't bestow on you an instant degree in pharmacotherapy, so you're going to need to talk to your doctor. Here are my guidelines for safe and effective use of medications:

1. Bring all the medicines you take (or a list of them) and their dosages to your doctor. This should include prescription, over-the-counter and herbal remedies. (If you have more than one doctor, decide which one will be your designated drug overseer.)
2. Make sure you thoroughly understand why you're taking the drug and what current and future benefits you should expect from it. If you're taking a drug for symptom relief, let your doctor know if it is making you feel better (or not).

324 / RELAX, THIS WON'T HURT

3. Check the list of possible side effects for each medication and report any you feel you might be experiencing.

4. Give your doctor an accurate and truthful accounting of your compliance with each drug regimen. This is not the time to fudge—if you're forgetting to take the medication or taking it only when *you* think you need it, your physician needs to know.

5. Make sure your doctor is aware of all your medical conditions, not just the ones she is treating you for.

6. Ask you doctor if your lists indicate possible contraindications or potential interactions or if you could get by with a lower dose.

7. If your medication routine is more complicated than a Chinese restaurant menu (in Chinese), ask your physician if there are ways to simplify it.

8. Find out how long you'll need to remain on each drug.

9. Take notes during your conversation with your doctor or take a friend or family member along to help you remember details.

10. Get all your medicines from one pharmacy.

And now a word about nonprescription drugs. The tendency is to feel that you can mix or match these as needed. But many over-the-counter products that are touted to help deal with somewhat different symptoms (from joint pain to headaches to difficulty sleeping) may all be chemically similar, and taking more than one product from the same class of drugs can lead to an overdose. The most common example is the nonsteroidal antiinflammatory drugs (NSAIDs), which can be associated with upper GI hemorrhage or even stroke. So include nonprescription drugs in any discussion you have with your pharmacist or doctor.

You may come away from reading all this feeling overdosed and overwhelmed. The natural tendency for both you and your doctor may be to scale back on dosages or omit certain drugs altogether. But underprescribing of medicines can lead to health problems as well. Studies have shown that beta-blockers and clot-busting medications (for heart problems) and warfarin (to prevent stroke) have traditionally been underprescribed to women over age 75. So if you have had a heart attack, are at severe risk for developing one or have atrial fibrillation, discuss the use of these drugs with your doctor. And if you end up in the emergency room with a suspected heart attack, you or your family should request anticlotting medicine, and don't accept age as a justification for its denial.

I KEEP GETTING BLADDER INFECTIONS. WHY?

The answer is estrogenically obvious: Long-term lack of this hormone leads to urogenital atrophy. This results in thinning of the vaginal lining, as well as shortening of the urethra (which carries urine from the bladder to the toilet), a relaxation of the pelvic muscles and a change in vaginal pH. And even if you've been diligently using estrogen, the receptors in your genital tract may have become less receptive to this hormone with time, and a milder form of this problem can occur. If the vaginal pH is off, overgrowth of the wrong bacteria is enhanced. Because the vaginal lining is thin and the urethra is short, these bacteria can easily ascend into the bladder, where they attach themselves to the bladder walls and multiply, resulting in infection. The classic symptoms—urinary frequency, pain and burning with urination—may be more subtle than they were when you were younger. You're more likely to become temporarily incontinent during the infection, and because your immunity may be weakened, there's a greater chance that you'll develop kidney infections or systemwide infection (sepsis). This is why bladder infections in your age group must be taken seriously and treated aggressively. That means a longer course of antibiotic therapy (10 to 14 days), and once the infection is treated, you should have a follow-up culture within a week to ensure that the antibiotic eradicated the offending organism. If your infections always seem to occur after intercourse, you should try taking a single dose of an antibiotic immediately after sex. The most commonly used are nitrofurantoin (Macrodantin) and trimethoprim-sulfamethoxazole (Septra). If you're using a pessary, this indwelling foreign body may be increasing bacterial growth and pushing bacteria into the bladder. Taking the pessary out at night or removing it permanently and having surgery to correct the prolapse are two alternatives that can promote bladder health. Or it may be necessary to take continuous low doses of an antibiotic if you are unable to do either. And if you are not on systemic estrogen or your doctor feels that the vaginal lining looks atrophic even with estrogen, local estrogen in the form of a cream or a ring may be worth trying. The old wives' tale about cranberry juice protecting against bladder infection has been studied and shown to really work for old wives—and young ones too. It diminishes the bacteria's ability to cling to the bladder wall. So try adding a daily glass of cranberry juice to your diet (diet juice may be equally effective).

If you've attempted all of the above and your infections still recur, you need more than just a fresh round of antibiotics. A kidney ultrasound or an intravenous pyelogram (IVP), in which dye is injected into the body and followed as it's excreted through the kidney, ureter and bladder, should be performed to rule out kidney stones, abnormal urinary tract anatomy and an abnormal pathway between the urinary tract and bowel. Cystoscopy, in which a viewing tube is inserted through the urethra, can also be used to check the bladder walls.

If this workup reveals no abnormalities, you may keep your infections under control by taking an antibiotic for several months. Your doctor needs to assess the pros and cons of this long-term therapy because it can make it difficult for you to fight off future infections.

It's possible that you don't have symptoms of a bladder infection, but a routine urinalysis shows bacteria. If this occurs several times, a culture should be done to confirm that bacteria are present—a condition known as *asymptomatic bacteriuria*, which is fairly common in elderly women. Whether this should be treated with long-term antibiotics is a subject of much debate. Proponents of therapy feel this prevents kidney infection and sepsis, while others believe that the bacteria cause less potential harm than the antibiotics. I tend to treat an initial silent infection and recheck the culture, and if the bacteria insidiously recur but there are no symptoms, I stop therapy.

I'M NOT REGULAR. WHAT SHOULD I DO ABOUT IT?

Irregularity is a euphemism that's commonly used to advertise laxatives, and I have to assume you've taken these ads to heart (or rather to bowel) and are complaining of constipation. But before I offer solutions, let's make sure that your definition of constipation and the medical definition of constipation are one and the same. If your idea of constipation is not having a bowel movement every day, then stop worrying. As long as you're not passing uncomfortable hard stool and you can go when you feel your bowel is full and have the urge, you're not constipated. But if your stool is uncomfortably hard or you can't pass it when you feel the need, then you are constipated. The prevalence of this problem increases after age 65, and women are more likely than men to suffer from it. The most common reason for constipation is one you can correct: a pattern of low fiber intake, low calorie intake and low fluid intake combined with too little exercise. If this sounds familiar, the therapy is the obvious. Increase all of the above. That means 20 to 35 grams of fiber per day (in the form of a fiber supplement if necessary), six to eight glasses of water, a sufficient caloric intake and regular walks or another form of exercise. It may help to develop a bowel routine. Following breakfast or lunch, take a walk to create an internal massage for your bowel and/or gently massage your lower abdomen. Then sit on the toilet and try to go but don't strain.

If this doesn't help or if your constipation is sudden and unexplained, you need to see your doctor and undergo colon testing, either barium X-ray or colonoscopy, in order to rule out cancer or diverticulitis. Other medical causes for constipation in older women include neurogenic disorders such as Parkinson's and stroke, low thyroid hormone, depression, weakness and use of certain medications. The list of drugs that can cause the problem is long: pain medications, antidepressants, antihistamines, anti-Parkinsonian drugs, GI antispasmodics, antipsychotics, anticonvulsants, antihypertensives, diuretics and aluminum antacids. Calcium and iron supplements are also potential culprits. Unfortunately, this probably includes just about every medication you might be taking. If corrective eating, exercise and good bowel habits don't prevail, stimulant laxatives (those containing castor oil, cascara or senna) may help you tolerate your drugs. But long-term use of any laxative can lead to pathologic changes in the colon, so be sure to tell your doctor if you're relying on these products. Mineral oil and stool softeners are useless against drug-induced constipation and their usefulness for general chronic constipation is debated, although they may help relieve short-term problems.

The "ir" in irregularity connotes a change in bowel habits, and in answering your question, I can't ignore the possibility that your problem might be diarrhea. Since I was very descriptive in describing constipation, I guess I should do the same for this other malady (although I'm sure that by the time you've reached this decade, you're well aware of what it is). Diarrhea is defined as an increase in frequency of defecation (more than three stools a day) associated with increased stool volume and fluid content and accompanied by urgency and pain. The most common cause of diarrhea in your age group is probably lactose intolerance, which affects up to a third of whites (and an even higher ratio of Jewish women) and two-thirds of women of Asian, Latin-American and African descent. You can test yourself for this problem by drinking a glass of room-temperature milk on an empty stomach. If you get pain, bloating, gas or diarrhea within two hours, you're lactose-intolerant. That doesn't mean you have to swear off milk products. If you consume small amounts with food, use lactose-reduced milk or take a lactose tablet before eating dairy, your symptoms should improve.

If your diarrhea came on suddenly, the cause is probably not lactose intolerance. You may have an infection. Switch to clear liquids such as broth, ginger ale or Gatorade with the onset of diarrhea. But make sure you consume a lot of them—two to three liters—so you don't end up with a fluid or electrolyte loss. After 24 hours, when you should feel better, you can return to solid food, but avoid fresh fruits and vegetables, fried or spicy foods, bran, candy and caffeinated and alcoholic beverages. When two to three days have passed, you can resume your normal diet.

If you don't begin to feel better within the first 24 hours after diarrhea starts, you may have a serious bacterial infection. This becomes more common with increasing age because anatomic and physiologic changes, chronic illnesses and increased drug use make your lower GI tract more susceptible to infection. Gastric acids that would normally kill bad bacteria in food are depleted, and slower movement of stool through the bowel allows bacteria and their toxins to remain in the gut and overgrow. This can result in debilitating diarrhea and even death, so don't wait to seek medical help. A diagnosis can be made with a stool culture (sometimes several are necessary); if an infection is found, antibiotics are in order. (This type of diarrhea is not to be confused with acute food poisoning, in which symptoms, including vomiting, tend to come on even more suddenly, within hours of ingesting contaminated food. Antibiotics won't cure this problem, but you may need intravenous fluids, so get immediate medical attention.)

If lactose intolerance, infection and food poisoning have been ruled out as the cause of your diarrhea, the next step is a full workup including a barium enema or colonoscopy to check for inflammatory bowel disease such as Crohn's and colitis (rarely first diagnosed in those over age 60), as well as tumors. If these too are negative, your diarrhea may be a result of a malabsorption syndrome, in which the intestine is unable to properly absorb fat, fat-soluble vitamins and, eventually, most major nutrients. This can be due to insufficient production of pancreatic enzymes or lesions in the intestinal walls. A hallmark symptom of malabsorption is mucousy stools (from unabsorbed fat), and this should always be reported to your doctor.

Finally, you may have intermittent constipation and diarrhea. This could be due to irritable bowel syndrome. It's often considered a disease of younger women, but it can affect the elderly almost as often. This is always a diagnosis of exclusion, and you should have all the tests I've mentioned above before you're told this is the origin of your irregularity. Treatment will depend on what's causing your diarrhea.

Obsession with regularity has made older people the target of many a joke. But irregularity is no joke and should be taken seriously.

WHAT TESTS DO I NEED?

Here are the examinations, tests and procedures I recommend for patients seventy and older:

Examination/test/procedure	How often
Complete physical	Annually
Blood pressure	Annually
Cholesterol test	Every five years until age 85
Fasting plasma glucose	Every three years
Thyroid hormone test	Every two years
Rectal exam	Annually
Fecal occult blood test	Annually; stop testing at 75 if your doctor recommends
Colorectal cancer screening	Every five to 10 years, depending on screening method used.
Urinalysis	Annually
STD testing	At your/your doctor's discretion
Pelvic exam & Pap smear	Annually; Pap at doctor's discretion after three negative tests
Clinical (physician) breast exam	Annually
Physician's skin exam	Annually
Mammogram	Annually
Eye exam	Every two years until age 80, then annually
Hearing test	Every two years until age 80, then annually
Electrocardiogram	Every five years
Bone mineral density	Once at age 70 if not performed earlier

Examination/test/procedure	How often
Immunizations	Tetanus booster every 10 years
Influenza vaccine	Annually
Pneumococcal vaccine	Once if you have never received it
Skin exam by dermatologist	Every two years
Skin self-exam	Annually

WHAT CAN GO WRONG AT MY AGE?

Stroke

Each year more than 700,000 people will have a stroke, and almost three-quarters of them will be over age 65. After 55 your risk of this condition doubles with each successive decade, and your lifetime risk of dying from a stroke is 1 in 12. Stroke is a brain injury, usually sudden, resulting from blockage of blood flow to the brain or bleeding within the brain. The medical term for this is a *cerebrovascular accident,* or CVA. Eighty percent of the time, the "accident" is an ischemic stroke that results from blocked blood flow. The blockage is either a clot that formed elsewhere in the body and traveled through the bloodstream to lodge in the brain or a blockage caused by plaque buildup within the brain. The other 20% of the time, stroke is caused by bleeding within the brain or into the spaces around it after a vessel inside the brain or on its surface ruptures. This is known as *hemorrhagic stroke.* Stroke is the third leading cause of death and the leading cause of serious disability among the elderly.

Although medicine has made tremendous progress in stroke treatment and rehabilitation, prevention is still the best cure. The first step is to reduce any controllable risk factors you have. These are the same risks you're probably already modifying to lessen your chance of heart attack: hypertension, smoking, high cholesterol, high homocysteine levels, diabetes and obesity. I've covered them in detail on page 293, but let me give you a sense of how reducing these risks will affect your chances of a stroke. Controlling high blood pressure with medication can reduce the risk of stroke by at least one-third even if it's just your systolic blood pressure (the top number) that's high; if diastolic pressure is also high, drug therapy that brings it down will reduce your stroke risk by 45%. Indeed, high blood pressure is the most important modifiable risk factor for stroke. The second is cigarette smoking. Five years after you stop smoking, your risk will equal that of someone who has never smoked. When it comes to cholesterol, the evidence is more preliminary, but it appears that cholesterol-lowering statin drugs decrease stroke incidence by about a third; however, it's not yet clear whether this reduction can be achieved in those over age 70 because most of the trials of these drugs did not include women in your age group. There's even more uncertainty when it comes to diabetes. This disease increases the risk of stroke by promoting atherosclerosis and disease of the small vessels of the brain. But there is no evidence that controlling blood sugar reduces this risk. Nevertheless, there are a lot of other good reasons to control blood sugar. Ditto for your weight, and although there have been no studies evaluating the effect of weight loss on stroke risk, it's reasonable to assume that maintaining a normal weight is a good idea. And if you're controlling your weight and blood pressure through exercise, all the better: It decreases the risk of both ischemic and hemorrhagic stroke.

In addition to these, there is another important risk factor: a cardiac arrhythmia called atrial fibrillation in which the heart beats irregularly so that the valves quiver. This makes it more likely that a clot will be released to the arteries going to your brain. The symptoms of atrial fibrillation include palpitations, dizziness, faintness, chest discomfort, shortness of breath and/or fatigue. Your doctor can confirm the diagnosis with an electrocardiogram. If you have atrial fibrillation, you should be aggressively treated because this condition increases your risk of stroke sixfold and accounts for more than a third of all strokes between ages 80 and 89. The treatment is an anticoagulant drug, and the best results are obtained with warfarin (Coumadin), which decreases stroke risk by 68%. Unfortunately, this therapy is underused in older people because of a concern about bleeding complications. Aspirin, which is the second choice after Coumadin, only decreases stroke risk by 21% but has a similar bleeding complication rate.

When your physician is checking your stroke risk factors, she should be listening not just to your heart but to the carotid arteries in your neck.

Blood flow disturbed by a partial occlusion is heard as a high-pitched *whoosh* known as a *carotid bruit*. If this is present, ultrasound and sometimes an angiogram should be done to measure blood flow in these vessels. If a blockage is found and it closes off more than 60% of the vessel, you may be a candidate for a plaque-removing surgical procedure called *carotid endarterectomy*. This can cut your risk of having a stroke in the next five years by as much as half.

Finally, your risk of stroke increases if you've had a heart attack—the ultimate sign of clogged arteries. And during or immediately following a heart attack, the chance of stroke is at its highest. Anticoagulant drugs given during the heart attack may help prevent this complication.

Our brains and the vessels supplying them often give out a "get me therapy" warning sign before the total shutdown of a true stroke. These warnings come in the form of transient ischemic attacks (TIAs), temporarily diminished blood flow to the brain that causes brief strokelike symptoms. They can be recurrent and always follow the same pattern. Symptoms include:

· sudden feeling of numbness or tingling
· temporary paralysis in muscles, including those in the face
· tremor or muscle spasm
· difficulty speaking
· confusion, disorientation or hallucinations
· sudden memory loss
· drowsiness
· double vision or gaps in vision
· unsteadiness

Since TIAs are the ultimate risk factor for stroke and indeed may be the beginning of one, they should always be investigated. Many people stop worrying because the symptoms go away, and attribute these signs to an off moment. Complacency can be fatal. This temporary shutoff signifies impending permanent shutoff of blood to the brain.

When symptoms first begin, it's not possible to predict if this is "just" a TIA or a full stroke. But in the latter case, there will be an increase in the severity and duration of the symptoms, to the point where paralysis of one side of the body, confusion, inability to speak and even unconsciousness occur. If the brain's breathing center or the component that controls the heart is knocked out, the stroke may be fatal.

Immediate diagnosis and institution of therapy are crucial to survival and minimizing permanent disability. A key ingredient to successful treatment is administration of a clot-busting medication called tissue plasminogen activator (TPA) within three hours of the onset of stroke. The complication of this therapy is hemorrhage, so a CT scan or MRI will be used to determine whether the stroke is ischemic or hemorrhagic. In the latter case, surgery can sometimes be performed to control the bleeding. There are many other things that can be done to minimize the damage done by a stroke and to make sure that another one does not occur in the future. The important thing to know is that stroke can be successfully treated and that with aggressive rehabilitation efforts, many people in your age group who experience this brain attack can go on to return to their homes and have a satisfactory quality of life.

Alzheimer's

This disease accounts for two-thirds of all cases of dementia in the elderly, and women are unfairly singled out: Alzheimer's is twice as likely to occur in women as in men. This is in part because women tend to live longer but also because, age for age, we are more vulnerable. Ninety-five percent of those who develop Alzheimer's do so after age 60. Five percent to ten percent of women over age 65 have the disease, and the prevalence increases steadily with age so that by 85, up to half of women may be affected. Memory loss—a reduction in the ability to learn and recall new information—is usually the first sign of this disorder. Unfortunately, we all suffer from occasional episodes of memory loss in this age of information overload. These common lapses that are casually referred to as "senior moments" may make early symptoms of the disease difficult to recognize. The progression of this disease is slow, taking place over 5 to 15 years. Initially someone with Alzheimer's might forget what she did recently and repeat questions or stories. She may also have problems finding the right words to express herself or have difficulty with routine tasks such as finding a number in the phone book. Disorientation can ensue, and someone with this disease might become lost in her own neighborhood, even her own home. With time, there can be difficulty carrying on a conversation. Personality changes occur, and the woman may become depressed, irritable, hostile, paranoid or delusional. Eventually, she becomes dependent on caregivers and no longer recognizes her family.

Alzheimer's disease is caused by the degeneration and death of cells in various portions of the brain. Neuron-connecting fibers become tangled and plaque made up of amyloid, a protein, is deposited in these areas. In addition, an enzyme necessary for production of acetylcholine, a vital neurotransmitter, is reduced. Some women are more at risk for Alzheimer's than others: About 20% of the time the disease appears to be genetic and in these cases there is a strong family history of the disease, especially before age 65. The gene that seems to increase susceptibility to this disease programs cells for production of a protein, apolipoprotein E4, which has been implicated in the brain-degeneration process.

High blood levels of apo E4 may soon be considered a marker for this disease or the risk of developing it. In the meantime, there is no one, certain diagnostic test for Alzheimer's. It is usually diagnosed based on symptoms, physical exam, family history and the exclusion of other causes of dementia. There are a handful of risk factors for this disease. The most important is probably a family history. Having a first-degree relative with dementia more than doubles one's risk; a family history of Down's syndrome also appears to be significantly linked. A personal history of depression, head trauma, thyroid disease, low educational level and exposure to solvents or aluminum may also increase risk.

There is no cure for this disease, but there are medications that may help improve some symptoms, especially in the early stages. Tacrine, a drug that inhibits enzymes that break down the neurotransmitter acetylcholine, is one of the first medications that seem to promise some improvement (and hope). But it has to be given four times a day and can cause temporary liver damage. Donepezil (Aricept), a once-a-day drug, has been marketed since 1997 and has fewer side effects. It raises the level of acetylcholine in the brain and has been shown to either cause improvement or halt the decline in 82% of Alzheimer's patients after six months of therapy. The results of longer therapy and the drug's effects on severely ill patients have not been reported, but they're expected to be promising. New drugs that work in a similar fashion are awaiting FDA approval.

Long-term use of estrogen may decrease the risk of Alzheimer's and when begun in women who already have the disease may improve cognition and social interaction. But (and there are a lot of buts when it comes to therapies for this disease) this finding is brought to you courtesy of trials that lasted no more than nine months.

If inflammation plays a role in Alzheimer's, anti-inflammatory drugs might help slow its development or progression. Indeed, a study has shown that use of NSAIDs over two years appears to cut the risk of this disease in half. Aspirin was less effective than other NSAIDs, and acetaminophen did nothing. Whether NSAIDs will help to treat the disease once it's developed is not yet known. There is, of course, concern that chronic use can cause GI bleeding. There are a few more "We think this may help" therapies. The antioxidant vitamin E, at doses of 2,000 international units per day, has been shown to slow progression of the disease after two years of therapy, especially when it was combined with deprenyl (Carbex), an MAO inhibitor. Vitamin E may sop up some of the free radicals that damage nerve cells, while the deprenyl increases the neurotransmitter dopamine. Both should be used with caution; high doses of E can cause GI upset and can also act as an anticoagulant.

Since one of the early and distressing symptoms of Alzheimer's is depression, antidepressants—especially SSRIs—may help. Herbal therapies have also been tried—gingko biloba is purported to increase blood flow to the brain, helping memory. When tested on Alzheimer's patients, it was found to be associated with modest improvement. It's certainly worth a try, and it won't hurt.

I wish I could report on more medications to reverse this disease we all justifiably fear. As a physician who treats women of every age, one of my goals is to prevent or delay the onset of Alzheimer's. So I offer estrogen replacement because when it comes to our brains, it may make a difference.

OSTEOARTHRITIS

If I were to X-ray every woman in your age group, I would find evidence of this joint disease in nearly everyone. This doesn't mean everyone feels the effects of degenerating joints, but those who do generally find it painful and disabling. This disorder has a gender predilection—in women it strikes the hands and knees; in men it tends to center in the hips. It can also be present in the feet, spine and pretty much everywhere else. Usually symptoms occur earlier in the weight-bearing joints. Osteoarthritis is caused by the disintegration of the cartilage that cushions bone surfaces, and subsequent new bone formation around the damaged joint. Initially the pain occurs when the joint is moved and may be relieved by rest, but eventually, no matter what you do, the pain remains constant. The severity of the pain does not always parallel the extent of joint damage that is visible on the X-ray. There is also stiffness, especially in the morning, but it tends to last a short time. When osteoarthritis affects the hands, it can cause thickenings, or nodes, to form between the joints of the fingers; with time this can progress to significant finger or hand deformity.

You meet the American College of Rheumatology's definition for having this disease if you have the following symptoms involving one or more joints:

Hands—painful, aching or stiff, with enlargement or deformity of two or more joints

Knee—pain, with X-rays showing abnormal bone projections (spurs), morning stiffness lasting less than 30 minutes and sensation of bone rubbing against bone on motion

Hip—pain and two or more other signs, which include normal blood sedimentation rate, X-rays showing bone projections or an X-ray showing narrowing of the joint space

You may have a genetic predisposition for this disorder. If your mother had osteoarthritis and developed characteristic finger nodules, your risk of also developing this disease increases twofold. It's threefold if your sister has it. Aside from the genetic and age links, risk factors for this disease include previous major joint trauma, repetitive joint use and joint overload due to athletic activities. Finally, obesity increases the risk of osteoarthritis of the knee and hips anywhere from two- to threefold depending on how overweight you are. Paradoxically, if you have osteoporosis, your risk of developing osteoarthritis may decrease.

Although osteoarthritis is associated with cartilage degeneration, it may actually start in the bony bed of the joint. The denser the bone, the stiffer it becomes, and over time it ceases to act as a shock absorber. Microfractures appear at the edges, and these in turn instigate cartilage damage. So now we're faced with the depressing bone fact that if we do everything possible to reduce bone loss, we can end up with joint loss. For once, I'm at a loss for words. I certainly can't recommend that women accept the former in order not to deal with the latter.

But I can suggest ways to control pain and preserve the function and mobility of your joints. (Unfortunately, there are no drugs to cure or stop the progression of this disorder.) You should begin with the nonpharmacological: local heat or ice, ultrasound and/or use of a transcutaneous electrical nerve stimulation (TENS) device to help relieve pain. Exercise is a must. I know that's contrary to the long-held belief that exercise will cause further joint damage and pain. The current rheumatologically correct advice is to treat this disorder *with* exercise. Evidence shows that your joints won't continue to function if you don't move them and strengthen the surrounding muscles. Resistance training, using light weights or even your own body weight, for just 15 minutes three times a week will substantially improve muscle strength after just three months. Low-impact aerobic exercise such as walking or swimming will also decrease your pain without joint injury. It's better to start with several short periods of exercise throughout the day rather than one continuous session.

If you have osteoarthritis of the knee and you are overweight, losing as little as 10 pounds can result in major symptom improvement. On the more medicinal side, if you need something for pain, begin with acetaminophen (Tylenol), at doses of up to 4 grams daily. But while on acetaminophen, avoid alcohol and have your doctor periodically check liver function tests. Many of my patients are also taking chondroitin sulfate and glucosamine, two natural supplements that are purported to relieve pain. The recommended dose is up to 1,500 mg of chondroitin sulfate and 500 to 1000 mg of glucosamine.

The next higher source of pain relief is the over-the-counter NSAIDs such as aspirin, ibuprofen and naprosyn. All of these with long-term use can cause GI bleeding and kidney problems, as can the stronger prescription NSAIDs such as oxaprozin (Daypro). The Cox-2 inhibitors such as celecoxib (Celebrex) and Vofecoxib (Vioxx) minimize some of these toxic reactions and are quickly becoming the drug of choice, particularly in older women with histories of ulcers and/or gastritis. Rubbing in capsaicin or methylsalicylate creams also helps relieve discomfort in the hands and knees. And if knee pain flares, your doctor may suggest a steroid shot. It usually works for several weeks, although some women may get longer-term relief. Another type of intrajoint injection, performed weekly with hyaluronic acid for three to five weeks, can work if steroid injections fail.

If these therapies cease to control your symptoms, you may need surgery. The least invasive is joint lavage followed by arthroscopy, in which a scope and instruments are inserted into the knee through very small incisions. Loose pieces of cartilage or bone are removed, and the joint is rinsed with saline. This joint cleansing can significantly improve mobility and pain. If all else fails, you may need more major surgery: total joint replacement. These amazing man- (or woman-) made joints have allowed many people to overcome the severe disability of this disease and literally move on with their lives.

MY TOP 10 LIST FOR STAYING HEALTHY IN YOUR SEVENTIES AND BEYOND

1. Don't automatically attribute new physical or mental symptoms to getting older.
2. Eat a variety of foods and make sure you're getting your five portions of fruits and vegetables.
3. Take a multivitamin and make sure you're getting 800 units of vitamin D and 1,500 milligrams of calcium from foods or supplements.
4. Continue to evaluate your need for estrogen replacement therapy.
5. Get some form of aerobic and strength-training exercise for a total of at least 30 minutes most days of the week. Exercise your mind too by engaging in productive activities such as volunteerism and hobbies.
6. Fall-proof your home.
7. Keep a list of every medication you take and go over it with your physician during your annual examination.
8. Seek immediate attention for any infection—everything from a skin sore to cold or flu.
9. Ask someone you trust to objectively assess your driving skills; give up your license if you're no longer safe behind the wheel.
10. Make sure your family and physician have and understand your advance directives (living will and durable power of attorney for health care).

YOUR GENETIC HISTORY

UP UNTIL NOW, I've dealt with your health concerns decade by decade. But there is one all-encompassing women's health issue that cannot be pigeonholed into a particular decade: your genetic history. Think of it as the foundation of a house. The stronger the material, the better it can weather environmental hazards and human abuse. But even if this foundation is fundamentally strong, careful tending is necessary to prevent structural damage. And if the foundation is weakened, the house can be bolstered with extra support and the right contractor.

To understand what your genetic foundation is built of, you need only to look at your family. Each of us shares 50 percent of our genes with our first-degree relatives—our parents, siblings and children (unless you're an identical twin, in which case you share 100% of your genes with your sibling). Twenty-five percent of your genes are reflected by your second-degree relatives (whether you like what you see or not). That's your grandparents, aunts, uncles, nieces and nephews. And farther down the line of ancestry, 12.5% of your genes are shared with your third-degree relatives: your great-grandparents and cousins.

So now that you know where to look for genetic clues, you need to know what to look for. The number of hereditary conditions and diseases is enormous, and I've covered many of these at various points in this book. The list includes obesity, cardiovascular disease, high blood pressure, high cholesterol, autoimmune disease, osteoporosis, Alzheimer's, Parkinson's and osteoarthritis. Many cancers are genetically linked—not just breast and ovarian but also skin, thyroid, colon, gastric, bladder and pancreatic. And there are a whole group of diseases we're most concerned about during pregnancy, including cystic fibrosis, sickle cell anemia, Tay-Sachs, Down's syndrome, thalassemia and muscular dystrophy. In order to know which of these inherited diseases are most likely to affect your health, you'll need to construct a family tree.

MAKING YOUR FAMILY TREE

Most of us consider genealogy to be a search for the origins of our names, our ancestral domiciles and, perhaps, previously unclaimed bequests. But just look at the root of the word: *gene*. What we learn about this basic blueprint for our being is the most important knowledge we can ever obtain in our search for our roots. In order to build your tree, start egocentrically with yourself. In pedigree nomenclature, women are represented by circles, men by squares. (I'll refrain from scoring any feminist points by commenting on these geometric forms.) Connect yourself with a short line to your spouse (if applicable) and then bring down one line between the two of you for each of your children. A line up from your personal circle connects you to your siblings and your parents. Connect your parents to their siblings (your aunts and uncles) and then put in their children (your cousins) in the same fashion. Confusing, I know—just refer to the diagram on the following page. The next step is to call members of your family to ascertain the causes of death for those who are deceased. If possible, determine whether these relatives had any other medical disorders. For example, Aunt Sophie on your mother's side might have died of a heart attack at 75, but she also broke her hip two years earlier. Or Grandpa Fred on your father's side died of "natural causes (he was old)" at 85, but it turns out that he was institutionalized for eight years before that because he had Alzheimer's disease. Not only do you need to know what diseases your relatives had and died from, but at what age this occurred. In general, the earlier the onset of disease, the more likely it has hereditary significance. Make sure you ask about factors that could have contributed to their demise, such as high cholesterol, high blood pressure and diabetes as well as alcoholism and smoking. The latter two may be the nongenetic cause of their disease but are a sign that you're genetically predisposed to addictive behavior.

Finally, I have to emphasize that we women must realize that a full 50%

of our genes derive from our father and his family. When it comes to female cancers such as breast and ovarian, many women erroneously believe that they need only consider the maternal side of their family, and they ignore the history of these cancers or other cancers that are genetically linked to breast and ovarian cancer on their paternal side. These include colon, prostate and pancreatic malignancies. Your male ancestors have equal rights in determining your genetic wrongs.

You're still not done with your ancestral homework. Unfortunately, most of your information is from relative (literally) hearsay. And since these relatives are rarely pathologists, their reporting and diagnoses may be broad, vague and sometimes inaccurate. Here's what I mean: Nearly every type of cancer in the abdominal cavity of a man is frequently referred to as "stomach cancer," while women's cancers are often termed "female problems." The former may have been colon cancer, the latter ovarian cancer. Or you could have been told a "dotty" relative had Alzheimer's when indeed she had Parkinson's and dementia or multiple strokes as the result of hypertension. And in this age of successful medical therapy, a female relative may have had a lumpectomy and radiation and is doing well, and the family thinks it's nothing and doesn't report it. But her breast cancer and age of diagnosis are paramount to your tree. So if your relatives can't give you appropriate medical details and confirmation of a diagnosis, it may be necessary to write to the hospital where a surgery or death took place and ask for copies of pathology reports or death certificates. You may need to ask your doctor to help you obtain these records. And don't forget that your tree has seasons and changes. It needs to be updated whenever a relative is diagnosed with a significant disease or dies.

It's also important to know the ethnicity and religious background of all your ancestors. Most noteworthy: If they were Jewish, were they from an Eastern European (Ashkenazi) background? And did female relatives die at an early age in concentration camps? If so, you would have no knowledge of what diseases their genes would have expressed had they lived longer. There are, unfortunately, too many of us who have truncated genetic histories due to the Holocaust and war. But I want to emphasize that lack of a history of diseases such as breast, ovarian and colon cancer in a small family made smaller by catastrophic events cannot reassure us that we have not inherited the genetic risk for these illnesses.

I've already focused in other parts of this book on the many diseases for which a genetic pedigree may increase risk. And I've outlined the tests you can have and the lifestyle changes you can make as well as the therapies that are available to prevent or at least delay the onset of these disorders. What I want to cover in this chapter is hereditary breast and ovarian cancer: the genetic tests that are currently available, who should have them, what the results mean and what if anything can or should be done about them.

HOW GENES CAN LEAD TO BREAST AND OVARIAN CANCER

I'm combining these cancers because when they're hereditary, they occur as the result of the same genetic changes. It could be argued that every disease is genetic in origin, the result of damage to the genetic structure of our cells that upsets the process of their multiplication, development and growth. Cancer is not caused by a single type of mutation, but rather by the "coincidence" of multiple genetic mishaps that affect the communication and interplay between genes. During cells' division, a gene may be poorly copied, but under normal conditions, the cell is destroyed under the guidance of tumor-suppressor genes. If the latter fail to protect from this mistake, mutated genes, or oncogenes, are allowed to take over and stimulate abnormal cells to multiply ceaselessly and uncontrollably. The inner directives of our cells are influenced by environmental factors and chemical carcinogens such as cigarette smoke, as well as viruses. The longer the period of insult, the more likely mutations will occur and be sustained. That's why the incidence of cancer increases with age. When the first mutation that sets this course is inherited rather than acquired by use and abuse, the cancer is deemed hereditary. When the mutations are due to nonhereditary damage, the cancer is termed *sporadic*.

It takes two genetic insults in order to trigger a malignancy. We inherit two copies of every gene, one from each parent. And if either one of these copies is abnormal, it will be present in every cell in your body. All it takes for hereditary cancer to develop in any tissue is for your remaining healthy copy of the gene to be damaged. In sporadic cancer, however, there must be two hits, one to each copy of the gene, to instigate the cancer. This double hit usually occurs in just one group of cells in one type of tissue, so that the cancer will be localized to that area until it spreads. The single-versus-double-hit phenomenon explains why individuals with inherited mutations are more likely to get cancer at a younger age and to develop it in several organs. Hence the connection between hereditary breast and ovarian cancer, as well as the association between these diseases and colon, endometrial and prostate cancer.

Inherited mutations in the genes known as BRCA1 and BRCA2 are responsible for most hereditary breast cancers. BRCA obviously stands for breast cancer. But these mutated genes are just as important for pre-disposing a woman to the development of ovarian cancer. To make this even more complicated, although these mutated genes are considered *autosomal dominant* (which means you have a 50% chance of inheriting the mutation if your parent has it), the effect of this mutated gene can skip a generation, so that neither of your parents develops the cancer. Your mother may have been fortunate, and in her case the mutated gene was never "expressed" (meaning it never triggered the condition). Or it's possible your mother had other genes that prevented the mutated gene from doing its harmful deed. Up to 44% of BRCA1 and BRCA2 mutation carriers will not develop breast cancer in their lifetimes. If the mutated gene comes from your father, he obviously won't have ovarian cancer, and it's unlikely he will develop breast cancer. So you'll have to look far-ther back, to your second- and third-degree relatives, or laterally to your siblings when considering your risk and whether to test for hereditary cancer.

Here's an abridged version of BRCA Genetics 101: Both genes cause production of proteins that aid in the repair of damaged DNA that, left to express itself, would lead to cancer. This is why they're called tumor sup-pressor genes. The BRCA1 gene is, in the world of genes, a very large one. More than 300 different mutations have been identified so far; some are probably nonsense mutations that don't affect the genes' behavior. But certain ones can lead to production of a shortened protein that doesn't work properly as a tumor suppressor. This results in a 56% to 87% lifetime risk of breast cancer and a 16% to 44% risk of ovarian cancer in women who have a significant family history of these cancers. But the breast can-cer risk in women who carry this gene may drop to "only" 36% if they have no significant family history.

Contrary to the above gloom-and-doom observations regarding the pres-ence of BRCA mutations, the type of ovarian cancer associated with the BRCA1 mutation may be less invasive than that which occurs sporadi-cally. Recent surveys have found that women with the inherited cancer survived 2.5 times longer than women with sporadic disease. However, mutation of BRCA1 also increases risk of colon, pancreatic and (in male relatives) prostate cancer.

The BRCA2 gene is twice as large as BRCA1. And so far, more than 100 mutations have been found. Once more, only a few have been observed in families with hereditary cancer. These mutations confer a life-time risk of breast cancer that is similar to that with a BRCA1 mutation, but a lower (10% to 15%) risk of ovarian cancer. In men who carry BRCA2, the risk of breast cancer is 5% to 10%. Once more, this is a poly-mishap gene; it also increases the risk of colon, pancreatic, stomach and prostate cancer. Recently a BRCA3 gene has been mapped. It's not yet clear what mutations in this gene can lead to.

Mutations in other genes can also contribute to hereditary breast and ovarian cancer. These include the genes associated with hereditary non-polyposis colon cancer, or Lynch syndrome II. Women who carry this gene have a three- to fourfold increase in their risk of ovarian cancer.

WHO SHOULD BE TESTED

One in 400 Americans is thought to carry a BRCA mutation, so screening the entire population is both impractical and unnecessary. Just because a single relative had breast cancer doesn't mean you should assume that you're a carrier. "Only" 7% of breast cancers and 10% of ovarian cancers result from an inherited mutation; the rest are sporadic. The prevailing opinion is that testing may be warranted if you have at least a 10% chance of testing positive for a mutation and if the result will help you make deci-sions about your own care or help other relatives decide about testing. According to the criteria of the American Society of Clinical Oncologists, you qualify for testing if you have any of the following:

- You have two or more first- or second-degree relatives on the same side of the family with early-onset (before age 50) breast cancer or ovarian can-cer at any age.
- You are personally diagnosed with early-onset breast cancer or ovarian cancer at any age and have at least one first- or second-degree relative with either of these diseases.
- You are a woman of Ashkenazi Jewish descent with a personal or family history of early-onset breast cancer or ovarian cancer at any age.
- You have a family history of male breast cancer.
- You have a first-, second- or third-degree relative who has tested positive for a mutation in BRCA1 or BRCA2.
- You have third-degree relatives on your father's side with early-onset breast or ovarian cancer, and a family history of other cancers suggests that your father may be a carrier.

The most comprehensive and expensive test, costing about $2,400, entails complete gene sequencing of BRCA1 and BRCA2 and allows for identification of all mutations. This process may pick up mutations that have not yet been identified and for which the significance is unknown. If at all possible, the first family member who should undergo testing is the one who has developed cancer. Should a mutation be found, you and other family members can be tested for that specific mutation. This single-site BRCA analysis will lower the cost (to around $400) and raise the accuracy of the genetic screening. A third testing option is the multisite-3 BRCA analysis, which detects three specific mutations in BRCA1 and BRCA2 that are more common among Ashkenazi individuals. This test runs about $450. (If this test is negative, many women will go on to have the comprehensive test.)

The actual BRCA testing requires that you have blood drawn. (Mutations are detected through an examination of your white blood cells.) But before you have this done, you should carefully go over your family and personal history, ideally with a genetic counselor. You have to understand that the test results can be unclear, showing mutations for which we cannot predict risk, or they can be false-negative (your particular familial BRCA mutation may not be identified). Also the percentages of risk we give you today may be changed as we get more information in the future. And finally, even if you're truly negative, you, like every other low-risk woman, can still go on to develop sporadic breast or ovarian cancer. Find out if genetic counseling is paid for by your insurance carrier. Many insurers will cover both counseling and testing if family history is deemed appropriate. One other insurance-related caveat: Current law prohibits a health insurer from denying you coverage based on genetic test results. But state laws vary in their protection, so inquire if this is an issue, not only with regard to obtaining insurance, but also when it comes to the price of a policy. Many of my patients pay for the test out of their own pocket and use fictitious names in order to avoid leaving a paper trail. But if they decide, based on their test results, to undergo any type of treatment, they may then be forced to reveal their genetic status.

There are also important psychological issues that you should confront. If your test is positive, you may feel depressed, angry and fearful about your future. But remember that it also allows you to take action and consider medical or surgical options. For many women, knowing that they don't have to passively wait for an uncertain cancer fate and that they can instead do something about it gives them a reassuring sense of control. Then there is the very disturbing knowledge that your children may also have inherited this gene. When and should they be tested? Here's where you really need the advice and help of a geneticist. If you receive a negative result, you can't totally relax. But it will prevent you from going through what might have been unnecessary prophylactic therapies or surgical removal of your otherwise normal ovaries or breasts.

HOW TO DEAL WITH TEST RESULTS

Once your blood is sent to the lab, it can take up to four weeks to receive the results. If they are negative, you should certainly continue your screening routine: monthly self-exams, yearly physician exams, yearly mammograms and, depending on your age and family history, the recommended colon testing. Discuss with your doctor whether you should continue high-risk ovarian testing. I would for my patients with a significant family history of this cancer, only because there may be other problem genes that we have not yet discovered and are not able to test for.

If you are found to have a gene mutation, the next step is to set up a surveillance plan. Make sure you become well acquainted with how your breasts feel by performing monthly self-exams, which you should have started at age 18. Have a doctor or nurse practitioner add their clinical expertise with a hands-on breast exam every 6 to 12 months beginning at age 25. Begin yearly mammograms at age 25 to 35. The younger age is advisable if your family history includes a young age of onset for breast cancer.

Ovarian surveillance is more difficult. Pelvic exam alone is inadequate, since it detects only 5% of ovarian cancers at an early stage. Your additional options include annual or semiannual serum CA-125 levels (see page 263) and pelvic vaginal ultrasounds combined with color Doppler to assess blood flow beginning between age 25 and 35.

Because a BRCA mutation can also increase your risk of colon cancer, you'll need to begin annual testing for fecal occult blood at age 40 and sigmoidoscopy every three to five years after age 50. It would be wise to have an initial colonoscopy at age 50 and, depending on the results, repeat it every 10 years. (If a family member had colon cancer at an early age, your screening should be earlier and more frequent.)

You may not want to rely on screening procedures alone. Probably the most important gain you acquire from knowing you have a BRCA mutation is that you can now set a course for risk reduction. The first step is to consider the use of chemoprophylaxis—medication to help prevent cancer. In a recent study, tamoxifen has been shown to reduce (or delay) onset of breast cancer in high risk women by 44% (see page 164). Although many of the women in the study were not tested for the BRCA gene mutation, or if they were, the results were not released, we have to assume that many of them would have tested positive. With more data, we will hopefully find that cancer prevention in BRCA carriers may be as high or higher than this preliminary 44 percent.

Ovarian cancer risk for all women is diminished by use of birth control pills (see page 42). For BRCA mutation carriers, that risk may be reduced by 60% after six years of birth control use. So if you're not trying to get pregnant, and while you're considering a later prophylactic removal of your ovaries, take birth control pills.

Since screening and early detection of ovarian cancer unfortunately remains inadequate, removal of both ovaries is currently recommended for women who are positive for the BRCA gene mutation, and possibly for those with hereditary nonpolyposis colorectal cancer. In the latter group, there is a high risk for both ovarian and uterine cancer, and a hysterectomy should probably be performed, together with removal of the ovaries. It's felt that you can wait until 35 or after you've finished childbearing (whichever comes first) to undergo ovary removal because the average age of diagnosis of hereditary ovarian cancer is 45 to 50. One in five ovarian cancers with BRCA1 or BRCA2 can occur before age 40. None have been noted before age 35, however. The procedure can be performed through a laparoscope, at which time the surgeon and pathologist should check for any signs of early cancer in the ovaries or abdomen. Unfortunately, this surgery is not a surefire guarantee. There is still a 2% to 11% chance of developing primary peritoneal carcinomatosis, in which cancer cells develop in the peritoneum, or lining, of the pelvic and abdominal cavity. These cells act and spread like metastatic ovarian cancer. This condition may be due to the fact that in some women, there were precancerous cells in the "normal" ovaries that were removed.

The issue that remains is what to do about estrogen replacement therapy once your ovaries are removed at such an early age. We don't know if estrogen contributes to breast cancer risk in women with BRCA mutations. All we have to go on is research showing that when estrogen is given to first-degree relatives of women with breast cancer, some of whom undoubtedly carry the mutation, there appears to be no increase in their risk. So many physicians, including myself, advocate the use of estrogen after prophylactic oopherectomy in a menopausal woman.

Although our methods of screening for early breast cancer are far superior to those used to detect ovarian cancer, once more, they aren't foolproof. And the knowledge that the risk of breast cancer is always there may be so overwhelming for some women that they, with their doctors' blessing, will choose to undergo prophylactic mastectomy. The question of defining to what extent this procedure will decrease future risk of breast cancer depends on how extensively the breast tissue is removed. A recent study of more than 600 women who underwent this procedure and were followed for 12 years found that their risk was reduced by almost 90%. Other studies have quoted a 1% to 19% cancer occurrence rate after mastectomy. Most of the women who developed cancer had subcutaneous mastectomies, in which breast tissue was removed and implants were inserted but the skin and nipple were left in place. We know that 10% of all breast cancers arise below the nipple, and this may be the site at which these women who had nipple-sparing procedures went on to develop cancer. If you have a BRCA mutation and decide to be as surgically safe as possible, you might want to consider a more complete removal with breast and nipple reconstruction. Deciding to have either of these procedures is emotionally wrenching, and no one can say for sure where you fall in this genetic fortunetelling free-for-all. The genetic experts and surgeons may give you the current statistics, but ultimately you have to look within yourself and decide if undergoing one of these irreversible surgeries will reassure your mind and soul that perhaps you have taken a positive action against the very real possibility of future breast and ovarian cancer.

EPILOGUE: AN APOLOGY

AS I LABORED through the writing of this book, I realized that what my publisher and I felt would be an attention-grabbing title could be considered glib. In fact, many things in medicine do hurt. And I don't want to diminish the intensity of the pain all of us suffer when given a life-altering diagnosis. I've personally experienced this at several points in my own life. When I was pregnant with my second daughter, I, the obstetrician, diagnosed my own rapidly growing pelvic tumor as I compulsively performed ultrasounds on myself. Once I shared my discovery with another physician (self-care only goes so far), there was a real concern that my tumor might be ovarian cancer. So midway through my second trimester, I assumed the role of a scared patient on an operating table, with my life and that of my unborn child in another surgeon's hands. Although this terrifying experience ended happily—the tumor was a fibroid, and I went on to deliver a healthy, full-term baby girl—there's no denying that it hurt, both emotionally and physically. What I went through changed the way I practice medicine. Even though I'm a surgeon, having experienced the fear and physical discomfort of surgery, I consider surgical intervention the last resort.

While reading this book you may have noticed that I often refer to what I do personally for my own health. Not only have I diligently tried to follow my own advice, I have avoided asking other women to do things that I don't do myself. I really make an effort to eat right, take my vitamins and calcium, exercise almost daily and get all my screening tests (yes, even colonoscopy). During perimenopause, I used birth control pills to regulate the hormonal fluctuations that were driving me and my family crazy. I also felt that I was protecting myself against future ovarian cancer. A year and a half ago I went off the Pill and started hormone replacement therapy because I felt I needed the protective effects of the type of estrogen in HRT. I'm thin, have a mild decrease in the bone density of my hip (although my spine is fine) and can't afford to have any changes in my short-term memory. I also can't deny the fact that I wanted the cosmetic effects that I feel estrogen bestows.

But being a good pupil—and what I hoped was an example for other women—did not guarantee me a good result. And when I had to face that, it hurt. During the preparation of this book I had to cope with a serious medical problem. While performing my annual mammogram, the radiographer who screens so many of my patients remarked that, as usual, my breasts were very dense, cystic and "hard to read." Although he had always proclaimed a strong belief that breast ultrasound should only be used to distinguish whether a palpable mass or abnormal mammographic finding is cystic or solid, he suggested that he use this test as an adjunct to my mammogram, "just this once." I'm very comfortable in the two-dimensional black, white and gray world of ultrasound. I spend considerable time using a vaginal probe ultrasound to "see" what I less exactly feel during a bimanual exam. So it was easy for me to interpret the sonographic images of my own breast tissue: lots of little, round, well-defined cysts and—wait, what was this?—a two-centimeter area with less whiteness but no clear border. The probe stopped and Dr. Brenner and I looked at one another. He tried to reassure me with an "it's probably nothing; we can double-check this with an MRI." But I knew that the latter test takes about three hours and would not definitively rule in or rule out cancer. So I looked at my watch, and noting that I had twenty minutes until I started seeing my afternoon patients, requested he do an immediate core biopsy to make sure that *nothing* was truly the appropriate term.

Muttering that "this was the problem with overenthusiastic ultrasound," he numbed the area with xylocaine and expertly performed a Mammotome biopsy. I felt almost triumphant. I'd gone through yet one more procedure for which I have referred patients and could now reassure them that it was no big deal. It scarcely hurt and afterward I was even able to comfortably get through five hours of patient exams. The next day, I was informed by the pathologist (also a friend) that there were atypical ductal cells—not many, not cancerous—but "at my convenience" these should be investigated with a wider excisional biopsy.

For the next six weeks there was no convenient time. I had a series on pregnancy to do for the *Today* show, I had a book deadline and I had planned to go to Washington to attend the Ford Theater show, which my husband produced. The latter turned into an exciting weekend when I even got to meet our president and first lady. It's amazing how easy it was for me to procrastinate and mentally dismiss that impending biopsy. But at the end of July 1999, I duly drove myself to the radiologist's office, telling my husband and myself that the procedure was no big deal, and he certainly didn't need to accompany me. Once more, the irregular area was imaged and the radiologist injected it with dye and inserted a small wire loop, which would allow the surgeon to locate and excise the abnormal tissue. A bandage held the loop in place, and I carefully drove to the outpatient facility at my hospital. Still feeling brave, I refused general anesthesia. (Actually, the bravery was really a misguided fear of losing control—what surgeon wants to be unconscious in the O.R.?) I also rationalized that, if I wasn't put under, I wouldn't have to recover and could use those extra hours of time off from my practice to write this book. So there I was lying on the O.R. table, chatting with my surgeon as he injected local anesthetic (that hurt), and then listening to the sounds of snipping and electric cautery. I discussed what he was doing as if I was a co-surgeon. When the pathologist arrived she showed me the "specimen" and reassured me that it looked grossly benign. I proudly marched out of the surgery center with my husband, who'd joined me there, went to a nearby deli (I hadn't eaten all morning) and, after the requisite chicken soup, drove home in my own car. The local anesthetic wore off that evening and I took one pain pill.

The following Monday when I spoke to the surgeon, I congratulated him on the ease with which we both had weathered the procedure. I wasn't expecting his reply: "Judy, there's florid atypical ductal hyperplasia [abnormal overgrowth of the ducts] and it continues onto the borders of the specimen. We don't think this is DCIS [ductal carcinoma in situ], but the pathologist wants to run more tests and send some slides for a second opinion."

I was no longer that clinical entity protected by a white coat and academic learning. I was now an upset and frightened woman. After the initial shock, I reached an almost immediate decision: If the borders weren't clear, we obviously hadn't cornered, or even defined, the abnormal breast tissue. Nothing had shown up in my mammogram—and perhaps never would, until it was invasive cancer. I had about an 8% chance of already possessing an obscured DCIS or early cancer in one or both breasts. And my mother had undergone a radical mastectomy for breast cancer at the age of 47. (Thankfully, she is fine 28 years later.)

I never felt that my femininity was defined by my breasts. (That's fortunate, because I'm very small.) And I didn't want to stop my hormone therapy, which I have enjoyed for the last year and a half. (Even the estrogen naysayers can't blame the atypical ductal cells on such a short course of therapy.) I made a very surgical decision to undergo bilateral (both breasts) subcutaneous mastectomy with immediate reconstruction. I did do my due diligence. I consulted an excellent oncologist, who gave me a hug and his blessing. I underwent testing for the three gene mutations that are associated with breast and ovarian cancer in women of Ashkenazi Jewish descent. (Happily for my ovaries and my daughters, the test was negative.) I consulted with a plastic surgeon who had done wonderful reconstruction on some of my patients who had similar surgeries. And then I set my surgery date, giving myself seven weeks to finish this book, get my practice in order and arrange to take two weeks off to recover.

The next period of time was awful. I had decided that this was a very private matter, so I continued to counsel my patients who had abnormal mammograms (and indeed in that period of time, five had a diagnosis of DCIS or breast cancer). I completed the book's genetics chapter, in which I discussed prophylactic mastectomy in what I hope was impartial and correct language. And I agonized over my decision.

On a Monday, I appeared on the *Today* show, talking about the importance of Pap smears. Then I flew back to Los Angeles. The next day, I spent seven hours in the O.R. as a patient, where I was put under for a procedure in which my breast tissue was removed and saline expanders were placed under my chest muscles. I entered the hospital under my husband's last name and no one except my staff, surgeons, anesthesiologists and a few members of my family and close friends knew I was there.

I had no idea—perhaps I repressed any idea I *did* have—that this would be such a grueling process. The post-operative pain was intense and I was, in my view at least, inexcusably weak. The two weeks that I had planned for complete recuperation were just not enough. (I compromised and went back to work half-time in the third week.) As I write this, four weeks post-surgery, I'm back to an almost normal energy level, but I am constantly aware of pressure in my chest. In a few months, when everything settles, including the expanders—which will ultimately give me a true B-size cup, something I admit to never having had—I'll have a second surgery.

I was very lucky. There was no DCIS or early cancer in either breast, only the extensive atypical ductal hyperplasia. This surgery probably reduced a 35% to 40% risk of my developing invasive cancer in the next five to 10 years to a negligible one.

My conspiracy of personal silence worked, and I could have continued counseling women on health care without sharing this experience. But as I resumed treating women and giving lectures, I felt like a fraud. I've always shared my personal medical issues with others; the premise being that I can't ask a woman to do something I won't do myself. I try to walk the walk I talk. So I'm getting this off my chest (an expression that I promise to never use again). I hope that in being honest, I help women who have or will need to cope with similar situations. I don't want to turn this book into a personal breast story. There is much more (at least 300 pages more) to our health than our breasts. So permit me to return to my original literary and medical intent.

I'm grateful that I had the knowledge and wherewithal to pursue the best of what medicine had to offer a woman in my situation. But when women have questions about their health and go looking for answers, too often the information they receive is inadequate. In my office, in my book and on the *Today* show I've sought to give all of us better access to and understanding of what medicine can do for women.

A friend of mine recently commented that the phrase "Relax, this won't hurt" has been usurped by the slightly more accurate phrase "This may cause some discomfort." But he says what the doctor really means is "This is going to hurt like the dickens." Somewhere in between these two extremes, we can prevent disease and benefit from the therapies medicine has to offer. I hope this book will help. No one wants to hurt.

Resources

Aging
National Council on the Aging
800-424-9046
www.ncoa.org

Alzheimer's Disease
Alzheimer's Association
800-272-3900
www.alz.org

Arthritis
Arthritis Foundation
800-283-7800
www.arthritis.org

Autoimmune Diseases
American Autoimmune-Related
Diseases Association
800-598-4668
www.aarda.org

Birth Defects
March of Dimes
888-MODIMES
www.modimes.org

Cancer
American Cancer Society
800-ACS-2345
www.ca.cancer.org

National Cancer Institute
800-4-CANCER
www.cancernet.nci.nih.gov

Contraception
Planned Parenthood
888-297-0152
www.plannedparenthood.org
www.teenwire.com (for teens)

Diabetes
American Diabetes
Association
800-AHA-DISC
www.diabetes.org

Endometriosis
Endometriosis Association
800-992-3636
www.endometriosisassn.org

Exercise
American College of Sports
Medicine
317-637-9200 (Indianapolis, IN)
www.acsm.org

Gynecologic Cancers
Gynecologic Cancer Foundation
800-444-4441
www.wcn.com

National Ovarian Cancer Coalition
888-OVARIAN
www.ovarian.org

Headache
American Council for Headache
Education
800-255-ACHE
www.achenet.org

Heart Disease
American Heart Association
800-AHA-USA1
www.amhrt.org

Incontinence
National Association for Continence
800-BLADDER
www.nafc.org

Infertility
Resolve
617-623-0744 (Somerville, MA)
www.resolve.org

Lung Disease
American Lung Association
800-LUNG-USA
www.lungusa.org

Lupus
Lupus Foundation of America
800-558-0121
www.lupus.org

Medications
Institute for Safe Medication
Practices
215-947-7797 (Warminster, PA)

Menopause
North American Menopause
Society
216-844-3334 (Cleveland, OH)

Multiple Sclerosis
MS Foundation
800-441-7055
www.msfax.org

Nutrition
American Dietetic Association
800-366-1655
www.eatright.org

Osteoporosis
National Osteoporosis
Foundation
202-223-2226 (Washington, DC)
www.nof.org

National Institutes of Health
Osteoporosis Resource Center
800-624-2663
www.osteo.org

Pregnancy
American College of Obstetricians
and Gynecologists
202-484-3321 (Washington, DC)
www.acog.org

Sexually Transmitted Diseases
Centers for Disease Control and
Prevention/American Social
Health Association
800-227-8922
www.ashastd.org

Skin Health
American Academy of
Dermatology
847-330-0101 (Schaumberg, IL)
www.aad.org

Women's Health (General)
National Women's Health
Information Center
800-994-WOMAN
www.4woman.gov

Index

dieting, diet, 27, 105, 175–80, 236, 318–19
   blood pressure and, 186
   breast pain and, 67
   diabetes and, 248
   estrogen replacement and, 203
   fat in, 161, 182, 186
   headaches and, 61
   heart disease and, 296–97
   osteoporosis and, 237, 238, 289–93
   pelvic pain and, 98–99
   PMS and, 31, 64
   pregnancy and, 91
   puberty and, 8
   soy protein in, 161, 162–63, 226–27
dilation and curettage (D&C), 29, 33, 91, 93, 111, 129, 269
diuretics, 31–32, 240, 310
diverticulosis, 302–3
dong quai, 226
dopamine, 181, 182
douching, 48, 50–51
drugs, 108
   for acne, 22
   after age 70, 321–24, 334–35, 337
   for Alzheimer's disease, 334–35
   antihypertensive, 186–87, 299
   antiobesity, 180–83
   for bladder problems, 276–77
   for breast pain, 67
   for depression, 32, 65, 71, 100, 105, 335
   fertility, 81–82, 138–39
   for headaches, 61–62
   for heart disease, 297–99
   for infertility, 81–82
   for menopause, 222–24
   for menstrual cramps, 10–11
   for multiple sclerosis, 57
   for osteoarthritis, 337
   for osteoporosis, 290–91
   for pelvic pain, 96, 99, 100, 101
   PMS and, 31–32
   sexual response curtailed by, 281–82
   for thyroid problems, 56, 57
   for vaginal infections, 48–49, 50
   for vulvar pain, 102, 103, 105
Dual Energy X-ray Absorbtiometry (DEXA), 288–89
ductal carcinoma in situ (DCIS), 230–31
dysmenorrhea, 10–11

eating disorders, 21, 23–25, 237
eggs (follicles), 4, 5, 10, 123–24
   diminished number of, 28–29
   donor, 80, 83, 138
   fertilization of, 5, 13
   see also ovulation
electrocardiograms (ECGs), 171, 246, 287, 299–300, 329
electron-beam CT (EBCT), 300
endocervical curettage (ECC), 111
endocrine system, 26
   see also specific glands
endometrial cancer, 28, 67, 73, 74, 110, 129, 258, 284
   hormone replacement and, 201–2, 206–7
   hysterectomy and, 144, 149, 150
endometriomas, 141
endometriosis, 33, 43–44, 81, 91–95, 126, 152, 263
   hysterectomy and, 147, 149, 150, 153
endometrium:
   perimenopause and, 132
   scarring of, 29, 269
endorphins, 30, 61
estrogen, 9, 27, 56, 57, 72, 123–24, 129, 152
   birth control pills and, 14, 15, 22, 28, 37–40, 70, 209–10
   breast cancer and, 159–62
   headaches and, 60–62, 189
   lack of, 193–97
   libido decrease and, 153, 154
   measuring of, 29
   perimenopause and, 130–34
   PMS and, 30, 60
   in puberty, 4–5, 7, 9
estrogen replacement therapy (ERT), 29, 152, 154, 186–87, 198–215, 220, 238, 261–62, 267, 281
   after age 70, 306, 308–9
   family history and, 204–5
   lifestyle factors and, 202–3
   low-dose, 212–13
   menopausal symptoms and, 198–99
   patches in, 211–12, 214–15, 241, 262
   pills in, 210–11, 215, 241
   types of, 209–14
   weight gain and, 219
evening primrose, 228
exercise, 27, 98, 194, 258
   blood pressure and, 185
   breast cancer and, 163

ovarian cysts (continued)
    adnexal, 141
    functional, 140
    nonfunctional, 141
    treatment of, 142–43
ovaries, 26, 27, 60
    failure of, 28–29
    in puberty, 3–4, 5, 7, 9, 10
    removal of, 144, 150–53, 264–65
overflow incontinence, 273, 275
overweight, 10, 171–83, 294
ovulation, 5, 10, 14, 27, 60, 95
    calculating the time of, 44–45, 80
    induction or enhancement of, 81–83
    lack of, 43, 56, 81
    Norplant and, 73
    pelvic pain and, 96–97

pancreas, 26, 124–25, 195, 247
Pap smear, 33, 55, 113, 171, 246, 329
    abnormal, 109–12
    HPV and, 35
    reliability of, 51–53
    in sixties, 259–61, 286
    in teens, 17–18, 21
Parkinson's disease, 306, 310
pelvic congestion syndrome, 100
pelvic exams, 55, 93, 113, 171, 246, 258,
    260–61, 286, 329
pelvic inflammatory disease (PID), 37,
    43, 51, 95, 96, 263
    contraception and, 69–70, 71, 74, 75,
    77
    IUDs and, 74, 75
pelvic pain, 92, 95–101
    accompanied by frequency, urgency,
        or pain during urination, 99
    central, with a previously diagnosed
        fibroid, 98
    constant achiness with periodic flare-
        ups, and pain at other body sites,
        100–101
    hysterectomy and, 147
    intermittent, bloating and, 98–99
    severe, unremitting, 96–98
    spasmodic, 99
    see also cramps, menstrual
pelvic prolapse, 147–48, 277–79, 283
pelvis, scarring of, 147, 149
PEPI (Post-menopausal Estrogen-
    Progestin Intervention trial)
    study, 216, 217, 262
perimenopause, 124, 129–33, 172, 197
pessaries, 279

phytoestrogens, 162–63
pituitary adenoma, 27–28, 80
pituitary gland, 4, 26–29, 56, 60, 70, 81
placenta previa, 90–91
Planned Parenthood, 16, 17, 18
pneumococcal vaccine, 287
polycystic ovarian syndrome (PCO), 10,
    28, 85, 129, 247
polyps, 33, 235, 269–70
Post-menopausal Estrogen-Progestin
    Intervention trial (PEPI) study,
    216, 217, 262
pregnancy, 7, 43–46
    after age 35, 80–81, 88–91, 137–38
    after birth control use, 43
    ectopic, 74, 96, 119, 141
    fertility problems and, 80–84, 137–38
    high-risk, 138
    multiple, 82, 83, 91, 138
    protection against, see contraception
    testing for, 16, 18, 29–30, 41
    unintended, 12, 13, 15, 64, 135–36
    weight gain and, 59, 173
premenstrual dysphoric disorder
    (PMDD), 23, 63–65
premenstrual syndrome (PMS), 23, 41,
    42, 56
    depression and, 30, 32, 63–65
    relief from, 30–32
prodrome, 61
progesterone, 45, 56, 57, 66, 123–24,
    152, 160
    in hormone replacement therapy, 29,
        201, 215–17, 262
    menstrual irregularities and, 10, 27,
        28, 60
    miscarriage and, 85, 87
    perimenopause and, 130, 132
    PMS and, 30
    in teen years, 5, 9, 10, 18
progesterone creams, 229
progestin, 72, 73
    in birth control pills, 14, 32, 37–42,
        70, 72
    in hormone replacement, 137, 201,
        202, 216
    in IUDs, 74, 75
prolactin, 28, 80
prostaglandins, 11, 30, 61
puberty, 3–10, 60
    early, 6–8
    hormones in, 4–5, 7, 9, 10, 23
    late, 6, 8–10
    normal, 5–6

JUDITH REICHMAN, M.D., is a gynecologist who practices and teaches at Cedars-Sinai Medical Center and UCLA in Los Angeles. She appears regularly on NBC TV's *Today* show as a contributor on women's health issues, and she co-wrote and hosted two acclaimed PBS series, *Straight Talk on Menopause* and *More Straight Talk on Menopause*. The author of two best-sellers, *I'm Too Young to Get Old* and *I'm Not in the Mood*, Dr. Reichman lives in Los Angeles with her husband and two daughters.